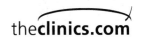

INFECTIOUS DISEASE CLINICS OF NORTH AMERICA

Update on Musculoskeletal Infections

GUEST EDITOR
John J. Ross, MD

CONSULTING EDITOR
Robert C. Moellering, Jr, MD

December 2005 • Volume 19 • Number 4

SAUNDERS

An Imprint of Elsevier, Inc.
PHILADELPHIA   LONDON   TORONTO   MONTREAL   SYDNEY   TOKYO

W.B. SAUNDERS COMPANY
A Division of Elsevier Inc.

Elsevier, Inc., 1600 John F. Kennedy Blvd., Suite 1800, Philadelphia, PA 19103-2899.

http://www.theclinics.com

INFECTIOUS DISEASE CLINICS Volume 19, Number 4
OF NORTH AMERICA ISSN 0891–5520
December 2005 ISBN 1-4160-2670-3
Editor: Carin Davis

The ideas and opinions expressed in *Infectious Disease Clinics of North America* do not necessarily reflect those of the Publisher. The Publisher does not assume any responsibility for any injury and/or damage to persons or property arising out of or related to any use of the material contained in this periodical. The reader is advised to check the appropriate medical literature and the product information currently provided by the manufacturer of each drug to be administered to verify the dosage, the method and duration of administration, or contraindications. It is the responsibility of the treating physician or other health care professional, relying on independent experience and knowledge of the patient, to determine drug dosages and the best treatment for the patient. Mention of any product in this issue should not be construed as endorsement by the contributors, editors, or the Publisher of the product or manufacturers' claims.

Infectious Disease Clinics of North America (ISSN 0891–5520) is published in March, June, September, and December (For Post Office use only: volume 19 issue 4 of 4) by Elsevier, Inc. Corporate and editorial offices: Elsevier, Inc., 1600 John F. Kennedy Blvd., Suite 1800, Philadelphia, PA 19103-2899. Accounting and circulation offices: 6277 Sea Harbor Drive, Orlando, FL 32887-4800. Periodicals postage paid at Orlando, FL 32862, and additional mailing offices. Subscription prices are $170.00 per year for US individuals, $285.00 per year for US institutions, $85.00 per year for US students, $200.00 per year for Canadian individuals, $345.00 per year for Canadian institutions, $225.00 per year for international individuals, $345.00 per year for international institutions, and $110.00 per year for Canadian and foreign students. To receive student rate, orders must be accompanied by name of affiliated institution, date of term, and the *signature* of program/residency coordinator on institution letterhead. Orders will be billed at individual rate until proof of status is received. Foreign air speed delivery is included in all *Clinics* subscription prices. All prices are subject to change without notice. POSTMASTER: Send address changes to *Infectious Disease Clinics of North America*, W.B. Saunders Company, Periodicals Fulfillment, Orlando, FL 32887-4800. **Customer Service: 1-800-654-2452 (US). From outside of the US, call 1-407-345-4000. E-mail: hhspcs@wbsaunders.com**

Infectious Disease Clinics of North America is also published in Spanish by Editorial Inter-Médica, Junin 917, 1er A 1113, Buenos Aires, Argentina.

Reprints. For copies of 100 or more, of articles in this publication, please contact the Commercial Reprints Department, Elsevier Inc., 360 Park Avenue South, New York, New York 10010-1710. Tel. (212) 633-3813, Fax: (212) 462-1935, email: reprints@elsevier.com

Infectious Disease Clinics of North America is covered in *Index Medicus, Current Contents/Clinical Medicine, Science Citation Alert, SCISEARCH, and Research Alert.*

Printed in the United States of America.

CONSULTING EDITOR

ROBERT C. MOELLERING, Jr, MD, Herrman L. Blumgart Professor of Medical Research, Harvard Medical School; and Physician-in-Chief and Chairman, Department of Medicine, Beth Israel Deaconess Medical Center, Boston, Massachusetts

GUEST EDITOR

JOHN J. ROSS, MD, Division of Infectious Diseases, Caritas Saint Elizabeth's Medical Center; Assistant Professor, Tufts University School of Medicine, Boston, Massachusetts

CONTRIBUTORS

ELIE F. BERBARI, MD, Assistant Professor of Medicine, Division of Infectious Diseases, Mayo Clinic College of Medicine, Rochester, Minnesota

LEONARD H. CALABRESE, DO, R. J. Fasenmyer Chair of Clinical Immunology, Department of Rheumatic and Immunologic Diseases, The Cleveland Clinic, Cleveland, Ohio

JASON H. CALHOUN, MD, FACS, Chair and J. Vernon Luck Distinguished Professor, Department of Orthopaedic Surgery, University of Missouri-Columbia, Columbia, Missouri

MICHAEL GARDAM, MSc, MD, CM, FRCPC, Director, Infection Prevention and Control; Medical Director, Tuberculosis Clinic, University Health Network; and Assistant Professor of Medicine, University of Toronto, Toronto, Ontario, Canada

SUSAN HADLEY, MD, Associate Professor of Medicine, Tufts University School of Medicine; Vice-Chief, Clinical Infectious Disease, Division of Geographic Medicine and Infectious Disease, Tufts-New England Medical Center, Boston, Massachusetts

PAUL D. HOLTOM, MD, Associate Professor of Clinical Medicine and Orthopaedics, Keck School of Medicine of University of Southern California, Los Angeles, California

LINDEN HU, MD, Associate Professor of Medicine, Tufts University School of Medicine; Associate Chief for Research, Division of Geographic Medicine and Infectious Diseases, Tufts-New England Medical Center, Boston, Massachusetts

JOHNNY HUARD, PhD, Director of the Growth and Development Laboratory of Children's Hospital of Pittsburgh; Associate Professor, Departments of Orthopaedic Surgery, Molecular Genetics and Biochemistry, and Bioengineering, University of Pittsburgh, Pittsburgh, Pennsylvania

SHELDON L. KAPLAN, MD, Professor and Vice-Chairman for Clinical Affairs, Department of Pediatrics, Baylor College of Medicine; Chief, Infectious Disease Service, Texas Children's Hospital, Houston, Texas

ADOLF W. KARCHMER, MD, Professor of Medicine, Harvard Medical School; Chief, Division of Infectious Diseases, Beth Israel Deaconess Medical Center, Boston, Massachusetts

RAKHI KOHLI, MD, MS, Assistant Professor of Medicine, Tufts University School of Medicine; Division of Geographic Medicine and Infectious Disease, Tufts-New England Medical Center, Boston, Massachusetts

YONG LI, MD, PhD, Growth and Development Laboratory of Children's Hospital of Pittsburgh; Assistant Professor, Department of Orthopaedics, University of Pittsburgh, Pittsburgh, Pennsylvania

SUE LIM, MD, FRCPC, Associate Hospital Epidemiologist, University Health Network, Toronto, Ontario, Canada

M. M. MANRING, PhD, Department of Orthopaedic Surgery, University of Missouri-Columbia, Columbia, Missouri

CAMELIA E. MARCULESCU, MD, Instructor of Medicine, Division of Infectious Disease, Medical University of South Carolina, Charleston, South Carolina

STANLEY J. NAIDES, MD, H. Thomas and Dorothy Willits Chair in Rheumatology; Professor of Medicine, Microbiology, and Immunology; and Pharmacology Chief, Division of Rheumatology, Penn State Milton S. Hershey Medical Center, Arthritis, Bone, & Joint Center, Hershey, Pennsylvania

DOUGLAS R. OSMON, MD, MPH, Associate Professor of Medicine, Division of Infectious Disease, Mayo College of Medicine, Rochester, Minnesota

MICHAEL J. PATZAKIS, MD, Professor and Chairman, The Vincent and Julia Meyer Chair, and Chief of Orthopaedic Surgery, Keck School of Medicine of University of Southern California, Los Angeles, California

DANIELLE LAUREN PETERSEL, MD, Fellow, Division of Rheumatology, Department of Medicine, University of Medicine and Dentistry of New Jersey, Robert Wood Johnson Medical School, New Brunswick, New Jersey

PETER A. RICE, MD, Professor of Medicine, Division of Infectious Diseases and Immunology, University of Massachusetts Medical School, Worcester, Massachusetts

JOHN J. ROSS, MD, Division of Infectious Diseases, Caritas Saint Elizabeth's Medical Center; Assistant Professor, Tufts University School of Medicine, Boston, Massachusetts

WEI SHEN, MD, MS, Growth and Development Laboratory of Children's Hospital of Pittsburgh; Graduate Student, Department of Bioengineering, University of Pittsburgh, Pittsburgh, Pennsylvania

RANDY SHERMAN, MD, Professor of Surgery, Orthopaedics and Neurosurgery; Chief, Division of Plastic and Reconstructive Surgery, Keck School of Medicine of University of Southern California, Los Angeles, California

IRENE G. SIA, MD, Assistant Professor of Medicine, Division of Infectious Diseases, Mayo Clinic College of Medicine, Rochester, Minnesota

LEONARD H. SIGAL, MD, Director-Immunology, Pharmaceutical Research Institute, Bristol-Myers Squibb, Princeton; Clinical Professor, Division of Rheumatology, Departments of Medicine and Pediatrics, University of Medicine and Dentistry of New Jersey, Robert Wood Johnson Medical School, New Brunswick, New Jersey

LORNE N. SMALL, MD, FRCPC, Fellow, Division of Geographic Medicine and Infectious Diseases, Tufts-New England Medical Center, Boston, Massachusetts

CHARALAMPOS G. ZALAVRAS, MD, Assistant Professor of Clinical Orthopaedics, Keck School of Medicine of University of Southern California, Los Angeles, California

CONTENTS

Adult osteomyelitis is difficult to treat, with considerable morbidity and cost. Bacteria reach bone through the bloodstream, from a contiguous focus of infection, from penetrating trauma, or from operative intervention. Appropriate treatment includes culture-directed antibiotic therapy and operative debridement of all necrotic bone and soft tissue. Treatment often involves a combination of antibiotics. Operative treatment is often staged and includes debridement, dead space management, soft tissue coverage, restoration of blood supply, and stabilization.

Osteomyelitis is one of the more common invasive bacterial infections in children leading to hospitalization and prolonged antibiotic administration. Over the past decade, increasing microbial virulence, diminishing antibiotic susceptibility, and advances in diagnostic molecular microbiology and imaging techniques have led to changes in the clinical management of children with suspected osteomyelitis, which are reviewed in this article.

Septic arthritis has increased in incidence in the United States in the past two decades, and increasingly affects an older population with a greater burden of chronic illness and a higher risk for drug-resistant organisms. Successful management depends on a high diagnostic suspicion, empiric antibiotic treatment, and joint drainage.

A bacteriologic diagnosis is more likely with inoculation into blood culture bottles than plating on solid media. As methicillin-resistant *Staphylococcus aureus* increases in prevalence in the community, empiric antibiotic regimens will increasingly need to be active against methicillin-resistant *S aureus*.

treatment with ceftriaxone or an advanced generation cephalosporin is warranted until signs and symptoms have regressed; continuation of treatment can usually be accomplished with a fluoroquinolone.

Reactive Arthritis
Danielle Lauren Petersel and Leonard H. Sigal

Reactive arthritis consists of sterile axial or peripheral articular inflammation, enthesitis, and extra-articular manifestations. Most patients are HLA-B27 positive, although determining the B27 status of an individual patient is irrelevant. Reactive arthritis is the result of prior genitourinary or gastrointestinal infection and the immune response to this infection; reactive arthritis does not represent active synovial infection. Diagnosis usually can be made by clinical examination and history. The current standard therapy is nonsteroidal anti-inflammatory drugs and physiotherapy, but molecular biologic treatment may ultimately become the mainstay in recalcitrant and severe reactive arthritis.

Prosthetic Joint Infections
Irene G. Sia, Elie F. Berbari, and Adolf W. Karchmer

Success in the treatment of infected orthopedic prosthesis requires the best surgical approach in combination with prolonged optimum targeted antimicrobial therapy. In choosing the surgical option, one must consider the duration of the infection, the functionality of the prosthesis, condition of the bone stock and soft tissue, the virulence and antimicrobial susceptibility of the pathogen, the general health and projected longevity of the patient, and the experience of the surgeon. If surgery is not possible, an alternative is long-term oral antimicrobial suppression to maintain a functioning prosthesis. Treatment must be individualized for a specific infection in a specific patient.

Management of Open Fractures
Charalampos G. Zalavras, Michael J. Patzakis,
Paul D. Holtom, and Randy Sherman

An open fracture is characterized by soft tissue disruption that results in communication of the fracture site with the outside environment. Open fractures are severe injuries with a potential for serious complications, such as infection and nonunion, and they constitute a challenging problem for the treating physician. During the past 3 decades, improved understanding of infection and fracture biology principles, new devices for fracture stabilization, and development of microsurgical procedures for reconstruction of the soft tissue envelope have considerably improved open fracture management, which aims to prevent infection at the fracture site, achieve fracture union, and restore function.

previously active and healthy young men. Pyomyositis in temperate countries is often regarded as an infection that occurs in hosts who are immunocompromised or otherwise debilitated. However, this distinction may be somewhat artificial, as tropical pyomyositis may be partly related to underlying infection with HIV or parasites, and temperate pyomyositis has been reported in healthy and athletic persons. This article discusses the pathogenesis, clinical presentation, diagnosis, and management of pyomyositis in the tropical and temperate settings.

Suppurative tenosynovitis and septic bursitis are closed space infections of the musculoskeletal system. Appropriate antibiotics in combination with incision and drainage are generally recommended. Aggressive surgical management is particularly important in tenosynovitis to prevent tendon necrosis. Empiric antibiotic coverage should be directed toward staphylococci and streptococci. Patient characteristics and epidemiologic exposures may provide clues to unusual causative organisms that are occasionally encountered, such as *Neisseria gonorrhoeae*, *Pasteurella multocida*, atypical mycobacteria, fungi, and protothecosis.

Antibiotics have greatly improved the outcome of musculoskeletal infections. The treatment of complicated musculoskeletal infections, however, continues to challenge orthopedic surgeons. Many researchers view gene therapy as a new weapon for conquering a variety of musculoskeletal disorders. This article introduces the concepts and strategies of gene therapy, the application of gene therapy in orthopedics, and the reasons why gene therapy could play a key role in the treatment of musculoskeletal infectious diseases.

RECENT ISSUES

INFECTIOUS
DISEASE CLINICS
OF NORTH AMERICA

Infect Dis Clin N Am 19 (2005) xiii–xiv

Preface

Update on Musculoskeletal Infections

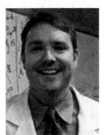

John J. Ross, MD
Guest Editor

Musculoskeletal infections are perhaps orphan conditions poised at the boundary between three disciplines: infectious diseases, orthopedic surgery, and rheumatology. However, these forlorn infections are likely to grow in importance and prevalence in North America as the population ages and the burden of risk factors such as underlying arthritis, diabetes mellitus, and immunosuppression increases. To complicate matters, drug-resistant bacteria such as methicillin-resistant *Staphylococcus aureus* are playing a greater role as pathogens in musculoskeletal infections. Outcomes are often poor. Osteomyelitis, especially in diabetic patients, can literally threaten life and limb. Septic arthritis of both prosthetic and native joints can permanently hamper mobility and locomotion. The limited ability of musculoskeletal tissue to regenerate may make these infections permanently disabling.

This issue of the *Infectious Disease Clinics of North America* attempts to define the state-of-the-art approach to such infections, including the problems and pitfalls associated with the management of mycobacterial, fungal, and borrelial musculoskeletal infection; the controversies associated with reactive arthritis; and the role of antibiotic prophylaxis in orthopedic surgery, as well as the management of open fractures. Finally, we explore the promise of the emerging technologies loosely lumped together under the category of gene therapy.

I wish to thank the contributors to this issue for lending their time, effort, and expertise. I realize my great fortune in working with such a talented, knowledgeable, and diverse group of rheumatologists, orthopedic surgeons, and infectious disease specialists. I also wish to express my gratitude to my family; to Carin Davis, Elsevier's editor extraordinaire, for her patience and

doi:10.1016/j.idc.2005.09.001
id.theclinics.com

diligence; and to Dr. Robert Moellering for the opportunity to edit this issue. Lastly, I wish to acknowledge my indebtedness to a trio of extraordi-
nary physicians who first sparked my interest in infectious diseases:
Michael G. Worthington, Jeffrey K. Griffiths, and Sherwood L. Gorbach.

John J. Ross, MD
Division of Infectious Diseases
Caritas St. Elizabeth's Medical Center
736 Cambridge Street
Boston, MA 02135, USA

E-mail address: jrossmd@cchcs.org

ELSEVIER
SAUNDERS

INFECTIOUS
DISEASE CLINICS
OF NORTH AMERICA

Infect Dis Clin N Am 19 (2005) 765–786

Adult Osteomyelitis

Jason H. Calhoun, MD*, M.M. Manring, PhD

*Department of Orthopaedic Surgery, University of Missouri-Columbia, DC053.00,
MC213, One Hospital Drive, Columbia, MO 65212, USA*

Adult osteomyelitis most commonly arises from open fractures, diabetic foot infections, or the surgical treatment of closed injuries. Patients usually have a history of prolonged debilitation and multiple surgical procedures. Treatment of osteomyelitis has improved considerably over the past quarter-century because of advances in diagnostic, surgical, and therapeutic techniques. The term "cure" is not used for osteomyelitis, because the infection may recur years after apparently successful treatment of the disease, if the patient suffers new trauma to the involved area, or the host response to the infection is suppressed. The goal of treatment is to arrest osteomyelitis, rather than achieve cure.

This article provides a broad discussion of adult osteomyelitis. The major classification systems are reviewed, with brief discussions of hematogenous, vertebral, contiguous-focus, and chronic osteomyelitis. Diagnosis is discussed, with particular attention on the role of different radiologic technologies. Finally, the focus is various approaches to treatment for different types of adult osteomyelitis, including cases involving special patient populations.

Classification systems

Physicians usually use one of two classification systems to describe osteomyelitis. Waldvogel and coworkers [1–3] classified bone infections as either hematogenous (derived from or transported by blood) or osteomyelitis secondary to a contiguous focus of infection. Contiguous-focus osteomyelitis is also subclassified as with or without vascular insufficiency. Either hematogenous or contiguous-focus osteomyelitis may be further classified as acute or chronic. Acute disease is defined as a suppurative

---

* Corresponding author.
  E-mail address: calhounj@health.missouri.edu (J.H. Calhoun).

0891-5520/05/$ - see front matter © 2005 Elsevier Inc. All rights reserved.
doi:10.1016/j.idc.2005.07.009   *id.theclinics.com*

infection with edema, vascular congestion, and small-vessel thrombosis. The vascular supply to the bone initially is compromised by injury or the infection extending into surrounding soft tissue. Large areas of dead bone (sequestra) may then be formed when both the medullary and periosteal blood supplies are sufficiently compromised. Bacteria may be particularly difficult to eradicate from necrotic and ischemic tissue, even with any combination of host response, antibiotic therapy, and surgery. Acute osteomyelitis evolves into the obstinate and often refractory problem of chronic osteomyelitis, characterized by a nidus of infected sequestra or scar tissue, with a surrounding ischemic soft tissue envelope [4].

An alternative classification system by Cierny and coworkers [5] and Mader and coworkers [6] considers the quality of the host, the bone's anatomic nature, treatment factors, and prognostic factors, yielding four anatomic disease types (stages 1–4) and three physiologic host categories (A, B, and C). Twelve discrete clinical stages of osteomyelitis (a matrix of four disease types and three host categories) are described through this system (Tables 1 and 2).

Stage 1 is medullary osteomyelitis, equating with early hematogenous osteomyelitis in which the primary lesion is endosteal. Although stage 1 usually can be treated in pediatric patients with antibiotics alone, adults commonly require cortical unroofing and intramedullary reaming. Another example of stage 1 osteomyelitis is an infected intramedullary rod in a stable bone; in this case, the infected rod must be removed, the medullary canal reamed, and culture-directed antibiotics given.

Stage 2 is superficial osteomyelitis. The infection in bone results from an adjacent soft tissue infection, which represents a true contiguous-focus lesion. At the base of a soft tissue wound an exposed, infected necrotic outer

Table 1
Cierny-Mader staging system

Anatomic type	Physiologic class
Stage 1: Medullary osteomyelitis	A Host: Normal host
Stage 2: Superficial osteomyelitis	B Host: Systemic compromise (Bs)
Stage 3: Localized osteomyelitis	Local compromise (Bl)
Stage 4: Diffuse osteomyelitis	Systemic and local compromise (Bls)
	C Host: Treatment worse than the disease

Systemic or local factors that affect immune surveillance, metabolism, and local vascularity

Systemic (Bs)	Local (Bl)
Malnutrition	Chronic lymphedema
Renal, hepatic failure	Venous stasis
Diabetes mellitus	Major vessel compromise
Chronic hypoxia	Arteritis
Immune disease	Extensive scarring
Malignancy	Radiation fibrosis
Extremes of age	Small vessel disease
Immunosuppression or neuropathy	Complete loss of sensation
Immune deficiency	Tobacco abuse

Table 2
Anatomic classification of adult long-bone osteomyelitis

Stage	Description	Etiology	Treatment
1 (medullary)	Necrosis limited to medullary contents and endosteal surfaces	Hematogenous	Antibiotics/host alteration (early); unroofing, intramedullary reaming (late)
2 (superficial)	Necrosis limited to exposed surfaces	Contiguous soft tissue infection	Antibiotics/host alteration (early); superficial debridement, coverage, possible ablation (late)
3 (localized)	Well-marginated and stable before and after debridement	Trauma, involving stages 1 and 2, Iatrogenic	Antibiotics/host alteration, debridement, dead space management, temporary stabilization, bone graft
4 (diffuse)	Circumferential or permeative; unstable before or after debridement	Trauma, involving stages 1–3, Iatrogenic	Antibiotics/host alteration, stabilization (ORIF, external fixation), debridement, dead space management, possible ablation

Abbreviation: ORIF, open reduction and internal fixation.

surface of bone is found. In stage 2, treatment is a superficial debridement and coverage with a local or microvascular flap, along with appropriate antibiotics.

Stage 3 is localized osteomyelitis, which is characterized by a full-thickness cortical sequestration that can be surgically removed without compromising bone stability. Stage 3 requires debridement, saucerization, antibiotics, and sometimes a bone graft to improve stability.

Stage 4 is diffuse osteomyelitis, a through and through section of the bone, usually requiring segmental resection. Occasionally, the patient may also have bone infection on both sides of a nonunion or joint. Diffuse osteomyelitis includes infections with a loss of bony stability (either before or after debridement). Stage 4 requires debridement, stabilization, dead-space management, second-stage reconstruction, and antibiotics.

Hosts are classified as A, B, or C. The class A host is a patient with normal physiologic, metabolic, and immunologic characteristics. B hosts are locally compromised, systematically compromised, or both. The goal of treatment for a B host is to remove the compromising factors that distinguish them from an A host. Finally, a C host is the patient for whom the consequences of treatment of bone infection are worse than the infection itself, or who is so ill that surgery is not possible.

Either classification system may be used according to the physician's experience and preference. The traditional Waldvogel system has the advantage of greater simplicity and familiarity, whereas the Cierny-Mader system is both specific, dictating treatment, and dynamic, altering therapy depending on patient response or change in status. The Waldvogel system is used throughout this article. The Cierny-Mader classes are referred to when appropriate.

Hematogenous osteomyelitis

Hematogenous osteomyelitis accounts for approximately 20% of cases of osteomyelitis in adults. The number of adult cases may be increasing, however, as the mean age of population rises in the United States and other developed countries [7]. For reasons not yet clear, it is more common in males, regardless of age. The vertebrae are the most common site of infection in adults, but hematogenous osteomyelitis also occurs in the long bones, pelvis, and clavicle [8].

Primary hematogenous osteomyelitis occurs mainly in infants and children. It is also found in the adult population. Infection usually begins in the diaphysis and may spread to the entire medullary canal (Fig. 1). Because the growth plate has matured and shares vessels with the metaphysis, extension into the joint may occur. Cortical penetration usually leads to a soft tissue abscess as the periosteum firmly adheres to the bone and may erode into the joint, causing a septic joint. Eventually, sinus tracts may form, connecting a sequestered nidus of infection to the skin through soft tissue extension. Secondary hematogenous osteomyelitis is more common and represents the reactivation of an infection originally experienced in infancy or childhood. Secondary hematogenous osteomyelitis in adults usually has a metaphyseal location.

A solitary pathogenic organism usually is recovered from bone. In adults, *Staphylococcus aureus* is the most common cause. Adults usually present

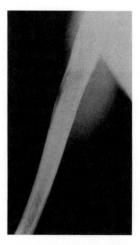

Fig. 1. Radiograph of a 28-year-old man shows hematogenous osteomyelitis in the diaphysis of the humerus. There is involvement of the intramedullary canal with cortical extension.

with pain and minimal constitutional symptoms, lasting 1 to 3 months in duration. Occasionally, patients present acutely, with chills, fever, swelling, and erythema over the affected bone or bones.

Vertebral osteomyelitis

Vertebral osteomyelitis is primarily a disease of adults, with most patients more than 50 years old. Generally, incidence increases progressively with each successive decade of life. Men are affected about twice as often as women. Before the development of antibiotics, vertebral osteomyelitis was fatal in about a quarter of all patients [9]. Mortality is now rare, but a delay in diagnosis may lead to devastating complications.

Pyogenic vertebral osteomyelitis usually has a hematogenous origin, with the arterial route as the most likely avenue of infection [10]. Commonly, segmental arteries supplying the vertebrae bifurcate to supply adjacent bony segments, and the disease commonly involves two adjacent vertebrae and the intervertebral disk. The lumbar region is affected in approximately 45% of patients, followed by the thoracic spine (35%) and the cervical spine (20%) [10]. Many sources of infection have been identified, including skin and soft tissue, the respiratory tract, infected intravenous sites, endocarditis, dental infection, and the genitourinary tract [11–13]. Most often, S aureus is the isolated organism, except in the case of intravenous drug users, in whom Pseudomonas aeruginosa is most commonly isolated [9,14,15].

Nearly all patients report localized pain and tenderness of the involved bone segments, slowly progressing over 3 weeks to 3 months. Fever and peripheral leukocytosis are present in approximately half of patients, and the erythrocyte sedimentation rate is usually elevated, providing a prognostic guide during treatment. Epidural and subdural abscesses, and sometimes meningitis, may result from posterior extension of the infection. Anterior or lateral extension may lead to paravertebral, retropharyngeal, mediastinal, subphrenic, or retroperitoneal abscesses. Motor and sensory defects are seen in as many as 15% of patients [9].

Contiguous-focus osteomyelitis without generalized vascular insufficiency

In contiguous-focus osteomyelitis, bacterial organisms may be directly inoculated into bone at the time of trauma, spread from a nearby soft tissue infection, or spread by nosocomial contamination. Common factors in this form of osteomyelitis include surgical reduction and internal fixation of fractures, prosthetic devices, open fractures, and chronic soft tissue infections. Although S aureus is the most commonly isolated organism, multiple pathogens are usually isolated from infected bone, frequently including gram-negative bacilli and anaerobic organisms. The infection usually occurs about 1 month after inoculation from trauma, surgery, or soft tissue infection. Patients present with low-grade fever, drainage, and pain. Loss of bone stability, necrosis, and soft tissue damage are frequent, leading to difficulties in treatment.

Contiguous-focus osteomyelitis with generalized vascular insufficiency

Most patients in this category suffer from diabetes mellitus, and the small bones of the feet are most commonly infected (Fig. 2). Inadequate tissue perfusion, which blunts local tissue response, may predispose patients to infection, which most often is caused by minor trauma to the feet. Multiple organisms are usually isolated from bone, most commonly coagulase-positive and -negative staphylococci, *Streptococcus* spp, *Enterococcus* spp, gram-negative bacilli, and anaerobic organisms.

The diagnosis of osteomyelitis can be challenging in patients with vascular compromise. Patients may present with a seemingly unrelated problem, such as an ingrown toenail, cellulitis, deep space infection, or perforating foot ulcer, and pain may be muted by peripheral neuropathy. Examination may show decreased dorsalis pedis and posterior tibial pulses, poor capillary refill, and decreased sensation. Osteomyelitis is present when bone is exposed in an ulcer bed before or after debridement, or if a probe of a foot ulcer encounters bone. Radiologic evidence is a late finding. The goal of treatment is generally to suppress infection and maintain the limb's integrity, keeping in mind that recurrent or new bone infections occur in most patients. Resection or amputation of the affected area is almost always needed.

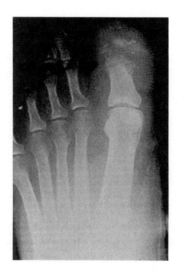

Fig. 2. Contiguous focus osteomyelitis in a 40-year-old male patient with diabetes mellitus. Bony destruction is visible around the proximal and distal phalanges of the first toe.

Chronic osteomyelitis

Both hematogenous and contiguous-focus osteomyelitis can become chronic. Chronic osteomyelitis is easily recognized when it occurs in a patient with a history of osteomyelitis who experiences a recurrence of pain, erythema, and swelling in association with a draining sinus. Diagnosis is more challenging in patients with a painful orthopedic prosthesis, a decubitus ulcer, a foot ulcer, or Charcot's foot associated with peripheral vascular disease or diabetes. The infection usually does not begin to regress until the nidus of the persistent contamination is removed. Unfortunately, antibiotic therapy alone is usually insufficient treatment of chronic osteomyelitis, although empiric or culture-directed antibiotics remove many of the symptoms. Arresting the infection is particularly challenging when the integrity of surrounding soft tissue is poor, the bone is unstable secondary to an infected nonunion, or there is an adjacent septic joint.

Patients typically present with chronic pain and drainage, and sometimes a low-grade fever. The sedimentation rate is usually elevated and the leukocyte count normal. The patient may present with a localized abscess, a soft tissue infection, or both if a sinus tract becomes obstructed. Rare complications of chronic osteomyelitis include squamous cell carcinoma at the site of tissue drainage and amyloidosis [16].

Diagnosis

Osteomyelitis can often be difficult to diagnose. The intensity of inflammation, infection duration and site, vascularity, the presence or absence of a foreign body, and the presence or absence of associated pathology all affect the accuracy of any test. No noninvasive test can definitively establish or exclude osteomyelitis in complicated cases. The difficulties with diagnosis were illustrated by Newman and coworkers [17] in a study of diabetic patients with foot ulcers. As determined by bone biopsy and culture, osteomyelitis was found to underlie 28 (68%) of 41 diabetic foot ulcers. Yet, only nine of the 28 cases had been diagnosed clinically by the referring physician. Most occurred in ulcers not exposing bone, and 64% had no evidence of inflammation on physical examination.

Diagnosis of long bone osteomyelitis rests on isolation of the pathogen from bone lesion or blood culture. In the case of hematogenous osteomyelitis, positive blood cultures often can eliminate the need for a bone biopsy, provided there is radiographic evidence of osteomyelitis. Sinus tract cultures are reliable for confirming S aureus, but they do not predict the presence or absence of gram-negative organisms that cause osteomyelitis [18,19]. Antibiotic treatment of osteomyelitis must be based on meticulous cultures taken at debridement surgery or from deep bone biopsies and antibiotic susceptibility tests [4]. Sedimentation rates and leukocyte counts often are elevated before therapy in acute disease, but the leukocyte count only rarely exceeds $15,000/mm^3$, and the count is usually normal in patients with chronic osteomyelitis [3]. Although a sedimentation rate that returns to normal in response to therapy is a favorable development, this laboratory determinant is not reliable in the compromised host, who may be constantly challenged by minor illnesses and peripheral lesions that can elevate the index.

Diagnosis of long bone osteomyelitis

Radiographic studies

In acute hematogenous osteomyelitis, radiographic changes accurately reflect the destructive process but lag at least 2 weeks behind the progress of the infection. The earliest visible changes include swelling of soft tissue, periosteal thickening or elevation, and focal osteopenia. Before the radiographs show lytic changes, at least 50% to 75% of the bone matrix must be destroyed. Likewise, clinical recovery may greatly outpace its radiographic detection, even when the patient is undergoing an appropriate antimicrobial regimen [20]. The diagnosis of acute osteomyelitis cannot be excluded if the plain films are negative. Osteomyelitis is the "great mimic," as healing fractures (Charcot's foot), cancers (osteosarcoma), and benign tumors (giant cell) can appear identical on radiographs. Further testing should be performed because early therapy is essential to reduce the formation of necrotic bone and the development of chronic osteomyelitis. In contiguous-focus and chronic osteomyelitis, radiographic changes are subtle, often found in association with other nonspecific radiographic findings, and require careful clinical correlation to achieve diagnostic significance.

Radionuclide studies

When the diagnosis of osteomyelitis is ambiguous, or more information is required to gauge the extent of bone and soft tissue inflammation, radionuclide scans may be obtained. These scans are not generally necessary for the diagnosis of long bone osteomyelitis, however, and they are all hampered by limited sensitivity and specificity. The technetium Tc 99m polyphosphate scan demonstrates increased isotope accumulation in areas of increased blood flow and reactive new bone formation [21]. In cases of hematogenous osteomyelitis later confirmed by bone biopsy, the radionuclide scan is usually positive as early as 48 hours after the initiation of the bone infection [22]. Negative technetium 99m scans in documented cases of osteomyelitis may reflect an impaired blood supply to the infected area [23].

Another class of radiopharmaceuticals used to diagnose osteomyelitis includes gallium citrate. It attaches to transferrin, which leaks from the bloodstream into areas of inflammation. Gallium scans show increased isotope uptake in infection, sterile inflammatory conditions, and malignancy [24]. One difficulty with the gallium scan is that it does not show bone detail particularly well, and may not distinguish well between bone and soft tissue inflammation. Comparison with a technetium 99m scan may help resolve this problem [25].

Less valuable are indium-labeled leukocyte scans, which are positive in approximately 40% of patients with acute osteomyelitis and 60% of patients with septic arthritis [26]. Negative indium-leukocyte scans are often taken from patients with chronic osteomyelitis, bony metastases, and degenerative arthritis.

CT

CT may also play a role in diagnosis of osteomyelitis, because increased marrow density occurs early in infection, and intramedullary gas has been reported in cases of hematogenous osteomyelitis [26,27]. CT may identify areas of necrotic bone and soft tissue, and assist in optimizing surgical debridement [26,28]. CT scans have one notable disadvantage: the scatter phenomenon when metal is near the area of bone infection. This results in significant loss of image resolution.

MRI

MRI is a useful tool for diagnosing musculoskeletal infection [29–31]; however, its limitations should be recognized. The spatial resolution offered by MRI makes it useful in differentiating bone and soft tissue infection, which often is a problem with radionuclide scans [32]. But MRI, unlike radionuclide studies, is not useful for whole-body examinations, and metal implants in the region of interest may produce focal artifacts. Also, differentiation of infection from neoplasm through MRI may be difficult, and clinical and radiographic confirmation is necessary [33].

Initial MRI screening usually consists of a T1-weighted and a T2-weighted spin-echo pulse sequence. Edema is dark and fat bright in the T1-weighted sequence (Fig. 3); these are reversed in the T2-weighted study. Osteomyelitis typically appears as a localized marrow abnormality with decreased intensity on T1-weighted images, and increased intensity on T2-weighted images. Occasionally, there may be decreased signal intensity on T2-weighted images. Surgical or posttraumatic scarring of marrow displays decreased signal intensity on T1-weighted images, with no change on T2-weighted images. Sinus tracts are seen as areas of high signal intensity on T2-weighted images, extending from the marrow and bone, through the soft tissues, and out of the skin. Cellulitis displays as diffuse areas of intermediate signal on T1-weighted images of soft tissue, with increased signal strength on T2-weighted images.

Diagnosis of vertebral osteomyelitis

Anteroposterior and lateral radiographic views of the spine reveal intervertebral disk space narrowing, with destruction and new bone formation at the anterior edge of the vertebral disk. Both CT and MRI

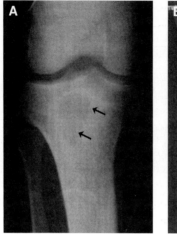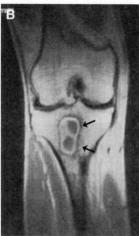

Fig. 3. (*A*) Arrows point to a typical lytic lesion in the upper tibia. (*B*) A T1-weighted MRI with contrast depicts the area of osteomyelitis.

can demonstrate evidence of osteomyelitis (early paravertebral soft tissue swelling and bone destruction), before changes are evident in radiographic studies [34–37]. Also valuable is the technetium Tc 99m polyphosphate scan, which often detects spinal abnormalities before radiographic changes can be seen [38]. A positive gallium scan suggests osteomyelitis, but may be difficult to interpret because of the high concentration of hematopoietic tissue in the vertebral bodies [39].

The pathogenic organism must be isolated from the bone for a definitive diagnosis of vertebral osteomyelitis. Generally, a bone biopsy is required, because blood cultures are usually sterile. Bone cultures are mandatory for bacteriologic diagnosis, except when blood cultures are positive and radiographic evidence of osteomyelitis is clearly present. The biopsy should be performed under fluoroscopy or CT scan, and the specimens should also be sent for fungal and mycobacterial stains and cultures and histologic examination. If the original cultures are negative, an open surgical biopsy should ideally be performed before empiric antibiotic therapy is begun.

Treatment

Appropriate therapy includes adequate drainage, thorough debridement, dead space management, wound protection, and specific antimicrobial coverage. If the host is compromised, an effort is made to correct or improve defects. Of particular significance are good nutrition and, if applicable, a smoking-cessation program in addition to dealing with specific abnormalities, such as diabetes. An attempt is made to improve the nutritional, medical, and vascular status of the patient and to provide optimal care for any underlying disease.

Antibiotics

Options and duration

The traditional duration of treatment in most stages (Cierny-Mader stages 1, 3, and 4) is 4 to 6 weeks. This duration is suggested by animal studies [40] and by observations that bone revascularization after debridement takes about 4 weeks. Trials of longer courses of intravenous or oral antibiotics (6 months or more) do not suggest any improvement compared with 6 weeks of therapy [41-43]. Outpatient intravenous therapy has been proved to reduce costs and improve quality of life. Options include a peripherally inserted central catheter, a Hickman catheter, or a Groshong catheter [44-47].

Clinicians have many options for oral antibiotic treatment (Table 3). Clindamycin, rifampin, trimethoprim-sulfamethoxazole, and fluoroquinolones have proved effective in the oral treatment of osteomyelitis. Clindamycin, a lincosamide antibiotic active against most gram-positive bacteria, has excellent bioavailability, and is currently given orally after initial intravenous treatment for 1 to 2 weeks [48,49]. Linezolid, which can be administered either orally or intravenously and is active against

Table 3
Antibiotics used in oral treatment of osteomyelitis

Drug	Spectrum	Adult dosage	Side effects and toxicity
Clindamycin	Staphylococci, anaerobic bacteria	300 mg four times daily	Antibiotic-associated diarrhea, pseudomembranous colitis
Cephalexin	Streptococci, staphylococci	500 mg four times daily	Rash
Rifampin	Staphylococci	600 mg daily	Hepatotoxicity
Ciprofloxacin	Enterobacteriaceae, *Pseudomonas aeruginosa*	750 mg twice daily	Hepatotoxicity, tendon damage
Levofloxacin	Streptococci, staphylococci, enterobacteriaceae	500 mg daily	Hepatotoxicity, tendon damage
Gatifloxacin	Streptococci, staphylococci, enterobacteriaceae	400 mg daily	Hepatotoxicity, tendon damage
Trimethoprim-sulfamethoxazole	Streptococci, staphylococci, enterobacteriaceae	160 TMP/800 SMX twice daily	Rash, Stevens-Johnson syndrome, hepatotoxicity
Linezolid	Gram-positive cocci, including MRSA	600 mg twice daily	Bone marrow toxicity, anemia, thrombocytopenia

Abbreviations: MRSA, Methicillin-resistant *staphylococcus aureus*; SMX, sulfamethoxazole; TMP, trimetho prim.

methicillin-resistant staphylococci, has been proved effective for treating serious infections, including osteomyelitis [50]. Oral quinolones for gram-negative organisms are often used in adult patients [51–53]. The second-generation quinolones (ciprofloxacin and ofloxacin) have poor activity against *Streptococcus* spp, *Enterococcus* spp, and anaerobic bacteria [54]. The third-generation quinolone levofloxacin has improved *Streptococcus* spp activity, but with minimal anaerobic coverage [55]. The newer fluoroquinolones gatifloxacin, moxifloxacin, and gemifloxacin cover many gram-positive and gram-negative organisms, and certain anaerobes [56]. Newer fluoroquinolones are not as active against *P aeruginosa* as ciprofloxacin.

None of the quinolones has reliable *Enterococcus* spp coverage. The currently available quinolones have variable *S aureus* and *Staphylococcus epidermidis* coverage, but resistance to the second- and third-generation quinolones is increasing [57]. Coverage of methicillin-sensitive *S aureus* should be obtained with another oral antibiotic, such as clindamycin or ampicillin-sulbactam. Quinolones can be given orally as soon as the patient is able to take them, thanks to their excellent oral absorption. Before changing to a nonquinolone oral regimen, the authors usually treat the patient with 2 weeks of parenteral antibiotic therapy. The decision to use oral versus parenteral antibiotics should be based on microorganism sensitivity results, patient compliance, infectious disease consultation, and the surgeon's experience. Combined parenteral and oral regimens are also used. Oral rifampin is used in combination with cell wall active antibiotics for synergistic killing in *S aureus* infections. Its use alone must be avoided because of the rapid emergence of resistant strains [58,59].

Ideally, treatment depends on the results of bone cultures. After cultures are obtained by bone biopsy or during debridement, a parenteral antimicrobial regimen is initiated to cover suspected pathogens. Once the organism is identified, the treatment may be modified according to sensitivity tests. If the patient is acutely ill, however, antibiotic treatment should not be delayed to wait for bone debridement.

Antibiotic treatment by stage

Stage 1 osteomyelitis in adults is usually treated with antibiotics and operative intervention. The patient is treated for 4 weeks with appropriate parenteral antimicrobial therapy, dated from initiation of therapy or after the last major operative debridement. If the initial medical management fails, and the patient is clinically compromised by a recurrent infection, bone or soft tissue debridement is necessary in conjunction with another 4-week course of antibiotics.

In stage 2 osteomyelitis, shorter courses of antibiotics usually are needed. With a 2-week course of antibiotics following debridement of the cortex and soft tissue coverage, an arrest rate of close to 100% in A hosts and 79% in B hosts has been described [60]. In stages 3 and 4 osteomyelitis, the patient should receive 4 to 6 weeks of antimicrobial therapy dated from the last major debridement surgery. Without adequate debridement, the failure rate is high no matter the duration of therapy. Even if necrotic tissue has been adequately debrided, the remaining tissue bed must be considered contaminated; it is important to treat the patient for at least 4 weeks with antibiotics. An arrest rate of 98% in A hosts and 80% (for stage 4) to 92% (for stage 3) in B hosts has been described [60].

Suppressive antibiotic therapy

When operative treatment of osteomyelitis is not feasible, suppressive antibiotic therapy, usually oral, is administered to control the disease and possibly correct the infection. Ideal drugs possess good bioavailability, low toxicity, and adequate bone penetration. The suppressive regimen should be culture directed.

Suppressive therapy has been extensively studied in the setting of infected orthopedic implants. Rifampin (in combination with other antibiotics), fusidic acid, ofloxacin, and trimethoprim-sulfamethoxazole have been administered to patients with infected implants [61–64]. In these studies, suppressive antibiotic treatment was administered for 6 to 9 months. After discontinuation of treatment, an arrest (ie, no recurrence of infection during the follow-up period) was achieved in 26 (67%) of 39 patients treated with trimethoprim-sulfamethoxazole [61], in 11 (55%) of 20 treated with fusidic acid and rifampin, and in 11 (50%) of 22 treated with rifampin and ofloxacin [63]. Suppressive therapy is traditionally administered for 6 months. If there is a recurrence of the infection after discontinuation, a new, lifelong suppressive regimen is administered.

Operative treatment

The principles of treating infection in bone include adequate drainage, extensive debridement of all necrotic tissue, dead space management, adequate soft tissue coverage, and restoration of blood supply [60,65]. A greater challenge is operative treatment in the compromised host. In some cases, the procedures required to arrest the disease are of such magnitude for the compromised host that treatment can lead to loss of function, limb, or life. Standard operative treatment of osteomyelitis is not feasible in all cases, and some patients, particularly severely compromised hosts, are often candidates for more radical treatment, such as amputation, or must receive only nonoperative treatment, such as antibiotic suppression.

Bone debridement

Debridement of bone is performed until punctate bleeding is noted, or the "paprika sign" [65]. After all necrotic tissue has been adequately debrided, the remaining tissue bed must still be considered contaminated. The importance of the extent of operative debridement has been investigated in both normal and compromised hosts [66]. B hosts treated with marginal resection (a clearance margin of less than 5 mm) had a higher rate of recurrence than did normal hosts. The extent of resection seems to be much more important in B hosts. In normal hosts a marginal resection may be acceptable.

Reconstruction and dead space management

Debridement often leaves a large bony defect, termed "dead space." This space is poorly vascularized, predisposing the persistence of infection. Appropriate management of any dead space created by debridement is required to arrest disease and maintain the integrity of the skeletal part. Dead bone and scar tissue must be replaced with durable vascularized tissue [65,67]. A free vascularized bone graft, usually obtained from the fibula or ilium, has been used to fill the dead space [68,69]. Local tissue flaps or free flaps may also be used [70–74]. As an alternative, cancellous bone grafts may be placed beneath local or transferred tissues where structural augmentation is needed. Open cancellous grafts without soft tissue coverage are useful when a free tissue transfer is not a treatment option and local tissue flaps are inadequate [75].

Antibiotic-impregnated acrylic beads may be used to sterilize and temporarily maintain a dead space (Fig. 4). The most commonly used antibiotics in beads are vancomycin, tobramycin, and gentamicin. The arrest rate of osteomyelitis ranges from 55%, in a study of 54 patients, to 96% in a study of 46 patients [76,77]. The beads usually are removed within 2 to 4 weeks and replaced with a cancellous bone graft [67,78–83]. Because most

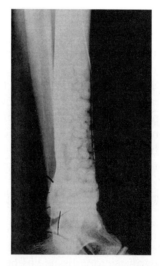

Fig. 4. Treatment of osteomyelitis of the distal tibia. After debridement surgery, polymethyl methacrylate beads impregnated with vancomycin and tobramycin were placed in the dead space. The beads were removed after 3 weeks, and the dead space was replaced with a cancellous bone graft.

beads act as a biomaterial surface to which bacteria preferentially adhere, infection has been associated with bead use [84]. For that reason, biodegradable antibiotic beads have also been used and have shown favorable antibiotic release kinetics [85]. Antibiotic-impregnated cancellous bone grafts were used in a clinical trial of 46 patients, with an arrest rate of 95% [86]. Clindamycin and amikacin have also been delivered directly into dead spaces with an implantable pump, obtaining very high local, and low systemic, levels of antibiotics [19,87].

Bone stabilization

Measures often must be taken to restore skeletal stability at the infection site. Plates, screws, rods, and external fixators may be used. External fixation is preferred over internal fixation because of the tendency of hardware to become secondarily infected. The Ilizarov external fixation method allows reconstruction of segmental defects and difficult infected nonunions [88]. This method is based on the technique of distraction osteogenesis, in which an osteotomy created in the metaphyseal region of the bone is gradually distracted to fill in the defect. The Ilizarov technique is used for difficult cases of osteomyelitis when stabilization and bone lengthening are necessary (Fig. 5). The method may also be used to compress nonunions and correct malunions. The technique is labor intensive, and requires an extended period of treatment; patients may experience an average of 8.5 months in the device [89]. In addition, the wires or pins usually become infected, and the device is painful. The arrest rate of osteomyelitis in the

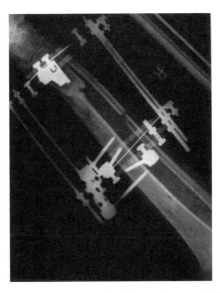

Fig. 5. Stage 4 (diffuse) osteomyelitis in an infected nonunion treated with an Ilizarov external fixator.

studies using this technique ranges between 75% in a study of 28 patients and 100% in a study of 13 patients [90,91].

Soft tissue coverage

Adequate soft tissue coverage of the bone is necessary to arrest osteomyelitis. Small soft tissue defects may be covered with a split-thickness skin graft. In the presence of a large soft tissue defect or an inadequate soft tissue envelope, local muscle flaps and free vascularized muscle flaps may be placed in one or two stages. Local muscle flaps and free vascularized muscle transfers improve the local biologic environment by bringing in a blood supply important for host defense mechanisms, antibiotic delivery, and osseous and soft tissue healing. Local and microvascular muscle flaps, and microvascular flaps alone, have been used in combination with antibiotics and operative debridement [72,92,93]. The arrest rate ranged from 90% in a study of 33 patients to 100% in a study of 18 patients [92]. Healing by so-called "secondary intention" should be discouraged, because scar tissue that fills the defect may later become avascular. Complete wound closure must be obtained whenever possible.

Hyperbaric oxygen therapy

Several clinical trials have shown that adjunctive hyperbaric oxygen therapy may be useful in the treatment of chronic osteomyelitis. One study included patients with recurring chronic osteomyelitis who had met the following criteria: an infection persisting longer than 1 month; at least one surgical debridement; and already having had hyperbaric oxygen therapy, surgery, and treatment with antibiotics. A total of 34 patients (85%) remained clinically free of disease, whereas six experienced recurrences of osteomyelitis [94]. In another study [95], the same criteria were used to evaluate hyperbaric oxygen therapy in 38 patients, and 34 remained free of clinical signs of osteomyelitis after 1 year follow-up. Although clinical trials are encouraging, the adjunctive role of hyperbaric oxygen in osteomyelitis is difficult to assess because of the multiple confounding variables of patient, surgery, organism, bone, and antibiotic. Animal studies have suggested that hyperbaric oxygen administered under standard treatment conditions is as effective as cephalothin in eradicating *S aureus* from bone infections [96]. Clearly, wound healing is a dynamic process, requiring adequate oxygen tension to succeed [97,98]. Hyperbaric oxygen therapy provides oxygen to promote collagen production, angiogenesis, and healing in the ischemic or infected wound.

Other clinical situations

Hemodialysis patients

Osteomyelitis sometimes occurs as a complication of hemodialysis. *S aureus* and *S epidermis* are common blood isolates in hemodialysis patients with indwelling cannulae that create portals for bacterial entry. Bone infections are probably hematogenous in origin, with the ribs and thoracic vertebral column the most common sites of involvement. Diagnosis of osteomyelitis is usually made 12 to 72 months after hemodialysis is initiated. The infection may not be recognized, because the clinical signs and radiographs may mimic renal osteodystrophy.

Sickle cell disease

It is often difficult to differentiate thrombotic marrow crisis from osteomyelitis in patients with sickle cell disease. A history of bone pain and fever, followed in 1 to 2 weeks by spiking fever, chills, and leukocytosis suggests osteomyelitis, and patients with sickle cell disease may present with multiple bone infection sites. Because the symptoms may mimic those of the marrow crisis, early cultures should be obtained to arrive at the correct diagnosis. Presumptive antibiotic therapy in sickle cell disease patients suspected of having osteomyelitis should include antibiotics with effectiveness against *Salmonella* spp, *S aureus*, and streptococci.

Heroin-addicted patients

Osteomyelitis is a complication of drug addiction. Fever is often absent, and clinical symptoms and signs of infection may be subtle, including localized pain. Infection is commonly found in the vertebrae, pubis, and clavicles, but can occur in any bone. The most commonly isolated pathogens are *S aureus*, *S epidermis*, gram-negative rods, and *Candida* spp. Initial radiographs often are normal, so multiple radiographs may be required. Bone cultures are mandatory to make a correct bacteriologic diagnosis, with the exception of when blood cultures are positive and radiographic evidence of osteomyelitis is clearly present.

Brodie's abscess

Brodie's abscess is a chronic localized bone abscess. A subacute case presents with fever, pain, and periosteal elevation, and chronic cases are often afebrile and present with long-standing dull pain. The distal part of the tibia is the most common site of involvement. The lesion, typically single, is most commonly located near the metaphysis. Approximately three quarters of patients are less than 25 years old. Surgical debridement and culture-specific antibiotics are often effective in arresting the condition [99,100].

Summary

Adult osteomyelitis remains difficult to treat, with considerable morbidity and costs to the health care system. Bacteria reach bone through the bloodstream, from a contiguous focus of infection, from penetrating trauma, or from operative intervention. Bone necrosis begins early, limiting the possibility of eradicating the pathogens, and leading to a chronic condition. Appropriate treatment includes culture-directed antibiotic therapy and operative debridement of all necrotic bone and soft tissue. Treatment often involves a combination of antibiotics. Operative treatment is often staged and includes debridement, dead space management, soft tissue coverage, restoration of blood supply, and stabilization. Clinicians and patients must share a clear understanding of the goals of treatment and the difficulties that may persist after the initial course of therapy or surgical intervention. Chronic pain and recurrence of infection still remain possible even when the acute symptoms of adult osteomyelitis have resolved.

References

[1] Waldvogel FA, Medoff G, Swartz MN. Osteomyelitis: a review of clinical features, therapeutic considerations and unusual aspects. 3. Osteomyelitis associated with vascular insufficiency. N Engl J Med 1970;282:316–22.

[2] Waldvogel FA, Papageorgiou PS. Osteomyelitis: the past decade. N Engl J Med 1980;303: 360–70.

[3] Lew DP, Waldvogel FA. Osteomyelitis. N Engl J Med 1997;336:999–1007.

[4] Cierny G III, Mader J. Adult chronic osteomyelitis. Orthopedics 1984;7:1557–64.

[5] Cierny G III, Mader JT, Penninck JJ. A clinical staging system for adult osteomyelitis. Clin Orthop 2003;414:7–24.

[6] Mader JT, Shirtliff M, Calhoun JH. Staging and staging application in osteomyelitis. Clin Infect Dis 1997;25:1303–9.

[7] Espersen F, et al. Changing pattern of bone and joint infections due to *Staphylococcus aureus*: study of cases of bacteremia in Denmark, 1959–1988. Rev Infect Dis 1991;13: 347–58.

[8] Lew DP, Waldvogel FA. Osteomyelitis. Lancet 2004;364:369–79.

[9] Sapico FL, Montgomerie JZ. Pyogenic vertebral osteomyelitis: report of nine cases and review of the literature. Rev Infect Dis 1979;1:754–76.

[10] Batson OV. The function of the vertebral veins and their role in the spread of metastases. 1940. Clin Orthop 1995;312:4–9.

[11] Lee YH, Kerstein MD. Osteomyelitis and septic arthritis: a complication of subclavian venous catheterization. N Engl J Med 1971;285:1179–80.

[12] Leonard A, et al. Osteomyelitis in hemodialysis patients. Ann Intern Med 1973;78:651–8.

[13] Watanakunakorn C. Vertebral osteomyelitis as a complication of *Pseudomonas aeruginosa* pneumonia. South Med J 1975;68:173–6.

[14] Sapico FL, Montgomerie JZ. Vertebral osteomyelitis in intravenous drug abusers: report of three cases and review of the literature. Rev Infect Dis 1980;2:196–206.

[15] Holzman RS, Bishko F. Osteomyelitis in heroin addicts. Ann Intern Med 1971;75:693–6.

[16] Gruber HE. Bone and the immune system. Proc Soc Exp Biol Med 1991;197:219–25.

[17] Newman LG, et al. Unsuspected osteomyelitis in diabetic foot ulcers: diagnosis and monitoring by leukocyte scanning with indium in 111 oxyquinoline. JAMA 1991;266: 1246–51.

[18] Mackowiak PA, Jones SR, Smith JW. Diagnostic value of sinus-tract cultures in chronic osteomyelitis. JAMA 1978;239:2772–5.

[19] Perry CR, Pearson RL, Miller GA. Accuracy of cultures of material from swabbing of the superficial aspect of the wound and needle biopsy in the preoperative assessment of osteomyelitis. J Bone Joint Surg Am 1991;73:745–9.

[20] Butt WP. The radiology of infection. Clin Orthop 1973;96:20–30.

[21] Jones AG, Francis MD, Davis MA. Bone scanning: radionuclidic reaction mechanisms. Semin Nucl Med 1976;6:3–18.

[22] Treves S, et al. Osteomyelitis: early scintigraphic detection in children. Pediatrics 1976;57: 173–86.

[23] Russin LD, Staab EV. Unusual bone-scan findings in acute osteomyelitis: case report. J Nucl Med 1976;17:617–9.

[24] Deysine M, et al. Diagnosis of chronic and postoperative osteomyelitis with gallium 67 citrate scans. Am J Surg 1975;129:632–5.

[25] Lisbona R, Rosenthall L. Observations of the sequential use of 99m Tc phosphate complex and 67 Ga imaging in osteomyelitis. Radiology 1977;123:123–9.

[26] Kuhn JP, Berger PE. Computed tomographic diagnosis of osteomyelitis. Radiology 1979; 130:503–6.

[27] Ram PC, et al. CT detection of intraosseous gas: a new sign of osteomyelitis. AJR Am J Roentgenol 1981;137:721–3.

[28] Seltzer SE. Value of computed tomography in planning medical and surgical treatment of chronic osteomyelitis. J Comput Assist Tomogr 1984;8:482–7.

[29] Ma LD, et al. CT and MRI evaluation of musculoskeletal infection. Crit Rev Diagn Imaging 1997;38:535–68.

[30] Erdman WA, et al. Osteomyelitis: characteristics and pitfalls of diagnosis with MR imaging. Radiology 1991;180:533–9.

[31] Tehranzadeh J, Wang F, Mesgarzadeh M. Magnetic resonance imaging of osteomyelitis. Crit Rev Diagn Imaging 1992;33:495–534.

[32] Unger E, et al. Diagnosis of osteomyelitis by MR imaging. AJR Am J Roentgenol 1988;150: 605–10.

[33] Modic MT, et al. Magnetic resonance imaging of musculoskeletal infections. Radiol Clin North Am 1986;24:247–58.

[34] Golimbu C, Firooznia H, Rafii M. CT of osteomyelitis of the spine. AJR Am J Roentgenol 1984;142:159–63.

[35] Post MJ, et al. Spinal infection: evaluation with MR imaging and intraoperative US. Radiology 1988;169:765–71.

[36] Jevtic V. Vertebral infection. Eur Radiol 2004;14(Suppl 3):E43–52.

[37] Tehranzadeh J, et al. Imaging of osteomyelitis in the mature skeleton. Radiol Clin North Am 2001;39:223–50.

[38] Adatepe MH, et al. Hematogenous pyogenic vertebral osteomyelitis: diagnostic value of radionuclide bone imaging. J Nucl Med 1986;27:1680–5.

[39] Hadjipavlou AG, et al. The effectiveness of gallium citrate Ga 67 radionuclide imaging in vertebral osteomyelitis revisited. Am J Orthop 1998;27:179–83.

[40] Norden CW, Dickens DR. Experimental osteomyelitis. 3. Treatment with cephaloridine. J Infect Dis 1973;127:525–8.

[41] Hedstrom SA. The prognosis of chronic staphylococcal osteomyelitis after long-term antibiotic treatment. Scand J Infect Dis 1974;6:33–8.

[42] Bell SM. Further observations on the value of oral penicillins in chronic staphylococcal osteomyelitis. Med J Aust 1976;2:591–3.

[43] Wagner DK, Collier BD, Rytel MW. Long-term intravenous antibiotic therapy in chronic osteomyelitis. Arch Intern Med 1985;145:1073–8.

[44] Hickman RO, et al. A modified right atrial catheter for access to the venous system in marrow transplant recipients. Surg Gynecol Obstet 1979;148:871–5.

[45] Couch L, Cierny G III, Mader JT. Inpatient and outpatient use of the Hickman catheter for adults with osteomyelitis. Clin Orthop 1987;219:226–35.

[46] Graham DR, et al. Infectious complications among patients receiving home intravenous therapy with peripheral, central, or peripherally placed central venous catheters. Am J Med 1991;91:95S–100S.

[47] Tice AD. Outpatient parenteral antimicrobial therapy for osteomyelitis. Infect Dis Clin North Am 1998;12:903–19.

[48] Rodriguez W, et al. Clindamycin in the treatment of osteomyelitis in children: a report of 29 cases. Am J Dis Child 1977;131:1088–93.

[49] Feigin RD, et al. Clindamycin treatment of osteomyelitis and septic arthritis in children. Pediatrics 1975;55:213–23.

[50] Birmingham MC, et al. Linezolid for the treatment of multidrug-resistant, gram-positive infections: experience from a compassionate-use program. Clin Infect Dis 2003;36: 159–68.

[51] Mader JT, Cantrell JS, Calhoun J. Oral ciprofloxacin compared with standard parenteral antibiotic therapy for chronic osteomyelitis in adults. J Bone Joint Surg Am 1990;72: 104–10.

[52] Mader J. Fluoroquinolones in bone and joint infections. In: Sanders WEJ, Sanders CC, editors. Fluoroquinolones in the treatment of infectious diseases. Glenview (IL): Physicians & Scientists; 1990. p. 71–86.

[53] Lew DP, Waldvogel FA. Quinolones and osteomyelitis: state-of-the-art. Drugs 1995; 49(Suppl 2):100–11.

[54] Schaberg DR, et al. Increasing resistance of enterococci to ciprofloxacin. Antimicrob Agents Chemother 1992;36:2533–5.

[55] Ernst ME, Ernst EJ, Klepser ME. Levofloxacin and trovafloxacin: the next generation of fluoroquinolones? Am J Health Syst Pharm 1997;54:2569–84.

[56] Saravolatz LD, Leggett J. Gatifloxacin, gemifloxacin, and moxifloxacin: the role of 3 newer fluoroquinolones. Clin Infect Dis 2003;37:1210–5.

[57] Blumberg HM, et al. Rapid development of ciprofloxacin resistance in methicillin-susceptible and -resistant Staphylococcus aureus. J Infect Dis 1991;163:1279–85.

[58] Norden CW. Experimental chronic staphylococcal osteomyelitis in rabbits: treatment with rifampin alone and in combination with other antimicrobial agents. Rev Infect Dis 1983; 5(Suppl 3):S491–4.

[59] Norden CW, et al. Chronic osteomyelitis caused by Staphylococcus aureus: controlled clinical trial of nafcillin therapy and nafcillin-rifampin therapy. South Med J 1986;79: 947–51.

[60] Cierny G III. Chronic osteomyelitis: results of treatment. Instr Course Lect 1990;39: 495–508.

[61] Stein A, et al. Ambulatory treatment of multidrug-resistant staphylococcus-infected orthopedic implants with high-dose oral co-trimoxazole (trimethoprim-sulfamethoxazole). Antimicrob Agents Chemother 1998;42:3086–91.

[62] Goulet JA, et al. Prolonged suppression of infection in total hip arthroplasty. J Arthroplasty 1988;3:109–16.

[63] Drancourt M, et al. Oral treatment of Staphylococcus spp. infected orthopaedic implants with fusidic acid or ofloxacin in combination with rifampicin. J Antimicrob Chemother 1997;39:235–40.

[64] Segreti J, Nelson JA, Trenholme GM. Prolonged suppressive antibiotic therapy for infected orthopedic prostheses. Clin Infect Dis 1998;27:711–3.

[65] Cierny G III, Mader JT. The surgical treatment of adult osteomyelitis. In: Evarts CMC, editor. Surgery of the musculoskeletal system. New York: Churchill Livingstone; 1983. p. 15–35.

[66] Gristina AG, et al. Adherent bacterial colonization in the pathogenesis of osteomyelitis. Science 1985;228:990–3.

[67] Mader JT, Ortiz M, Calhoun JH. Update on the diagnosis and management of osteomyelitis. Clin Podiatr Med Surg 1996;13:701–24.

[68] Minami A, Kaneda K, Itoga H. Treatment of infected segmental defect of long bone with vascularized bone transfer. J Reconstr Microsurg 1992;8:75–82.

[69] Han CS, et al. Vascularized bone transfer. J Bone Joint Surg Am 1992;74:1441–9.

[70] Ruttle PE, et al. Chronic osteomyelitis treated with a muscle flap. Orthop Clin North Am 1984;15:451–9.

[71] May JW Jr, et al. Treatment of chronic traumatic bone wounds. Microvascular free tissue transfer: a 13-year experience in 96 patients. Ann Surg 1991;214:241–50 [discussion: 250–2].

[72] Anthony JP, Mathes SJ, Alpert BS. The muscle flap in the treatment of chronic lower extremity osteomyelitis: results in patients over 5 years after treatment. Plast Reconstr Surg 1991;88:311–8.

[73] Irons GB Jr, Wood MB. Soft-tissue coverage for the treatment of osteomyelitis of the lower part of the leg. Mayo Clin Proc 1986;61:382–7.

[74] Anthony JP, Mathes SJ. Update on chronic osteomyelitis. Clin Plast Surg 1991;18:515–23.

[75] Papineau LJ, et al. Chronic osteomyelitis: open excision and grafting after saucerization. Int Orthop 1979;3:165–76.

[76] Cho SH, et al. Antibiotic-impregnated cement beads in the treatment of chronic osteomyelitis. Bull Hosp Joint Dis 1997;56:140–4.

[77] Modi SP, Eppes SC, Klein JD. Cat-scratch disease presenting as multifocal osteomyelitis with thoracic abscess. Pediatr Infect Dis J 2001;20:1006–7.

[78] Scott DM, Rotschafer JC, Behrens F. Use of vancomycin and tobramycin polymethylmethacrylate impregnated beads in the management of chronic osteomyelitis. Drug Intell Clin Pharm 1988;22:480–3.

[79] Wilson KJ, et al. Comparative evaluation of the diffusion of tobramycin and cefotaxime out of antibiotic-impregnated polymethylmethacrylate beads. J Orthop Res 1988;6:279–86.

[80] Adams K, et al. In vitro and in vivo evaluation of antibiotic diffusion from antibiotic-impregnated polymethylmethacrylate beads. Clin Orthop 1992;278:244–52.

[81] Calhoun JH, Mader JT. Antibiotic beads in the management of surgical infections. Am J Surg 1989;157:443–9.

[82] Henry SL, et al. Antibiotic-impregnated beads. Part I: Bead implantation versus systemic therapy. Orthop Rev 1991;20:242–7.

[83] Popham GJ, et al. Antibiotic-impregnated beads. Part II: Factors in antibiotic selection. Orthop Rev 1991;20:331–7.

[84] Neut D, et al. Biomaterial-associated infection of gentamicin-loaded PMMA beads in orthopaedic revision surgery. J Antimicrob Chemother 2001;47:885–91.

[85] Liu SJ, et al. In vivo release of vancomycin from biodegradable beads. J Biomed Mater Res 2002;63:807–13.

[86] Chan YS, et al. Antibiotic-impregnated autogenic cancellous bone grafting is an effective and safe method for the management of small infected tibial defects: a comparison study. J Trauma 2000;48:246–55.

[87] Perry CR, Davenport K, Vossen MK. Local delivery of antibiotics via an implantable pump in the treatment of osteomyelitis. Clin Orthop 1988;226:222–30.

[88] Green SA. Osteomyelitis: the Ilizarov perspective. Orthop Clin North Am 1991;22:515–21.

[89] Calhoun JH, et al. The Ilizarov technique in the treatment of osteomyelitis. Tex Med 1991; 87:56–9.

[90] Cattaneo R, Catagni M, Johnson EE. The treatment of infected nonunions and segmental defects of the tibia by the methods of Ilizarov. Clin Orthop 1992;280:143–52.

[91] Morandi M, Zembo MM, Ciotti M. Infected tibial pseudarthrosis: a 2-year follow up on patients treated by the Ilizarov technique. Orthopedics 1989;12:497–508.

[92] May JW Jr, Gallico GG III, Lukash FN. Microvascular transfer of free tissue for closure of bone wounds of the distal lower extremity. N Engl J Med 1982;306:253–7.

[93] Weiland AJ, Moore JR, Daniel RK. The efficacy of free tissue transfer in the treatment of osteomyelitis. J Bone Joint Surg Am 1984;66:181–93.

[94] Morrey BF, et al. Hyperbaric oxygen and chronic osteomyelitis. Clin Orthop 1979;144: 121–7.

[95] Davis JC, et al. Chronic non-hematogenous osteomyelitis treated with adjuvant hyperbaric oxygen. J Bone Joint Surg Am 1986;68:1210–7.

[96] Mader JT, et al. Therapy with hyperbaric oxygen for experimental osteomyelitis due to *Staphylococcus aureus* in rabbits. J Infect Dis 1978;138:312–8.

[97] Hunt TK, Pai MP. The effect of varying ambient oxygen tensions on wound metabolism and collagen synthesis. Surg Gynecol Obstet 1972;135:561–7.

[98] Hunt TK, Zederfeldt B, Goldstick TK. Oxygen and healing. Am J Surg 1969;118:521–5.

[99] Miller WB Jr, Murphy WA, Gilula LA. Brodie abscess: reappraisal. Radiology 1979;132: 15–23.

[100] Dunn EC, Singer L. Operative treatment of Brodie's abscess. J Foot Surg 1991;30:443–5.

ELSEVIER
SAUNDERS

Infect Dis Clin N Am 19 (2005) 787–797

INFECTIOUS
DISEASE CLINICS
OF NORTH AMERICA

Osteomyelitis in Children

Sheldon L. Kaplan, MD[a,b],*

[a]*Department of Pediatrics, Baylor College of Medicine, One Baylor Plaza,
Houston, TX 77030, USA*
[b]*Infectious Disease Service, Texas Children's Hospital, Feigin Center MC 3-2371,
Suite 1150, 1102 Bates, Houston, TX 77030, USA*

Osteomyelitis is one of the more common invasive bacterial infections in children leading to hospitalization and prolonged antibiotic administration. Over the past decade, increasing microbial virulence, diminishing antibiotic sensitivity, and advances in diagnostic molecular microbiology and imaging techniques have led to changes in the clinical management of children with suspected osteomyelitis.

Pathogenesis

Most cases of osteomyelitis in children arise hematogenously, occurring characteristically in the metaphysis of long bones, such as the femur, tibia, and humerus [1]. Preceding blunt trauma to the site of the bone infection is quite common, but the role of trauma in the pathogenesis of osteomyelitis in children remains unclear [2]. Presumably, small hematomas in the metaphysis may permit microbial seeding after transient bacteremia. Penetrating injuries or surgical manipulation with such devices as spinal instrumentation are mechanisms for direct inoculation of bacteria into bone [3]. The least common pathway for osteomyelitis developing in children is local invasion from a contiguous focus of infection.

Microbiology

By far the most common bacterial pathogen causing osteomyelitis in children is *Staphylococcus aureus* in all age groups [1]. Some investigators have attributed the prominence of *S aureus* to virulence factors, such as the

---

* Texas Children's Hospital, Feigin Center MC 3-2371, Suite 1150, 1102 Bates, Houston, TX 77030.
E-mail address: skaplan@bcm.tmc.edu

0891-5520/05/$ - see front matter
doi:10.1016/j.idc.2005.07.006   *id.theclinics.com*

collagen adhesin encoded by the *cna* gene [4]. *S aureus* isolates from most children seen at Texas Children's Hospital with acute osteomyelitis, however, do not carry the *cna* gene [5]. Group A streptococcus (especially complicating varicella) [6], *Streptococcus pneumoniae* [7], and the emerging pathogen *Kingella kingae* [8] are the next most common organisms in infants and children. Group B streptococcus and gram-negative enterics are important agents in the neonatal period. *Salmonella* species are the most common cause of osteomyelitis in children with hemoglobinopathies [9] and *Pseudomonas aeruginosa* is particularly associated with puncture wounds of the calcaneus, metatarsal, and tarsal bones [10]. *Haemophilus influenzae* type b infection is now rare from the success of the *H influenzae* type b conjugate vaccine. In almost half of children with acute osteomyelitis, a bacterial etiology is never established [11]. Chronic osteomyelitis is most commonly caused by *S aureus* and gram-negative enterics. Polymicrobial etiologies are found in a high proportion of children with osteomyelitis secondary to trauma or infected contiguous soft tissue [12].

Clinical manifestations

The clinical manifestations of acute osteomyelitis in infants and children are well known and are not reviewed in depth in this article [1]. Osteomyelitis tends to be more diffuse in infants because of low anatomic barriers to limit spread of infection; concomitant septic arthritis, soft tissue infection, and pseudoparalysis of the involved extremity are common. In older children, infection is usually more focal. Fever and bacteremia are much more common in children with osteomyelitis than in adults.

Virulence of community-acquired methicillin-resistant Staphylococcus aureus

New manifestations of acute osteomyelitis are associated with clones of community-acquired methicillin-resistant *S aureus* (CA-MRSA) carrying the genes encoding Panton-Valentine leukocidin (*pvl*). Typically, only one site of infection is noted in children with acute hematogenous osteomyelitis caused by *S aureus*. Bocchini and coworkers [13], however, report that 15% of children with acute osteomyelitis caused by *pvl* + *S aureus* isolates have multiple sites of infection. In addition, myositis, pyomyositis, and intra-osseous or subperiosteal abscesses are more commonly seen in association with *pvl* + isolates than for *pvl*− isolates [12]. Up to 10 sites of bone infection have been seen with CA-MRSA isolates. Furthermore, chronic osteomyelitis is more likely to be present at the time of diagnosis or at follow-up with *pvl* + isolates than with *pvl*− isolates [14].

Severe life-threatening infections in adolescents in association with CA-MRSA osteomyelitis are also more frequent [15]. These patients with bacteremia and multiple sites of osteomyelitis quickly become severely ill and require admission to the pediatric intensive care unit, most because of pulmonary involvement. Vascular complications, such as deep venous thromboses and septic pulmonary emboli, seem to be more common with CA-MRSA infections than was recognized in the past with *S aureus* osteomyelitis (Fig. 1) [14,16,17].

Pneumococcal and streptococcal disease

In a large series of children with pneumococcal bone infections from a multicenter study, the mean age of 21 children with bone infections was 12 ± 22.4 months [7]. Only four (19%) of the children had a history of antecedent trauma to the affected area. As with *S aureus*, the large bones were most commonly involved, but the calcaneus was infected in three, and the ileum or a rib in one each. Ten children with osteomyelitis of a long bone had septic arthritis of an adjacent joint.

In the most recent series of osteomyelitis caused by *Streptococcus pyogenes*, the mean age of the patients was 49.4 ± 38.7 months (range: 4–129 months) [6]. The mean ages of children with either *S pneumoniae* or *S pyogenes* osteomyelitis were younger than the age of children with *S aureus* osteomyelitis. As with *S pneumoniae*, osteomyelitis of cuboidal bones is more common with *S pyogenes* than with *S aureus*.

Vertebral osteomyelitis and diskitis

For vertebral osteomyelitis, the mean age in a series of 14 children was 7.5 years (range: 2–13 years), which was significantly older than the 36

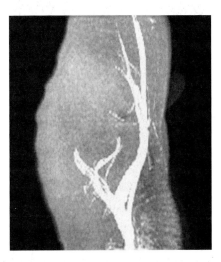

Fig. 1. MR angiogram demonstrating occlusion of the popliteal vein behind the distal femur in adolescent boy with CA-MRSA osteomyelitis of the proximal tibia, complicated by deep venous thrombophlebitis.

children with diskitis (mean: 2.8 years; range: 7 months to 16 years) [18]. Preceding trauma was noted in only 2 of the 14 children. Back pain was the most common presenting complaint and the lumbosacral area was most commonly involved (64%), followed by the thoracolumbar area (29%). The mean duration of symptoms was 33 days (range: 5 days to 3 months).

Diagnosis

Laboratory investigations

When the history and physical examination suggest acute osteomyelitis, laboratory and diagnostic imaging evaluation are required to confirm the diagnosis. Standard laboratory indicators of inflammation, such as the total white blood cell count, erythrocyte sedimentation rate, and C-reactive protein, are all generally elevated. The C-reactive protein is most commonly increased, and was elevated in all (98%) but one of 44 children compared with an elevated erythrocyte sedimentation rate in 92% (35 of 38) in one series [19]. Both the erythrocyte sedimentation rate and the C-reactive protein at the initial evaluation, and the maximum value during hospitalization, were significantly higher in children with pvl + S aureus isolates, compared with children with pvl− S aureus isolates [13]. Blood cultures are positive in 50% to 60% of patients [2,20]. Bone aspiration under CT or ultrasound guidance may reveal an etiologic agent when the blood cultures are negative [20].

Polymerase chain reaction may become an important diagnostic technique for determining the etiology of osteomyelitis when blood or bone cultures are negative. Polymerase chain reaction is already useful for cases caused by Bartonella henselae or K kingae [21]. Placing bone aspirates or synovial fluid into blood culture bottles enhances the yield of isolating K kingae, and may also serve as a medium for detecting 16S rRNA of K kingae by polymerase chain reaction.

Imaging studies

Plain radiographs early in the clinical course usually show soft tissue swelling and obliteration of tissue planes, but bone abnormalities, such as periosteal elevation or lytic lesions, are typically not identified until 10 to 14 days into the course. Plain films do help in demonstrating fractures or bone malignancies, which are included in the differential diagnosis of osteomyelitis. Technetium-labeled methylene diphosphate bone scan is about 90% sensitive in detecting osteomyelitis, and is especially useful if multifocal osteomyelitis is a concern, or the site of infection is poorly localized [22–24]. Periosteal abscesses can be detected readily by ultrasound, which is useful for helping to distinguish infection from infarction in bone of children with sickle cell disease [25].

MRI is now the most sensitive modality for detecting changes in bone consistent with acute osteomyelitis [24]. Bone marrow edema is seen as low signal intensity (dark) on T1-weighted images and high signal intensity (bright) on T2-weighted images (Fig. 2) [26]. Abscesses are best demonstrated with intravenous gadolinium contrast on the T1-weighted images with fat suppression. These changes are not specific, so findings must be interpreted within the clinical context [26]. In addition to bone abnormalities, myositis or pyomyositis contiguous to the site of osteomyelitis is readily detected. In the author's patients with *pvl* + *S aureus* isolates, 28 (62%) of 45 had surrounding myositis or pyomyositis on MRI, compared with 6 (31.6%) of 19 with *pvl*– isolates ($P = .05$) [13]. In addition, 34 (76%) of 45 of the group with *pvl* + isolates had subperiosteal or intraosseal abscesses, compared with 9 (47%) of 19 in the group with *pvl*– strains. MRI is especially useful for children with pelvic or vertebral osteomyelitis. Furthermore, MRI allows the orthopedic surgeon to plan the optimal surgical management for the patient. The disadvantages of MRI are the increased time required for scanning, the need for sedation in younger children, and the cost compared with CT.

Treatment

Empiric regimens for osteomyelitis in children

The selection of antibiotics for the empiric treatment of acute osteomyelitis in children should always include an agent directed against *S aureus*. Choosing a particular antistaphylococcal agent is now more complicated, however, in the era of CA-MRSA [27–29]. In the past, nafcillin

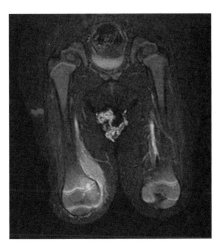

Fig. 2. Signal abnormality in the medial aspect of the distal right femoral metaphysis on the inversion recovery sequence of MRI of a child with CA-MRSA osteomyelitis.

or oxacillin had been the standard agent, or was included in a combination of antibiotics for empiric treatment. This is no longer appropriate where CA-MRSA isolates are common. In some regions of the United States, methicillin-resistant rates among community S aureus isolates are 75% or more [27]. Physicians must have some knowledge of the local rates of MRSA among community S aureus isolates, such as information derived from hospital or commercial laboratories processing S aureus isolates from local outpatients.

Some experts recommend that once the rate of methicillin-resistance among community S aureus isolates is ≥10%, antibiotics effective against CA-MRSA should be administered from the onset of treatment. Vancomycin is the gold standard for treating MRSA infections, and the addition of gentamicin, rifampin, or both for synergy may be helpful in children requiring intensive care unit admission. Recently, the value of adding rifampin to vancomycin for MRSA has been questioned [30]. In most areas of the country, 90% or more CA-MRSA isolates are susceptible to clindamycin. Clindamycin is an effective antibiotic for the treatment of acute osteomyelitis caused by CA-MRSA when the S aureus isolate is fully susceptible [15]. Microbiology laboratories, however, must screen for inducible macrolide-lincosamide-streptogramin resistance using the "D-test" [31]. Serious infections caused by S aureus isolates with inducible-clindamycin resistance should not be treated with clindamycin, because the risk of inducing resistance in vivo with resultant treatment failure is substantial [31,32]. When local clindamycin resistance rates among community S aureus isolates exceed 10% to 15%, clindamycin is not recommended for initial empiric treatment.

Vancomycin and clindamycin are also active against almost all isolates of S pyogenes and S pneumoniae, the other two main causes of acute hematogenous osteomyelitis in otherwise normal children [33,34]. Neither has in vitro activity against K kingae. In the normal child with osteomyelitis thought to have developed hematogenously, I prefer to initiate a single antibiotic. In our area with a very high rate of CA-MRSA, clindamycin or vancomycin is the agent of choice. Where CA-MRSA is unlikely, nafcillin or oxacillin is the agent of choice. If no organism is isolated and the child is clearly improving, a pathogen susceptible to clindamycin, vancomycin, or nafcillin is likely.

Oral step-down therapy

Once an organism is isolated and antibiotic susceptibilities are determined, antibiotic treatment may be modified. Nafcillin or oxacillin is the agent of choice for treating methicillin-susceptible S aureus. The main issues with prolonged nafcillin or oxacillin are the development of neutropenia related to bone marrow suppression, hypersensitivity reactions, and elevation in liver transaminases. Cephalexin or dicloxacillin are the primary oral antistaphylococcal β-lactam antibiotics used to complete therapy, after the patient has responded to a period of intravenous treatment [35–37].

Clindamycin is an excellent agent for treating methicillin-susceptible *S aureus* in patients allergic to or intolerant of nafcillin [38,39]. Clindamycin is also an important option for the treatment of CA-MRSA osteomyelitis caused by susceptible strains [14]. In either setting, clindamycin may be administered orally following appropriate intravenous treatment. Common adverse events with clindamycin are diarrhea and rash. Pseudomembranous enteritis secondary to *C difficile* toxin is the major concern with clindamycin, but this seems to be relatively uncommon in children even after prolonged administration [40].

Trimethoprim-sulfamethoxazole and tetracyclines

Other therapeutic options for CA-MRSA infections are less well studied for osteomyelitis. Virtually all CA-MRSA isolates are susceptible to trimethoprim-sulfamethoxazole, but there is little information on the use of trimethoprim-sulfamethoxazole in the treatment of invasive MRSA infections, especially osteomyelitis [41,42].

Long-acting tetracyclines, such as minocycline or doxycycline, have good in vitro activity against most CA-MRSA isolates. In a recent study, 24 adults with MRSA infections were treated with doxycycline or minocycline for greater than 50% of the total treatment duration [43]. Skin and soft tissue infections were the most common sites (67%), but four had osteomyelitis. Two of the four with osteomyelitis were considered cured. These investigators also reviewed the literature, and found four other patients with osteomyelitis treated with minocycline and rifampin. They concluded that doxycycline or minocycline might be reasonable oral alternatives for patients with skin and soft tissue MRSA infections, but that data are insufficient to recommend their routine use in osteomyelitis or bacteremia. Minocycline or doxycycline may only be considered in children over 8 years of age, because of the risk of stunted bone and tooth growth.

Linezolid

Linezolid is an oxazolidinone antibiotic, with excellent in vitro activity against MRSA isolates. It is approved for pediatric use. In a large comparative trial, linezolid was equivalent to vancomycin for the treatment of infections caused by resistant gram-positive bacteria [44]. In a subset analysis of children with MRSA infections in this and another trial of linezolid for skin and soft tissue infections, linezolid was effective for a variety of MRSA infections, including nosocomial pneumonia and bacteremia, but osteomyelitis was not included [45].

Although linezolid has not been evaluated in a formal manner for treatment of osteomyelitis, it has been used successfully in a compassionate use program [46]. Linezolid was administered to patients with multidrug-resistant gram-positive infections who were intolerant to other potentially effective antibiotics, or who could not tolerate long-term intravenous antibiotic therapy. Fifty-five patients with a mean age of 58 years were evaluable for clinical assessment. Twenty-eight patients had long bone osteomyelitis. MRSA was the primary pathogen in 25 of 55 patients overall. At short-term follow-up a median of 21 days after the last dose, 16 (70%) of 23 patients with MRSA osteomyelitis were considered cured. Linezolid is an important oral agent for completing therapy for osteomyelitis caused by MRSA isolates resistant to clindamycin. Unfortunately, the suspension of linezolid is not very palatable for young children. Although linezolid is expensive, the oral route is convenient and cost effective, compared with home intravenous therapy with vancomycin.

The major side effects of linezolid are gastrointestinal disturbances, rashes, and elevated liver transaminases. A fall in hemoglobin or platelets may occur in adults receiving linezolid greater than 14 days [47]. In children, myelosuppression associated with linezolid is minimal in the first 2 weeks of therapy [48]. Long-term linezolid use in adults has been associated rarely with a peripheral neuropathy, and optic neuritis [49]. Lactic acidosis has also been reported in a few adults who received linezolid for prolonged periods [50].

Daptomycin

Daptomycin is a cyclic lipopeptide, with rapid bactericidal activity against MRSA in vitro [51]. Daptomycin is only available in an intravenous formulation. It is approved for the treatment of complicated skin and soft tissue infections in adults [52]. Daptomycin is inferior to ceftriaxone for the treatment of community-acquired pneumonia in adults, and currently is not approved for the treatment of pneumonia [51]. The lack of efficacy of daptomycin in pneumonia may relate to low concentrations of daptomycin in the bronchial-alveolar lining fluid and lung parenchyma, and inhibition of daptomycin by surfactant [51,53]. There are no pharmacokinetic data in children, so appropriate dosing for daptomycin in pediatrics is not known [54]. In addition, a substantial percentage of moderately ill children with *S aureus* osteomyelitis have pulmonary involvement, in which case daptomycin does not seem to be appropriate therapy as a single agent [55]. The role of daptomycin in the treatment of MRSA osteomyelitis in children is unclear.

β-Lactam antibiotics

Aqueous penicillin G is the agent of choice for treating osteomyelitis caused by group A streptococcus or penicillin-susceptible *S pneumoniae*. Amoxicillin or penicillin VK is the optimal agent for completing therapy with an oral agent. For pneumococcal isolates with resistance to penicillin, cefotaxime or ceftriaxone is recommended [7]. *K kingae* is susceptible to most β-lactam antibiotics, including nafcillin or oxacillin, and the second- and third-generation cephalosporins. Ceftazidime or antipseudomonal penicillins, plus an aminoglycoside, are typically administered for *Pseudo-*

monas osteochondritis. For *Salmonella* osteomyelitis, ampicillin is used for susceptible isolates. Cefotaxime or ceftriaxone are recommended for ampicillin-resistant isolates.

Antibiotics treatment is provided for a minimum of 21 days based on the study by Dich and coworkers [56]. I generally recommend treating until the C-reactive protein and erythrocyte sedimentation rate are both within a normal range, which typically requires 4 to 6 weeks of total therapy.

Surgical therapy

A drainage procedure is indicated if a subperiosteal or intraosseous abscess is present in patients with acute hematogenous osteomyelitis. This can often be accomplished through interventional radiology. Surgical debridement is more critical for optimal treatment of osteomyelitis associated with contiguous infections, direct inoculation, or chronic osteomyelitis [10,12]. Hyperbaric oxygen may be a useful adjunctive treatment measure in the management of chronic osteomyelitis that is refractory to standard approaches [57].

References

[1] Krogstad P. Osteomyelitis and septic arthritis. In: Feigin RD, Cherry JD, Demmler GJ, et al, editors. Textbook of pediatric infectious diseases. 5th edition. Philadelphia: WB Saunders; 2004. p. 713–36.
[2] Stott NS. Review article: paediatric bone and joint infections. J Orthop Surg 2001;9:83–90.
[3] Richards BS. Delayed infections following posterior spinal instrumentation for the treatment of idiopathic scoliosis. J Bone Joint Surg Am 1995;77:524–9.
[4] Elasri MO, Thomas JR, Skinner RA, et al. *Staphylococcus aureus* collagen adhesin contributes to the pathogenesis of osteomyelitis. Bone 2002;30:275–80.
[5] Mishaan AM, Mason EO Jr, Martinez-Aguilar G, et al. Emergence of a predominant clone of community-acquired *Staphylococcus aureus* among children in Houston, Texas. Pediatr Infect Dis J 2005;24:201–6.
[6] Ibia EO, Imoisili M, Pikas A. Group A β-hemolytic streptococcal osteomyelitis in children. Pediatrics 2003;112:e22–6.
[7] Bradley JS, Kaplan SL, Tan TQ, et al. Pediatric pneumococcal bone and joint infections. Pediatrics 1998;102:1376–82.
[8] Yagupsky P, Dagan R. *Kingella kingae*: an emerging cause of invasive infections in young children. Clin Infect Dis 1997;24:860–6.
[9] Burnett MW, Bass JW, Cook BA. Etiology of osteomyelitis complicating sickle cell disease. Pediatrics 1998;101:296–7.
[10] Jacobs RF, McCarthy RE, Elser JM. Pseudomonas osteochondritis complicating puncture wounds of the foot in children: a 10-year evaluation. J Infect Dis 1989;160:657–61.
[11] Floyed RL, Steele RW. Culture-negative osteomyelitis. Pediatr Infect Dis J 2003;22:731–5.
[12] Dubey L, Krasinski K, Hernanz-Schulman M. Osteomyelitis secondary to trauma or infected contiguous soft tissue. Pediatr Infect Dis J 1988;7:26–34.
[13] Bocchini CE, Hulten KG, Mason Jr. EO, et al. Panton-Valentine leukocidin genes are associated with enhanced inflammatory response and local disease in acute hematogenous *Staphylococcus aureus* osteomyelitis in children. Pediatrics, in press.

[14] Martinez-Aguilar H, Avalos-Mishaan A, Hulten K, et al. Community-acquired, methicillin-resistant and methicillin-susceptible *Staphylococcus aureus* musculoskeletal infections in children. Pediatr Infect Dis J 2004;23:701–6.

[15] Gonzalez BE, Martinez-Aguilar G, Hulten KG, et al. Severe Staphylococcal sepsis in adolescents in the era of community-acquired methicillin-resistant *Staphylococcus aureus*. Pediatrics 2005;115:642–8.

[16] Gonzalez BE, Hulten KG, Hammerman W, et al. Deep venous thrombophlebitis in patients with *Staphylococcus aureus* invasive infections [Abstract #525]. Presented at the Pediatric Academic Societies' 2005 Meeting. Washington, May 15, 2005.

[17] Gorenstein A, Gross E, Houri S, et al. The pivotal role of deep vein thrombophlebitis in the development of acute disseminated staphylococcal disease in children. Pediatrics 2000; 106:E87.

[18] Fernandez M, Carrol CL, Baker CJ. Discitis and vertebral osteomyelitis in children: an 18-year review. Pediatrics 2000;105:1299–304.

[19] Unkila-Kallio L, Kallio MJT, Eskola J, et al. Serum C-reactive protein, erythrocyte sedimentation rate, and white blood cell count in acute hematogenous osteomyelitis in children. Pediatrics 1994;93:59–62.

[20] Karwowska A, Davies HD, Jadavji T. Epidemiology and outcome of osteomyelitis in the era of sequential intravenous-oral therapy. Pediatr Infect Dis J 1998;17:1021–6.

[21] Moumile K, Merckx J, Glorion C, et al. Osteoarticular infections caused by *Kingella kingae* in children: contribution of polymerase chain reaction to the microbiologic diagnosis. Pediatr Infect Dis J 2003;22:837–9.

[22] Darville T, Jacobs RF. Management of acute hematogenous osteomyelitis. Pediatr Infect Dis J 2004;23:255–7.

[23] Kaiser S, Jorulf H, Hirsch G. Clinical value of imaging techniques in childhood osteomyelitis. Acta Radiol 1998;39:523–31.

[24] Connolly LP, Connolly SA, Drubach LA, et al. Acute hematogenous osteomyelitis of children: assessment of skeletal scintigraphy-based diagnosis in the era of MRI. J Nucl Med 2002;43:1310–6.

[25] Rifai A, Nyman R. Scintigraphy and ultrasonography in differentiating osteomyelitis from bone infarction in sickle cell disease. Acta Radiol 1997;38:139–43.

[26] Chung T. Magnetic resonance imaging in acute osteomyelitis in children. Pediatr Infect Dis J 2002;22:869–70.

[27] Kaplan SL, Hulten KG, Gonzalez BE, et al. Three-year surveillance of community-acquired *Staphylococcus aureus* infections in children. Clin Infect Dis 2005;40:1785–91.

[28] Herold BC, Immergluck LC, Maranan MC, et al. Community-acquired methicillin-resistant *Staphylococcus aureus* in children with no identified predisposing risk. JAMA 1998;279: 593–8.

[29] Buckingham SC, McDougal LK, Cathey LD, et al. Emergence of community-associated methicillin-resistant *Staphylococcus aureus* at a Memphis, Tennessee children's hospital. Pediatr Infect Dis J 2004;23:619–24.

[30] Shelburne SA, Musher DM, Hulten K, et al. In vitro killing of community-associated methicillin-resistant *Staphylococcus aureus* with drug combinations. Antimicrob Agents Chemother 2004;48:4016–9.

[31] Lewis JS II, Jorgensen JH. Inducible clindamycin in staphylococci: should clinicians and microbiologists be concerned? Clin Infect Dis 2005;40:280–5.

[32] Frank AL, Marcinak JF, Mangat PD, et al. Clindamycin treatment of methicillin-resistant *Staphylococcus aureus* infections in children. Pediatr Infect Dis J 2002;21: 530–4.

[33] Hasenbein ME, Warner JE, Lambert KG, et al. Detection of multiple macrolide- and lincosamide-resistant strains of *Streptococcus pyogenes* from patients in the Boston area. J Clin Microbiol 2004;42:1559–63.

[34] Mason EO Jr, Wald ER, Bradley JS, et al. Macrolide resistance among middle ear isolates of *Streptococcus pneumoniae* observed at eight United States pediatric centers: prevalence of M and MLS_B phenotypes. Pediatr Infect Dis J 2003;22:623–7.

[35] Tetzlaff TR, McCracken GH, Nelson JD. Oral antibiotic therapy for skeletal infections of children. J Pediatr 1978;92:485–90.

[36] Bryson YJ, Connor JD, LeClerc M. High dose dicloxacillin treatment of acute staphylococcal osteomyelitis in children. J Pediatr 1979;94:673–5.

[37] Prober CG, Yeager AS. Use of the serum bactericidal titer to assess the adequacy of oral antibiotic therapy in the treatment of acute hematogenous osteomyelitis. J Pediatr 1979;95: 131–5.

[38] Feigin RD, Pickering LK, Anderson D, et al. Clindamycin treatment of osteomyelitis and septic arthritis in children. Pediatrics 1975;55:213–23.

[39] Kaplan SL, Mason EO Jr, Feigin RD. Clindamycin versus nafcillin or methicillin in the treatment of *Staphylococcus aureus* osteomyelitis in children. South Med J 1982;75:138–42.

[40] Michelow IC, McCracken GH Jr. Antibacterial therapeutic agents. In: Feigin RD, Cherry JD, Demmler GJ, et al, editors. Textbook of pediatric infectious diseases. 5th edition. Philadelphia: WB Saunders; 2004. p. 2987–3029.

[41] Markowitz N, Quinn EL, Saravolatz LD. Trimethoprim-sulfamethoxazole compared with vancomycin for the treatment of *Staphylococcus aureus* infection. Ann Intern Med 1992;117: 390–8.

[42] Adra M, Lawrence KR. Trimethoprim-sulfamethoxazole for treatment of severe *Staphylococcus aureus* infections. Ann Pharmacother 2004;38:338–41.

[43] Ruhe JJ, Monson T, Bradsher RW, et al. Use of long-acting tetracyclines for methicillin-resistant *Staphylococcus aureus* infections: case series and review of the literature. Clin Infect Dis 2005;40:1429–34.

[44] Kaplan SL, Deville JG, Yogev R, et al. Linezolid versus vancomycin for treatment of resistant gram-positive infections in children. Pediatr Infect Dis J 2003;22:677–85.

[45] Kaplan SL, Afghani B, Lopez P, et al. Linezolid for the treatment of methicillin-resistant *Staphylococcus aureus* infections in children. Pediatr Infect Dis J 2003;22:S178–85.

[46] Rayner CR, Baddour LM, Birmingham MC, et al. Linezolid in the treatment of osteomyelitis: results of compassionate use experience. Infection 2004;32:8–14.

[47] Gerson SL, Kaplan SL, Bruss JB, et al. Hematologic effects of linezolid: summary of clinical experience. Antimicrob Agents Chemother 2002;46:2723–6.

[48] Meissner HC, Townsend T, Wenman W, et al. Hematologic effects of linezolid in young children. Pediatr Infect Dis J 2003;22:S186–92.

[49] Tan TQ. Update on the use of linezolid. Pediatr Infect Dis J 2004;23:955–6.

[50] Palenzuela L, Hahn NM, Nelson RP Jr, et al. Does linezolid cause lactic acidosis by inhibiting mitochondrial protein synthesis? Clin Infect Dis 2005;40:e113–6.

[51] Carpenter CF, Chambers HF. Daptomycin: another novel agent for treating infections due to drug-resistant gram-positive pathogens. Clin Infect Dis 2004;38:994–1000.

[52] Arbeit RD, Maki D, Tally FP, et al. The safety and efficacy of daptomycin for the treatment of complicated skin and skin-structure infections. Clin Infect Dis 2004;38:1673–81.

[53] Silverman JA, Mortin LI, Vanpraagh AD, et al. Inhibition of daptomycin by pulmonary surfactant: in vitro modeling and clinical impact. J Infect Dis 2005;191:2149–52.

[54] Bradley JS. Newer antistaphylococcal agents. Curr Opin Pediatr 2005;17:71–7.

[55] Gonzalez BE, Hulten KG, Dishop MK, et al. Pulmonary manifestations in children with invasive community-acquired *Staphylococcus aureus* infections. Clin Infect Dis 2005;41:583–90.

[56] Dich PQ, Nelson JD, Haltalin KC. Osteomyelitis in infants and children: a review of 163 cases. Am J Dis Child 1975;129:1273–8.

[57] Waisman D, Shupak A, Weisz G, et al. Hyperbaric oxygen therapy in the pediatric patient: the experience of the Israeli Naval Medical Institute. Pediatrics 1998. Available at: http://www.pediatrics.org/cgi/content/full/102/5/e53.

ELSEVIER
SAUNDERS

Infect Dis Clin N Am 19 (2005) 799–817

INFECTIOUS
DISEASE CLINICS
OF NORTH AMERICA

Septic Arthritis

John J. Ross, MD

Division of Infectious Diseases, Caritas Saint Elizabeth's Medical Center,
736 Cambridge Street, Boston, MA 02135, USA

Septic arthritis is a true rheumatologic emergency, mandating immediate joint drainage and antibiotics. Unfortunately, the incidence of septic arthritis in the United States is increasing, the average patient is older and more vulnerable, antibiotic resistance is rising, and the diagnosis at presentation remains problematic. Two virulent pathogens, methicillin-resistant *Staphylococcus aureus* (MRSA) and group B streptococcus, are increasing in importance, whereas gonococcal arthritis, which has more benign outcomes, is now rare in most centers. The diagnosis of septic arthritis at presentation may be markedly imprecise. Synovial fluid white blood cell (WBC) counts in septic arthritis are notoriously variable. A synovial fluid WBC value of $>50,000$ cells/mm^3 is a commonly used threshold for empiric antibiotic therapy. Many patients with synovial leukocytosis of this magnitude have crystalline arthritis, however, whereas at least one third of infected joints have synovial fluid WBCs below 50,000 cells/mm^3. The yield of synovial fluid culture is maximized with inoculation into blood cultures, compared with plating on solid media. If the diagnosis is unclear, it is reasonable to treat empirically, given the risk of irreparable joint damage with delayed diagnosis. Whether arthroscopic irrigation and debridement is superior to bedside arthrocentesis has not been determined in prospective trials. These issues regarding the pathogenesis, presentation, bacteriology, diagnosis, and treatment of septic arthritis are reviewed in detail.

Pathogenesis

Septic arthritis is most often a consequence of occult bacteremia. Synovium is highly vascular, but lacks a protective basement membrane, making it vulnerable to bacteremic seeding [1]. Minute breaks in skin or

E-mail address: jrossmd@cchcs.org

doi:10.1016/j.idc.2005.07.004
id.theclinics.com

mucous membranes may allow staphylococci and streptococci initial access to the bloodstream. Gram-negative septic arthritis probably arises from bacteremia from the gastrointestinal or urinary tracts. Occasionally, septic arthritis results from penetrating trauma, such as bite wounds, stepping on nails, or errant injection drug use. This is the most common means of infection of the small joints of the hands and feet [2]. Rarely, arthroscopy or therapeutic joint injection with corticosteroids may be complicated by septic arthritis.

Gram-positive organisms are responsible for most cases of septic arthritis. Enteric gram-negative rods account for 43% of community-acquired bacteremias, but cause only 10% of septic arthritis [3,4]. This likely relates to the superior ability of gram-positive organisms to bind connective tissue and extracellular matrix proteins. *S aureus*, the commonest cause of septic arthritis, produces several surface adhesins that bind extracellular matrix proteins, known as "microbial surface components recognizing adhesive matrix molecules." Staphylococcal strains defective in microbial surface components recognizing adhesive matrix molecules are less arthritogenic in animal models [5].

Joint damage in septic arthritis results from bacterial invasion, host inflammation, and tissue ischemia. Bacterial enzymes and toxins are directly injurious to cartilage. Cartilage may suffer "innocent bystander" damage, as host neutrophils release reactive oxygen species and lysosomal proteases. Cytokines activate host matrix metalloproteinases, leading to autodigestion of cartilage [6]. Ischemic injury also plays a role. Cartilage is avascular, and highly dependent on diffusion of oxygen and nutrients from the synovium. As purulent exudate accumulates, joint pressure increases, and synovial blood flow is tamponaded, resulting in cartilage anoxia [7].

Risk factors

The foremost risk factor for septic arthritis is pre-existing joint disease. Up to 47% of patients have prior joint problems [2]. A high index of suspicion for septic arthritis should be maintained in patients with other rheumatologic conditions, such as rheumatoid arthritis, osteoarthritis, gout, pseudogout, recent trauma, prior joint surgery, and systemic lupus erythematosus. Of these, rheumatoid arthritis is the most common, and is associated with worse outcomes.

Rheumatoid arthritis patients are at high risk for septic arthritis from the combination of joint damage, immunosuppressive medications, and skin breakdown. Periarticular infection may result in sinus tracts, bursitis, and rupture of synovial cysts. Polyarticular disease is common, functional outcomes are worse, and mortality is high in rheumatoid arthritis patients with septic joints [8,9]. Diagnosis is often delayed because of the confusion of septic arthritis for a flare of rheumatoid arthritis. In gouty patients with septic arthritis, inflammation results in shedding of synovial microtophi, obscuring the diagnosis. All patients with apparent gouty joints should also have routine Gram stain and culture performed to exclude concomitant septic arthritis [10,11].

Two other broad categories of risk for septic arthritis are conditions causing loss of skin integrity, such as psoriasis, eczema, skin ulcers, and injection drug abuse, and conditions associated with compromised immunity, such as diabetes mellitus, renal failure, cirrhosis, and immunosuppressive drugs. A recently described risk factor is anti-inflammatory therapy with tumor necrosis factor blockers. Lethal infection and unusual organisms, such as *Listeria, Salmonella*, and *Actinobacillus ureae*, have been reported [12–15]. A significant proportion of patients with septic arthritis, however, up to 22% in some studies, have no medical risk factors and no underlying joint disease [16].

A review of cases of septic arthritis from the National Hospital Discharge Survey revealed that the average age of septic arthritis patients had risen from 37 years in 1979 to 51 in 2002. In recent years, patients had more comorbid medical conditions, had septic arthritis in the setting of complicated hospitalizations, and were more likely to have infection with antibiotic-resistant organisms. Overall in-hospital mortality was 2.6%, and was similar from 1979 to 2002 (unpublished data).

Clinical presentation

The diagnosis of septic arthritis presents no difficulty in the classic patient with fever; rigors; and a warm, swollen, and exquisitely painful joint. Unhappily, however, the clinical and laboratory diagnosis of septic arthritis is often highly imprecise. High-grade fever is only present in 58% [16], although 90% have at least low-grade fever [17]. Serum leukocytosis is present in only 50% to 60% of patients [16,17]. Joint pain is blunted in the immunosuppressed, such as the rheumatoid arthritis patient on cortico-steroids, leading to delayed diagnosis and greater complications [9,18].

Predictors of mortality in a multivariate analysis include age ≥ 65 years, confusion at presentation, and polyarticular disease. Predictors of joint damage include age ≥ 65 years, diabetes mellitus, and infection with β-hemolytic streptococci [16].

Joint distribution

The knee is the principal target of bacterial septic arthritis. Forty-five percent of septic arthritis cases in adults involve the knee [2]. Presumably, this is a consequence of the imperfect human adaptation to bipedal locomotion. The enormous stresses about the knee particularly predispose it to injury [19]. Other large joints of the appendicular skeleton, including the hip (15%), ankle (9%), elbow (8%), wrist (6%), and shoulder (5%), are commonly involved in adults [2]. Polyarticular disease is seen in about 10%

to 20% of cases; it is more common with gonococcal, pneumococcal, group B streptococcal, and gram-negative septic arthritis. Polyarticular septic arthritis is usually asymmetric, and involves an average of four joints. At least one knee is involved in 72% of cases. Major risk factors are steroid therapy, rheumatoid arthritis, lupus, and diabetes mellitus [20].

Septic arthritis of cartilaginous joints

Involvement of cartilaginous joints of the axial skeleton is infrequent, except in intravenous drug users [21]. Sacroiliac septic arthritis is generally seen in younger patients, although cases in the elderly are sporadically observed (Fig. 1). Patients present with buttock pain and fever. It may be difficult to localize the pain on examination. The FABERE test (*F*lexion, *AB*duction, *E*xternal *R*otation, and *E*xtension) stresses the sacroiliac joint. It is performed on the supine patient by placing the ipsilateral medial malleolus on the opposite knee. The ipsilateral knee is depressed, with pressure exerted on the opposite superior iliac spine. Pain is elicited in sacroiliitis, although the FABERE test is not specific for infection [22,23].

Infection of the pubic symphysis presents with fever; suprapubic and hip pain; and a waddling, antalgic gait. Pubic symphysis septic arthritis is rare, occurring in patients with well-defined risk factors: intravenous drug use; pelvic malignancy or surgery (Fig. 2); and athletes, such as soccer players, with overuse injuries of the hip adductors and pubic periostitis [24]. Sternoclavicular septic arthritis is discussed later.

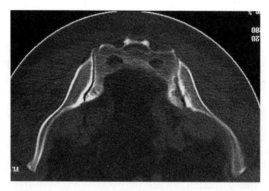

Fig. 1. Sacroiliac septic arthritis in a 71-year-old woman, previously healthy except for venous stasis ulceration, presenting with sudden onset of right buttock pain and fever. Pelvic CT 4 weeks after the onset of symptoms demonstrates sclerosis, widening, and erosion of the right sacroiliac joint. CT scan previously obtained 8 days after the onset of symptoms had been normal. Low-grade *Staphylococcus aureus* bacteremia was present. Transesophageal echocardiography was unremarkable. Clinical cure was achieved with 4 weeks of intravenous antibiotics and 2 weeks of oral antibiotic therapy.

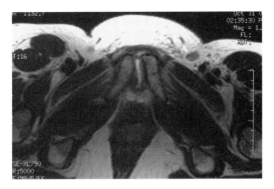

Fig. 2. Pubic symphysis septic arthritis in a 36-year-old woman with fever, suprapubic pain, and *Streptococcus pneumoniae* bacteremia following cesarian section. T2-weighted MRI shows edema of the pubic symphysis, pubic bones, hip adductors, and adjacent soft tissue. Fluid is present within the pubic symphysis. No other source of pneumococcal bacteremia was found. (Courtesy of Linden T. Hu, MD.)

Bacteriology

Staphylococcus aureus

The most common cause of septic arthritis is *S aureus*, which accounts for 44% of cases (Table 1). Only 46% have an underlying focus of staphylococcal infection, such as cellulitis [25]. In the remainder, septic

Table 1
Organisms isolated in 2407 cases of septic arthritis

Organism	No. Isolates (%)
Staphylococcus aureus	1066 (44.3)
Streptococcus pyogenes	183 (7.6)
Streptococcus pneumoniae	156 (6.5)
Haemophilus influenzae	104 (4.3)
Mycobacterium tuberculosis	101 (4.2)
Escherichia coli	91 (3.8)
Coagulase-negative staphylococci	84 (3.5)
Neisseria gonorrhoeae	77 (3.2)
Streptococcus agalactiae	69 (2.9)
Pseudomonas aeruginosa	36 (1.5)
Neisseria meningitidis	28 (1.2)
Salmonella sp	25 (1)
Other gram-negative rods	110 (4.6)
Other β-hemolytic streptococci	104 (4.3)
Polymicrobial	33 (1.4)
Fungi	4 (0.2)
Miscellaneous	136 (5.7)

Adapted from Ross JJ, Saltzman CL, Carling P, et al. Pneumococcal septic arthritis: review of 190 cases. Clin Infect Dis 2003;36:319–327; with permission.

arthritis presumably arises as a consequence of transient bacteremia from a skin or mucous membrane source. Outcomes may be poor. Mortality ranges from 7% to 18%, and osteomyelitis or loss of joint function occurs in up to 27% to 46% [16,17]. The ability of *S aureus* to induce a vigorous host immune response by superantigen production may contribute to arthritis severity and mortality [26].

MRSA may be increasing in importance in septic arthritis. In the last 5 years at Caritas St. Elizabeth's Medical Center and Tufts-New England Medical Center, 25% of septic arthritis was caused by MRSA (unpublished data). All cases in the series were associated with chronic illness, older age, and health care exposure. Community-acquired MRSA septic arthritis, however, has occurred in some regions of the United States [27].

β-Hemolytic streptococci

Group B streptococci (*Streptococcus agalactiae*) have emerged as invasive pathogens in the elderly, especially those with diabetes, cirrhosis, and neurologic disease [28]. At one center, group B streptococci increased from 1% of septic arthritis cases in the 1980s, to 6% in the 1990s [29]. In two other recent series, group B streptococci caused 10% of septic arthritis [30,31]. Bacteremia was seen in 66%, polyarticular disease in 32%, and mortality was 9% [30]. Functional outcomes are typically poor in septic arthritis because of group B streptococci and other β-hemolytic streptococci [16]. The sternoclavicular and sacroiliac joints may be involved with disproportionate frequency [30], although this could be the result of reporting bias. Other β-hemolytic streptococci, particularly group A streptococci (*Streptococcus pyogenes*), may cause an equally virulent form of septic arthritis in adults, although with lesser frequency.

Pneumococcus

Streptococcus pneumoniae caused 6% of septic arthritis in one literature review, possibly skewed upward by the high rates in a few series [4,32,33]. As with septic arthritis caused by group B streptococci, pneumococcal septic arthritis is notable for a high frequency of bacteremia and polyarticular disease. Only 50% have an underlying focus of pneumococcal disease, such as pneumonia. Mortality in adults is high (19%), although functional outcomes are good in 95% of survivors. Drug resistance may be an increasing problem [4].

Gonococcal arthritis

Neisseria gonorrhoeae, once the leading cause of septic arthritis in young adults in the United States, has dwindled in importance since the 1980s. Safer sex in the AIDS era led to a 64% decline in gonorrhea from 1985 to 1997 [34]. Recent increases in high-risk sexual behavior in young gay men, however, and rising rates of fluoroquinolone-resistant gonorrhea, suggest that epidemic gonorrhea could return to the United States.

Gonococcal septic arthritis is a distinct clinical syndrome, with a good prognosis. Seventy-five percent of cases occur in women; menses and pregnancy increase the risk of disseminated gonococcal infection [35]. Seventy-two percent of cases are polyarticular [25]. Patients may experience a fleeting and migratory polyarthritis, or a more conventional septic arthritis picture of several hot, swollen, and exquisitely tender joints. Knee involvement is most common. The characteristic hemorrhagic pustules of disseminated gonococcal infection are found in 42% of patients, and tenosynovitis in 21%. Urinary signs or symptoms are present in only 32%. Gonococci are recovered from joint fluid in less than 50% of cases. This is probably largely because of the difficulty in recovering these fastidious organisms from cultures, but may also indicate that some cases of gonococcal arthritis are immune-mediated [35]. Complete recovery is the rule with appropriate therapy, and sequelae are rare.

Enteric gram-negative rods

Gram-negative rods cause approximately 10% of adult septic arthritis. Two major groups are at risk: elderly patients with comorbid medical conditions, and young intravenous drug users [36,37]. Outcomes are typically better in the latter group. Older series suggested that the mortality of gram-negative septic arthritis was 25%, with poor functional outcomes in 79% of survivors [17]. More recent data suggest that outcome of gram-negative septic arthritis in older patients may be relatively good with prompt diagnosis and aggressive therapy, with mortality rates of only 5%, and poor functional outcomes in 32%. Perhaps surprisingly, an underlying source of gram-negative septic arthritis, such as a urinary tract infection, is only found in 50% of older patients [38]. Gram-negative bacilli have waned in importance as a cause of septic arthritis in injection drug users in recent years (see later).

Meningococcal arthritis

It was recognized in the nineteenth century that arthritis was a frequent complication during meningococcal epidemics, and that joint fluid might be serous or purulent [39]. The incidence of arthritis in invasive meningococcal disease is as high as 14%. The usual presentation is a monoarthritis or oligoarthritis, involving the knee and other large joints. In most cases, arthritis develops several days into antibiotic therapy, and the joint fluid is sterile. Synovial fluid immune complexes have been detected in several of these patients, suggesting an immunologic basis of arthritis [40,41]. Less commonly, patients present with an isolated septic joint (primary meningococcal arthritis), or an arthritis-dermatitis syndrome akin to disseminated gonococcal infection [42]. Outcomes in meningococcal arthritis are usually excellent, with complete preservation of joint function [40].

Coagulase-negative staphylococci and postarthroscopic septic arthritis

Most isolates of coagulase-negative staphylococci from native joints are contaminants, but they can be true joint pathogens after arthroscopy, anterior cruciate ligament reconstruction, and other orthopedic procedures. Septic arthritis after arthroscopy is more likely with intra-articular corticosteroids, longer operating times, multiple prior procedures, and chrondroplasty or soft tissue debridement. Coagulase-negative staphylococcal joint infection tends to present in an indolent fashion, with low-grade fever, normal peripheral leukocyte counts, and mild to moderate joint symptomatology. Two weeks of parenteral antibiotics are usually curative for postarthroscopic septic arthritis [43]. Septic arthritis complicating anterior cruciate ligament reconstruction is treated with aggressive arthroscopic irrigation and debridement, followed by antibiotics for 6 weeks. Grafts can usually be retained, if they appear intact on arthroscopic inspection [44].

Septic arthritis in specific populations or after unusual exposures

Tuberculosis

Tuberculous septic arthritis is discussed elsewhere in this issue.

Brucellosis

Brucellosis is a common cause of subacute or chronic arthritis in countries where unpasteurized dairy products are consumed. In the United States, most cases are seen in immigrants from Latin America and the Middle East. The sacroiliac joint is involved in up to 54% of patients, for unclear reasons. Spondylitis occurs in 7%. Other patients present with monoarthritis or oligoarthritis, with lower extremity predominance. It has been suggested that brucellar arthritis may be reactive [45]. Brucellosis is diagnosed by blood culture or serology. The highest cure rates were reported with the combination of doxycycline for 45 days and streptomycin for 14 days [46].

Rat-bite fever (Streptobacillus moniliformis)

In Europe and Asia, a rat bite or scratch, or ingestion of food and drink contaminated with murine feces, may result in rat-bite fever. Patients present with a febrile systemic illness, arthralgias or arthritis, and an acral rash often involving the palms and soles. Inflammation at the bite wound is not prominent, and the patient may be oblivious to the bite if it occurs during sleep [47]. The causative organism, *S moniliformis*, is a fastidious gram-negative rod, and diagnosis requires the use of enriched media or polymerase chain reaction. Sodium polyanethol sulfonate in commercial blood culture systems inhibits streptobacilli. Fatal cases of rat-bite fever in healthy individuals have recently been reported in the United States [48].

In Asia, rat-bite fever is caused by a spirochete, *Spirillum minus*. The illness, known as sodoku, is distinct from streptobacillary infection: eschar formation and lymphangitis at the bite site are usual, fevers are prolonged and relapsing without antibiotics, rash spares the palms and soles, and arthritis is uncommon [49]. *S moniliformis* and *S minus* are both sensitive to penicillin.

Foreign body synovitis and plant thorn injuries

Penetrating joint injuries involving thorny plants, sea urchin spines, wood splinters, and other foreign bodies may cause a chronic synovitis. This arthritis is usually allergic in nature. The plant pathogen *Pantoea agglomerans*, however, has been implicated in several cases of thorn injuries [50]. There is also a report of *Nocardia asteroides* infection in this setting [51]. Thorn fragments and other synovial foreign bodies are best localized by ultrasound. Treatment is arthrotomy, complete resection of foreign matter, and appropriate antibiotics based on joint cultures.

Human and animal bites

Human bites cause polymicrobial infection, involving aerobic bacteria, such as staphylococci; α- and β-hemolytic streptococci; oral gram-negative rods, such as *Eikenella corrodens*; and oral anaerobes, including *Prevotella*, *Fusobacterium*, and *Peptostreptococcus* species [52]. Animal bites have a similar bacteriology, with *Pasteurella multocida* as an important additional pathogen [53,54]. Treatment relies on drainage and debridement of devitalized tissues, careful assessment for tenosynovitis, and use of ampicillin-sulbactam, or a regimen with similar aerobic and anaerobic activity.

Melioidosis

The gram-negative rod *Burkholderia pseudomallei* commonly cause pneumonia and sepsis in rural Southeast Asia and tropical Australia during the wet season. Like tuberculosis, melioidosis may present with late reactivation, hence the sobriquet "Vietnamese time bomb." It grows readily on blood agar, but can be confused with *Burkholderia cepacia* or *Pseudomonas* sp. It is an important cause of septic arthritis in endemic areas, with a poorly understood propensity for upper extremity involvement [55]. Melioidotic septic arthritis is treated with joint drainage and a 6-month course of doxycycline and trimethoprim-sulfamethoxazole, with or without ceftazidime.

Whipple's disease

The multisystem disorder, Whipple's disease, is caused by the fastidious actinomycete *Tropheryma whippelii*. In 63% of cases, a migratory, non-destructive, peripheral arthritis is the initial manifestation, preceding the onset of abdominal pain, diarrhea, malabsorption, and weight loss by a mean of 8 years in one series. Because patients often have HLA-B27 positivity, the arthritis may be mistakenly treated with immunosuppressive medication, precipitating gastrointestinal symptoms [56,57]. Fever, lymph-adenopathy, hyperpigmentation, and cardiac and neurologic involvement may also be prominent. Diagnosis is usually made on the basis of small bowel biopsy, although polymerase chain reaction of synovial fluid may also be useful [58]. Two weeks of parenteral ceftriaxone is recommended as initial therapy, followed by oral trimethoprim-sulfamethoxazole for at least 1 year [59].

Mycoplasmas and ureaplasmas

True septic arthritis caused by mycoplasmas and ureaplasmas is unusual, occurring almost exclusively in the setting of hypogammaglobulinemia or organ transplantation. Diagnosis depends on polymerase chain reaction or cultivation on special media. Good outcomes have been reported with the combination of doxycycline and quinolones over weeks to months [60–62].

Intravenous drug users

Before 1983, *Pseudomonas aeruginosa* caused 64% of reported septic arthritis in intravenous drug users, with *S aureus* responsible for only 10%. After 1983, the roles of these pathogens were reversed: *P aeruginosa* resulted in only 9% of septic arthritis in intravenous drug users, whereas *S aureus* caused 71% [21]. This switch is explained by shifting patterns of intravenous drug use. In 1983, in response to an epidemic of pentazocine abuse, the manufacturer coformulated it with the narcotic antagonist naloxone. With oral administration, naloxone is rapidly inactivated, but with injection, it negates the intoxicating effect of pentazocine. Thereafter, heroin supplanted pentazocine as the drug of choice among injection drug users [63].

Intravenous drug users often inject drugs with the most convenient water supply, such as puddles in alleys or toilet water. In one study, 81% of injection drug users reported injecting in public toilets in the past 6 months, and 80% in the street [64]. Unlike pentazocine, which dissolves in water at room temperature, heroin must be heated to dissolve, typically by boiling in a spoon held over a flame. This process of "cooking" reduces contamination with environmental bacteria, such as *Pseudomonas* sp. The risk of staphylococcal infection is equivalent, however, with heroin and pentazocine abuse. Cooking does not diminish the risk of staphylococcal infection, because the bacterial source is likely a colonized skin site, rather than environmental water [65].

Septic arthritis in intravenous drug users often affects joints containing intra-articular cartilage, such as the pubic symphysis, and the sternoclavicular and sacroiliac joints. These joints are uncommonly infected in other patients with septic arthritis [21,24,66]. The progressive sclerosis and calcification with aging of these joints may decrease the risk of infection in the predominantly older population at highest risk of septic arthritis, compared with the younger patients who acquire septic arthritis from intravenous drug use. The sternoclavicular joint may account for up to 17% of septic arthritis in intravenous drug users. This joint is likely infected from phlebitis or valvulitis of the underlying subclavian vein, after injection of contaminated drugs into the upper extremity. CT or MRI should be obtained routinely in patients with sternoclavicular septic arthritis, given the high frequency of complications requiring surgery, such as chest wall abscess or mediastinitis [66].

Children

In pediatric septic arthritis, knee involvement is not as dominant as in adults. The knee and hip are infected in one third of cases each in children [67]. Staphylococci and streptococci are responsible for most cases. *Haemophilus influenzae* type b septic arthritis is now uncommon because of the protection provided by conjugate vaccines [68].

Kingella kingae, one of the fastidious gram-negative rods of the HACEK group, has recently been recognized as an important cause of septic arthritis, osteomyelitis, and intervertebral diskitis in children less than 2 years of age. *Kingella* septic arthritis is often preceded by pharyngitis or stomatitis. Seasonality of infection has been observed, perhaps related to viral infection or other cofactors. There is one report of an outbreak of invasive *Kingella* infections in a day care. Routine inoculation of pediatric synovial fluid specimens into aerobic blood culture bottles has been recommended, instead of direct plating of specimens on solid media, to improve recovery of *Kingella* [69–72].

Community-acquired MRSA is a major pediatric pathogen in several regions of the United States. In a recent study from Rhode Island, 40% of skin and soft tissue infections in children were caused by MRSA [73]. In Houston, community-acquired MRSA caused 53% of all community-acquired staphylococcal musculoskeletal infections in children, including 50% of cases of staphylococcal septic arthritis [74]. Sequelae, such as decreased joint range of motion and limping gait, may be more common with MRSA infection [75].

Prosthetic joints

The diagnosis and management of prosthetic joint infection are reviewed elsewhere in this issue.

Diagnosis: problems and pitfalls

Gram stain and culture of synovial fluid should be routinely obtained in any case of undiagnosed arthritis. Gram staining of synovial fluid, however, is insensitive for the diagnosis of septic arthritis. Gram stains are positive in 71% of gram-positive septic arthritis [17], 40% to 50% of cases of gram-negative septic arthritis [36–38], and less than 25% of cases of gonococcal septic arthritis [1].

It is recommended to treat patients empirically for septic arthritis when synovial fluid WBC counts exceed 50,000 cells/mm^3, although gout and pseudogout commonly cause WBC counts of this magnitude [76]. Unfortunately, lower WBC counts do not exclude septic arthritis. In one recent study, one third of patients with septic arthritis had synovial fluid WBCs of less than 50,000 cells/mm^3 [31], and in one older study, 50% of patients with septic arthritis had synovial fluid WBC counts less than 28,000 cells/mm^3 [77]. Immunosuppressed patients may lack synovial leukocytosis altogether. Synovial chemistry tests, such as glucose and protein, are not useful in the diagnosis of septic arthritis [78].

Blood cultures should be obtained in all patients with suspected septic arthritis. At least one third of patients with septic arthritis have associated bacteremia. In up to 14% of patients, a bacteriologic diagnosis is made only on the basis of blood cultures [25,79]. Serologic testing for Lyme disease should be obtained from patients with undiagnosed inflammatory arthritis in endemic areas, particularly if Gram stain and culture of synovial fluid are negative.

The diagnosis of gonococcal septic arthritis may be elusive. Less than 50% of synovial fluid cultures are positive, even when appropriately subcultured onto chocolate agar. The diagnosis is usually based on a clinical syndrome compatible with disseminated gonococcal infection, and isolation of N gonorrhoeae from cultures of the cervix, urethra, rectum, or oropharynx. Bacteremia is uncommon in disseminated gonococcal infection, despite the frequency of polyarticular involvement [1,25,35].

Many cases of suspected septic arthritis have negative cultures of synovial fluid on solid media. There are many possible explanations for this phenomenon: the clinical diagnosis of septic arthritis is mistaken; synovial fluid is obtained after the initiation of antibiotics; small numbers of bacteria are present, perhaps because of brisk neutrophil phagocytosis; the quantity of synovial fluid plated is inadequate; or infecting bacteria may have fastidious growth requirements. Many of these problems may be overcome by inoculation of synovial fluid into blood culture bottles. Antibiotics and other bacterial inhibitors, such as complement, may be diluted in blood culture bottles; lytic agents present in most blood culture media, such as saponin, may release intracellular bacteria; larger amounts of synovial fluid can be inoculated into blood cultures; and blood cultures better support the growth of fussy organisms, such as *Kingella* and nutritionally variant streptococci. Several studies have shown a higher yield for pathogens, and fewer contaminants, with inoculation of synovial fluid into blood cultures, compared with solid media [80–82].

Therapy and outcomes

When a joint has become distended with pus, if it is freely opened and copiously irrigated, it may forthwith undergo a startling improvement and, if the patient survives, may completely recover and retain absolutely free movement.

Howard Marsh, 1902 [83]

Because synovial fluid tests lack precision for diagnosing septic arthritis, the threshold for starting antibiotics should be low. Patient epidemiology may help tailor empiric therapy toward likely organisms. Because septic arthritis is so rapidly destructive, however, broad-spectrum antibiotics are usually warranted until culture data are available. If Gram stains of synovial fluid are negative, cefazolin is a reasonable initial choice for empiric coverage of suspected septic arthritis in patients at low risk of MRSA and gonorrhea, providing staphylococcal, streptococcal, and some gram-negative coverage [84]. Patients at higher risk of gram-negative infection, such as the elderly and immunocompromised, could be treated with cefepime as a broad-spectrum single-agent active against streptococci, methicillin-sensitive S aureus, and gram-negative bacilli.

Intravenous drug users with septic arthritis may be covered empirically with vancomycin and an antipseudomonal β-lactam for MRSA and Pseudomonas sp. Vancomycin is also reasonable empiric therapy for other patients with MRSA risk factors, such as hemodialysis, diabetes, recent nursing home admission, or recent or current hospitalization [85]. Certain areas of North America have experienced outbreaks of community-acquired MRSA infection, and it is reasonable to initiate empiric therapy for MRSA in patients with septic arthritis in these regions [86]. There are favorable but limited data supporting the use of linezolid, daptomycin, and pristinamycin as alternative agents for MRSA septic arthritis [87–89].

Combination therapy with vancomycin and cefepime, or another agent with broad gram-negative activity, should be administered for critically ill patients with septic arthritis. Septic arthritis associated with human or animal bites should be treated with agents active against oral flora, such as ampicillin-sulbactam. Sexually active patients with clinical syndromes suggestive of disseminated gonococcal infection should receive ceftriaxone. Recommendations for empiric antibiotic therapy of suspected septic arthritis are summarized in Table 2.

Once the causative organism has been identified, therapy should be narrowed. Resistant gram-negative bacilli, such as Pseudomonas sp, are best treated with the combination of a β-lactam drug with an aminoglycoside or

Table 2
Empiric antibiotic therapy of suspected septic arthritis

Gram stain of synovial fluid	Antibiotic therapy
Gram-positive cocci	
No risk factors for MRSA (see text)	Cefazolin, 2 g IV q 8 h
MRSA risk factors or β-lactam allergy	Vancomycin, 1 g IV q 12 h
Gram-negative cocci (presumptive *Neisseria sp*)	Ceftriaxone, 1 g IV q 24 h
Gram-negative rods	Cefepime, 2 g IV q 8 h or piperacillin-tazobactam, 4.5 g IV q 6 h
No organisms on gram stain	
Previously healthy, low MRSA risk	Cefazolin, 2 g IV q 8 h
MRSA risks present	Vancomycin, 1 g IV q 12 h plus cefepime, 2 g IV q 8 h or piperacillin-tazobactam, 4.5 g IV q 6 h

Abbreviation: MRSA, methicillin-resistant *Staphylococcus aureus*.

a quinolone. Data on duration of therapy are scanty. In general, the authors recommend courses of therapy for septic arthritis of at least 3 weeks, which may include a period of step-down oral therapy. Gonococcal septic arthritis can be treated with 2 weeks of ceftriaxone. Because osteomyelitis is common in infections of cartilaginous joints, such as the sternoclavicular and sacroiliac joints, antibiotic courses of 4 to 6 weeks are recommended [66].

Historical series of septic arthritis have shown that a large proportion of patients with suspected septic arthritis have negative joint fluid cultures. These patients have similar clinical and epidemiologic features compared with those with bacteriologically confirmed septic arthritis. It is probably reasonable to complete a short course of oral antibiotic therapy in these patients [90].

Joint drainage

Even in the preantibiotic era, some patients with septic arthritis had good outcomes with aggressive joint irrigation alone. Today, septic arthritis is managed with antibiotics combined with joint drainage by arthroscopy, arthrocentesis, or arthrotomy. Joint drainage decompresses the joint; improves blood flow; and removes bacteria, toxins, and proteases. Arthrocentesis should be repeated daily until effusions resolve and cultures are negative. There is general agreement that surgical drainage is indicated for septic arthritis of the hip, failure to respond after 5 to 7 days of antibiotics and arthrocentesis, and soft tissue extension of infection. The shoulder joint should be drained either surgically or under radiologic guidance [91,92]. Retrospective data suggest that patients with rheumatoid arthritis have better functional outcomes with surgical management [8].

No good data show a superiority of surgical drainage over arthrocentesis. In fact, one meta-analysis, and a more recent retrospective study, demonstrated better functional outcomes with arthrocentesis compared with surgery, although mortality was higher in patients treated with arthrocentesis [16,93]. Selection bias probably explains these differences. Critically ill patients are poor surgical candidates, whereas otherwise stable patients with severe septic arthritis are more likely to undergo surgical drainage. Randomized, clinical trials of arthrocentesis compared with surgical or arthroscopic drainage are needed.

A recent study showed a significant benefit of dexamethasone therapy in preventing disability in children with septic arthritis, but no data exist to recommend its use in adults [94].

Aggressive rehabilitation is essential to prevent joint contractures and muscle atrophy. Patients should be mobilized as soon as pain allows. Although early reviews recommended joint immobilization in the acute phase of infection [1], in animal models of septic arthritis, more cartilage degeneration and adhesions were seen in immobilized animals, compared with animals treated with continuous passive motion devices [95].

Summary

Septic arthritis has increased in incidence in the United States in the past two decades, and increasingly affects an older population with a greater burden of chronic illness and a higher risk for drug-resistant organisms. Successful management depends on a high diagnostic suspicion, empiric antibiotic treatment, and joint drainage. A bacteriologic diagnosis is more likely with inoculation into blood culture bottles than plating on solid media. As MRSA increases in prevalence in the community, empiric antibiotic regimens increasingly need to be active against MRSA.

References

[1] Goldenberg DL, Reed JI. Bacterial arthritis. N Engl J Med 1985;312:764–71.
[2] Kaandorp CJ, Dinant HJ, van de Laar MA, et al. Incidence and sources of native and prosthetic joint infection: a community based prospective survey. Ann Rheum Dis 1997;56: 470–5.
[3] Haug JB, Harthug S, Kalager T, et al. Bloodstream infections at a Norwegian university hospital, 1974–1979 and 1988–89: changing etiology, clinical features, and outcome. Clin Infect Dis 1994;19:246–56.
[4] Ross JJ, Saltzman CL, Carling P, et al. Pneumococcal septic arthritis: review of 190 cases. Clin Infect Dis 2003;36:319–27.
[5] Patti JM, Bremell T, Krajewska-Pietrasik D, et al. The *Staphylococcus aureus* collagen adhesin is a virulence determinant in experimental septic arthritis. Infect Immun 1994;62: 152–61.
[6] Shirtliff ME, Mader JT. Acute septic arthritis. Clin Microbiol Rev 2002;15:527–44.
[7] Stevens CR, Williams RB, Farrell AJ, et al. Hypoxia and inflammatory synovitis: observations and speculation. Ann Rheum Dis 1991;50:124–32.
[8] Gardner GC, Weisman MH. Pyarthrosis in patients with rheumatoid arthritis: a report of 13 cases and a review of the literature from the past 40 years. Am J Med 1990;88:503–11.
[9] Blackburn WD, Dunn TL, Alarcón GS. Infection versus disease activity in rheumatoid arthritis: eight years' experience. South Med J 1986;79:1238–41.

[10] Ilahi OA, Swarna U, Hamill RJ, et al. Concomitant crystal and septic arthritis. Orthopedics 1996;19:613–7.
[11] Yu KH, Luo SF, Liou LB, et al. Concomitant septic and gouty arthritis: an analysis of 30 cases. Rheumatology (Oxford) 2003;42:1062–6.
[12] Baghai M, Osmon DR, Wolk DM, et al. Fatal sepsis in a patient with rheumatoid arthritis treated with etanercept. Mayo Clin Proc 2001;76:653–6.
[13] Rachapalli S, O'Daunt S. Septic arthritis due to Listeria monocytogenes in a patient receiving etanercept. Arthritis Rheum 2005;52:987.
[14] Katsarolis I, Tsiodras S, Panagopoulos P, et al. Septic arthritis due to Salmonella enteritidis associated with infliximab use. Scand J Infect Dis 2005;37:304–6.
[15] Kaur PP, Derk CT, Chatterji M, et al. Septic arthritis caused by Actinobacillus ureae in a patient with rheumatoid arthritis receiving anti-tumor necrosis factor-alpha therapy. J Rheumatol 2004;31:1663–5.
[16] Weston VC, Jones AC, Bradbury N, et al. Clinical features and outcome of septic arthritis in a single UK Health District 1982–1991. Ann Rheum Dis 1999;58:214–9.
[17] Goldenberg DL, Cohen AS. Acute infectious arthritis. Am J Med 1976;60:369–77.
[18] Edwards SA, Cranfield T, Clarke HJ. Atypical presentation of septic arthritis in the immunosuppressed patient. Orthopedics 2002;25:1089–90.
[19] Jones A, Doherty M. ABC of rheumatology: osteoarthritis. BMJ 1995;310:457–60.
[20] Dubost JJ, Fis I, Denis P, et al. Polyarticular septic arthritis. Medicine (Baltimore) 1993;72:296–310.
[21] Brancos MA, Peris P, Miro JM, et al. Septic arthritis in heroin addicts. Semin Arthritis Rheum 1991;21:81–7.
[22] Vyskocil JJ, McIlroy MA, Brennan TA, et al. Pyogenic infection of the sacroiliac joint: case reports and review of the literature. Medicine (Baltimore) 1991;70:188–97.
[23] Zimmermann B III, Mikolich DJ, Lally EV. Septic sacroiliitis. Semin Arthritis Rheum 1996;26:592–604.
[24] Ross JJ, Hu LT. Septic arthritis of the pubic symphysis: review of 100 cases. Medicine (Baltimore) 2003;82:340–5.
[25] Sharp JT, Lidsky MD, Duffy J, et al. Infectious arthritis. Arch Intern Med 1979;139:1125–30.
[26] Bremell T, Tarkowski A. Preferential induction of septic arthritis and mortality by superantigen-producing staphylococci. Infect Immun 1995;63:4185–7.
[27] Fridkin SK, Hageman JC, Morrison M, et al. Methicillin-resistant Staphylococcus aureus disease in three communities. N Engl J Med 2005;352:1436–44.
[28] Farley MM. Group B streptococcal disease in nonpregnant adults. Clin Infect Dis 2001;33:556–61.
[29] Dubost JJ, Soubrier M, De Champs C, et al. No changes in the distribution of organisms responsible for septic arthritis over a 20 year period. Ann Rheum Dis 2002;61:267–9.
[30] Nolla JM, Gomez-Vaquero C, Corbella X, et al. Group B streptococcus (Streptococcus agalactiae) pyogenic arthritis in nonpregnant adults. Medicine (Baltimore) 2003;82:119–27.
[31] Li SF, Henderson J, Dickman E, et al. Laboratory tests in adults with monoarticular arthritis: can they rule out a septic joint? Acad Emerg Med 2004;11:276–80.
[32] Ryan MJ, Kavanagh R, Wall PG, et al. Bacterial joint infections for England and Wales: analysis of bacterial isolates over a four year period. Br J Rheumatol 1997;36:370–3.
[33] Ispahani P, Weston VC, Turner DPJ, et al. Septic arthritis due to Streptococcus pneumoniae in Nottingham, United Kingdom, 1985–1998. Clin Infect Dis 1999;29:1450–4.
[34] Centers for Disease Control and Prevention. Gonorrhea—United States, 1998. MMWR Morb Mortal Wkly Rep 2000;49:538–42.
[35] O'Brien JP, Goldenberg DL, Rice PA. Disseminated gonococcal infection: a prospective analysis of 49 patients and a review of pathophysiology and immune mechanisms. Medicine (Baltimore) 1983;62:395–406.

[36] Goldenberg DL, Brandt KD, Cathcart ES, et al. Acute arthritis due to gram-negative bacilli: a clinical characterization. Medicine (Baltimore) 1974;53:197–208.

[37] Bayer AS, Chow AW, Louie JS, et al. Gram-negative bacillary septic arthritis: clinical, radiographic, therapeutic, and prognostic features. Semin Arthritis Rheum 1977;7: 123–32.

[38] Newman ED, Davis DE, Harrington TM. Septic arthritis due to gram negative bacilli: older patients with good outcome. J Rheumatol 1988;15:659–62.

[39] Osler W. The arthritis of cerebro-spinal fever. Boston Med Surg J 1898;139:641–3.

[40] Schaad UB. Arthritis in disease due to *Neisseria meningitidis*. Rev Infect Dis 1980;2:880–8.

[41] Goedvolk CA, von Rosenstiel IA, Bos AP. Immune complex associated complications in the subacute phase of meningococcal disease: incidence and literature review. Arch Dis Child 2003;88:927–30.

[42] Rompalo AM, Hook EW III, Roberts PL, et al. The acute arthritis-dermatitis syndrome: the changing importance of *Neisseria gonorrhoeae* and *Neisseria meningitidis*. Arch Intern Med 1987;147:281–3.

[43] Armstrong RW, Bolding F, Joseph R. Septic arthritis following arthroscopy: clinical syndromes and analysis of risk factors. Arthroscopy 1992;8:213–23.

[44] Indelli PF, Dillingham M, Fanton G, et al. Septic arthritis in postoperative anterior cruciate ligament reconstruction. Clin Orthop 2002;398:182–8.

[45] Gotuzzo E, Alarcon GS, Bocanegra TS, et al. Articular involvement in human brucellosis: a retrospective analysis of 304 cases. Semin Arthritis Rheum 1982;12:245–55.

[46] Solera J, Rodriguez-Zapata M, Geijo P, et al. Doxycycline-rifampin versus doxycycline-streptomycin in treatment of human brucellosis due to *Brucella melitensis*. Antimicrob Agents Chemother 1995;39:2061–7.

[47] Thong BY, Barkham TM. Suppurative polyarthritis following a rat bite. Ann Rheum Dis 2003;62:805–6.

[48] Centers for Disease Control and Prevention (CDC). Fatal rat-bite fever—Florida and Washington, 2003. MMWR Morb Mortal Wkly Rep 2005;53:1198–202.

[49] Washburn RG. *Spirillum minus* (rat-bite fever). In: Mandell GL, Bennett JE, Dolin R, editors. Mandell, Douglas, and Bennett's principles and practice of infectious diseases. 6th edition Philadelphia: Elsevier; 2005. p. 2810.

[50] Kratz A, Greenberg D, Barki Y, et al. *Pantoea agglomerans* as a cause of septic arthritis after palm tree thorn injury; case report and literature review. Arch Dis Child 2003;88:542–4.

[51] Freiberg AA, Herzenberg JE, Sangeorzan JA. Thorn synovitis of the knee joint with *Nocardia* pyarthrosis. Clin Orthop 1993;287:233–6.

[52] Talan DA, Abrahamian FM, Moran GJ, et al. Clinical presentation and bacteriologic analysis of infected human bites in patients presenting to emergency departments. Clin Infect Dis 2003;37:1481–9.

[53] Talan DA, Citron DM, Abrahamian FM, et al. Bacteriologic analysis of infected dog and cat bites. N Engl J Med 1999;340:85–92.

[54] Chevalier X, Martigny J, Avouac B, et al. Report of 4 cases of *Pasteurella multocida* septic arthritis. J Rheumatol 1991;18:1890–2.

[55] Kosuwon W, Taimglang T, Sirichativapee W, et al. Melioidotic septic arthritis and its risk factors. J Bone Joint Surg Am 2003;85:1058–61.

[56] Feurle GE, Marth T. An evaluation of antimicrobial treatment for Whipple's Disease: tetracycline versus trimethoprim-sulfamethoxazole. Dig Dis Sci 1994;39:1642–8.

[57] Mahnel R, Kalt A, Ring S, et al. Immunosuppressive therapy in Whipple's disease patients is associated with the appearance of gastrointestinal manifestations. Am J Gastroenterol 2005; 100:1167–73.

[58] Lange U, Teichmann J. Whipple arthritis: diagnosis by molecular analysis of synovial fluid–current status of diagnosis and therapy. Rheumatology (Oxford) 2003;42:473–80.

[59] Mahnel R, Marth T. Progress, problems, and perspectives in diagnosis and treatment of Whipple's disease. Clin Exp Med 2004;4:39–43.

[60] Asmar BI, Andresen J, Brown WJ. *Ureaplasma urealyticum* arthritis and bacteremia in agammaglobulinemia. Pediatr Infect Dis J 1998;17:73–6.

[61] O'Sullivan MV, Isbel NM, Johnson DW, et al. Disseminated pyogenic *Mycoplasma pneumoniae* infection in a renal transplant recipient, detected by broad-range polymerase chain reaction. Clin Infect Dis 2004;39:e98–9.

[62] Mian AN, Farney AC, Mendley SR. *Mycoplasma hominis* septic arthritis in a pediatric renal transplant recipient: case report and review of the literature. Am J Transplant 2005;5:183–8.

[63] Baum C, Hsu JP, Nelson RC. The impact of the addition of naloxone on the use and abuse of pentazocine. Public Health Rep 1987;102:426–9.

[64] Darke S, Kaye S, Ross J. Geographic injecting locations among injecting drug users in Sydney, Australia. Addiction 2001;96:241–6.

[65] Tuazon CU, Sheagren JN. Increased rate of carriage of *Staphylococcus aureus* among narcotic addicts. J Infect Dis 1974;129:725–7.

[66] Ross JJ, Shamsuddin H. Sternoclavicular septic arthritis: review of 180 cases. Medicine (Baltimore) 2004;83:139–48.

[67] Krogstad P, Smith AL. Osteomyelitis and septic arthritis. In: Feigin RD, Cherry JD, editors. Textbook of pediatric infectious disease. 4th edition. Philadelphia: WB Saunders; 1998. p. 683–704.

[68] Luhmann JD, Luhmann SJ. Etiology of septic arthritis in children: an update for the 1990s. Pediatr Emerg Care 1999;15:40–2.

[69] Yagupsky P, Dagan R, Howard CB, et al. Clinical features and epidemiology of invasive *Kingella kingae* infections in southern Israel. Pediatrics 1993;92:800–4.

[70] Yagupsky P, Peled N, Katz O. Epidemiological features of invasive *Kingella kingae* infections and respiratory carriage of the organism. J Clin Microbiol 2002;40:4180–4.

[71] Centers for Disease Control and Prevention. Osteomyelitis/septic arthritis caused by *Kingella kingae* among day care attendees—Minnesota, 2003. MMWR Morb Mortal Wkly Rep 2004;53:241–3.

[72] Centers for Disease Control and Prevention. *Kingella kingae* infections in children—United States, June 2001-November 2002. MMWR Morb Mortal Wkly Rep 2004;53:244.

[73] Dietrich DW, Auld DB, Mermel LA. Community-acquired methicillin-resistant *Staphylococcus aureus* in southern New England children. Pediatrics 2004;113:e347–52.

[74] Martinez-Aguilar G, Avalos-Mishaan A, Hulten K, et al. Community-acquired, methicillin-resistant and methicillin-susceptible *Staphylococcus aureus* musculoskeletal infections in children. Pediatr Infect Dis J 2004;23:701–6.

[75] Wang CL, Wang SM, Yang YJ, et al. Septic arthritis in children: relationship of causative pathogens, complications, and outcome. J Microbiol Immunol Infect 2003;36:41–6.

[76] Fye KH. Arthrocentesis, synovial fluid analysis, and synovial biopsy. In: Klippel JH, editor. Primer on the rheumatic diseases. 12th edition. Atlanta: Arthritis Foundation; 2001. p. 138–44.

[77] McCutchan HJ, Fisher RC. Synovial leukocytosis in infectious arthritis. Clin Orthop 1990; 257:226–30.

[78] Shmerling RH, Delbanco TL, Tosteson AN, et al. Synovial fluid tests. What should be ordered? JAMA 1990;264:1009–14.

[79] Cooper C, Cawley MI. Bacterial arthritis in an English health district: a 10 year review. Ann Rheum Dis 1986;45:458–63.

[80] Yagupsky P, Press J. Use of the isolator 1.5 microbial tube for culture of synovial fluid from patients with septic arthritis. J Clin Microbiol 1997;35:2410–2.

[81] Hughes JG, Vetter EA, Patel R, et al. Culture with BACTEC Peds Plus/F bottle compared with conventional methods for detection of bacteria in synovial fluid. J Clin Microbiol 2001; 39:4468–71.

[82] Hepburn MJ, Fraser SL, Rennie TA, et al. Septic arthritis caused by *Granulicatella adiacens*: diagnosis by inoculation of synovial fluid into blood culture bottles. Rheumatol Int 2003;23: 255–7.

[83] Marsh H. Septic arthritis: the Bradshaw Lecture, 1902. London: Smith, Elder & Co; 1903.

[84] Fass RJ. Treatment of osteomyelitis and septic arthritis with cefazolin. Antimicrob Agents Chemother 1978;13:405–11.

[85] Salgado CD, Farr BM, Calfee DP. Community-acquired methicillin-resistant *Staphylococcus aureus*: a meta-analysis of prevalence and risk factors. Clin Infect Dis 2003;36:131–9.

[86] Naimi TS, LeDell KH, Como-Sabetti K, et al. Comparison of community-acquired and health-care associated methicillin-resistant *Staphylococcus aureus* infection. JAMA 2003; 290:2976–84.

[87] Howden BP, Ward PB, Charles PG, et al. Treatment outcomes for serious infections caused by methicillin-resistant *Staphylococcus aureus* with reduced vancomycin susceptibility. Clin Infect Dis 2004;38:521–8.

[88] Finney MS, Crank CW, Segreti J. Use of daptomycin to treat drug-resistant gram-positive bone and joint infection [abstract 427]. In: Programs and abstracts of the 42nd Annual Meeting of the Infectious Diseases Society of America. Boston: Infectious Diseases Society of America; 2004. p. 120.

[89] Ng J, Gosbell IB. Successful oral pristinamycin therapy for osteoarticular infections due to methicillin-resistant *Staphylococcus aureus* (MRSA) and other *Staphylococcus spp.* J Antimicrob Chemother 2005;55:1008–12.

[90] Gupta MN, Sturrock RD, Field M. Prospective comparative study of patients with culture proven and high suspicion of adult onset septic arthritis. Ann Rheum Dis 2003;62:327–31.

[91] Pioro MH, Mandell BF. Septic arthritis. Rheum Dis Clin North Am 1997;23:239–58.

[92] Smith JW, Piercy EA. Infectious arthritis. Clin Infect Dis 1995;20:225–31.

[93] Broy SB, Schmid FR. A comparison of medical drainage (needle aspiration) and surgical drainage (arthrotomy or arthroscopy) in the initial treatment of infected joints. Clin Rheum Dis 1986;12:501–22.

[94] Odio CM, Ramirez T, Arias G, et al. Double blind, randomized, placebo-controlled study of dexamethasone therapy for hematogenous septic arthritis in children. Pediatr Infect Dis J 2003;22:883–9.

[95] Salter RB. The biologic concept of continuous passive motion of synovial joints: the first 18 years of research and its clinical application. Clin Orthop 1989;242:12–25.

ELSEVIER
SAUNDERS

INFECTIOUS
DISEASE CLINICS
OF NORTH AMERICA

Infect Dis Clin N Am 19 (2005) 819–830

Mycobacterial Osteomyelitis and Arthritis

Michael Gardam, MSc, MD, CM, FRCPC[a,b,*],
Sue Lim, MD, FRCPC[b]

[a]Tuberculosis Clinic, Toronto Western Hospital, Toronto, ON, Canada
[b]University Health Network, 200 Elizabeth Street, 3ES-430, Toronto General Hospital,
Toronto, ON M5G 2C4, Canada

Mycobacterium tuberculosis is by far the most common cause of mycobacterial osteomyelitis and arthritis worldwide [1]. Once a rarity, the incidence of nontuberculous mycobacteria (NTM) disease dramatically increased in the 1980s and 1990s, in parallel with the advancing AIDS epidemic. Pulmonary and disseminated disease, however, still account for most cases. Although musculoskeletal infection with *M tuberculosis* and NTM shares several characteristics, such as bone destruction and relatively slow symptom onset, there are significant differences in their epidemiology and treatment, as discussed later.

Tuberculous osteomyelitis plays a unique role in tuberculosis epidemiology, allowing medical historians to assess the presence of *M tuberculosis* in skeletal remains. Several techniques, including histologic and pathologic examination, radiography, and polymerase chain reaction, have detected tuberculosis bone disease in Egyptian mummies [2–4]. Genetic material from *M tuberculosis* has been identified using polymerase chain reaction techniques in Iron Age Southeast Asian skeletons [5], and European skeletal remains from the Dark Ages and Middle Ages [6,7]. These studies and others suggest that *M tuberculosis* has had an intimate relationship with *Homo sapiens* for millennia. Indeed, it has been proposed that the *M tuberculosis* bacillus has been present for 15,000 years [8].

---

* Corresponding author. University Health Network, 200 Elizabeth Street, 3ES-430, Toronto General Hospital, Toronto, ON M5G 2C4, Canada.
E-mail address: michael.gardam@uhn.on.ca (M. Gardam).

0891-5520/05/$ - see front matter © 2005 Elsevier Inc. All rights reserved.
doi:10.1016/j.idc.2005.07.008
id.theclinics.com

Pathophysiology

Tuberculous osteomyelitis and arthritis are generally believed to arise from foci of bacilli lodged in bone during the original mycobacteremia of primary infection. Alternatively, tuberculous bacilli may travel from the lung to the spine by Batson's paravertebral venous plexus, or by lymphatic drainage to the para-aortic lymph nodes. In most otherwise healthy individuals, the cellular immune response is able to contain the bacilli present in these sites, but not eradicate them. Given its rich vascular supply, the growth plate of long bones is the most frequent site of infection. The growth plate is in close proximity to the joint space, hence tuberculous arthritis is believed to result from an initial bone focus that extends into the joint.

Atypical mycobacterial osteomyelitis and arthritis in nonimmunocompromised individuals is secondary to direct inoculation rather than hematogenous dissemination, either from trauma or surgery [9,10]. NTM also have a predilection for causing infections associated with foreign bodies, such as prosthetic joints [11–13], although *M tuberculosis* may also cause prosthetic joint infections [14]. Hematogenous dissemination with resultant multifocal disease, including bone and joint involvement, can occur in immunocompromised individuals, and is best described in individuals with AIDS [15].

A large United States–based study of all bone and joint tuberculosis over a 4-year period revealed that the most common site of bony tuberculosis was the spine (40%); followed by weight-bearing joints (hip and knee); and lastly, other sites [16]. A British study from the same decade found a similar rate of spinal disease (43%) [17]. The proportion of spinal disease was found to be greater than 50% in more recent studies, which may be caused by demographic differences in the study populations [18,19]. The predilection for spinal disease may be explained by the fact that the vertebrae are extremely well vascularized, even in adulthood. Spinal disease is most frequently located in the lower thoracic and lumbar spine, with thoracic disease being more common in children and adolescents, whereas lumbar disease is found more commonly in adults [20–22]. Most cases of tuberculous bone and joint disease are isolated to one area, but multifocal disease has also been described [23].

Spinal tuberculosis typically involves the initial destruction of the anteroinferior part of the vertebrae. Bacilli may then spread beneath the anterior spinal ligament and involve the anterosuperior aspect of the adjacent inferior vertebra, giving rise to the typical "wedge-shaped" deformity. Further spread may result in adjacent abscesses [24]. The radiographic features of tuberculous osteomyelitis and arthritis are discussed further later.

Chronic granulomatous infection of bone by NTM is a rare but recognized clinical syndrome, and usually occurs in the setting of direct inoculation of the organism following trauma, surgical incisions, puncture wounds, or injections [25].

Epidemiology

Several factors influence the development of tuberculous osteomyelitis and arthritis (Table 1). In a large United States population-based study, age over 65 years was shown to be a significant risk factor for the development of bone and joint tuberculosis [26]. Although children up to 14 years in age were more likely to develop extrapulmonary tuberculosis than older age groups, they were overall less likely to develop bone and joint disease. This same study also showed that bone and joint tuberculosis was twofold higher in women than men. The association with older age and female gender has also been shown in a more recent study [18].

Several studies have shown that immigration affects the relative proportion of bone and joint disease in a population. A recent Dutch study showed that being of African or East Asian origin was a significant risk factor for the development of bone and joint tuberculosis compared with native Dutch [18]. The Somali population was found to be at greatest risk. Similar findings were described in a Danish study [19] and an earlier British study, although most immigrants in the British study were from the Indian subcontinent rather than Africa [17]. In the United States study, which was the largest of the group, foreign birth was not a significant risk factor for the development of bone and joint tuberculosis [26]. This finding may have been explained by the effect of the AIDS epidemic among American-born tuberculosis cases, resulting in increased extrapulmonary disease in this group.

The impact of race and ethnicity on rates of bone and joint tuberculosis when controlled for foreign birth is less clear. In the Rieder study, bone and joint tuberculosis was more closely associated with foreign birth than race, which was divided into Hispanic, black, Native American, and Asian groups, although neither variable reached significance [26].

NTM were first recognized as pathogens in the 1950s, when several large series of pulmonary disease were reported [27–29]. Most NTM organisms are ubiquitous, and have been isolated from water and soil [30,31]. There is marked geographic variability in the prevalence of disease and the specific NTM responsible for disease [32]. A history of trauma or puncture wounds, or osteomyelitis in a geographic setting where a particular NTM is known to be endemic, should raise clinical suspicion of a possible NTM bone infection.

Table 1
Risk factors for mycobacterial bone and joint infections

Risk factors for the development of bone and joint tuberculosis	Risk factors for the development of atypical mycobacterial bone and joint infections
Age >65	Trauma
Female gender	Surgery
Country of origin	Compromised immune status

Clinical presentation

The symptoms of tuberculous bone and joint infections are nonspecific, and the clinical course is often indolent, usually leading to significant delays in diagnosis, and resultant bone or joint destruction. Only about 50% of patients with bone and joint tuberculosis have chest radiographs suggestive of tuberculous infection, further obscuring the diagnosis. Pain or local swelling is the most frequent presenting complaint [33,34]. Fever and weight loss are present in only a minority of patients. Cutaneous fistulae, abscesses, and obvious joint deformity may also be present, should the disease have been active for a long time. Like some other forms of extrapulmonary tuberculosis, such as lymph node disease, local symptoms are typically more prominent than systemic constitutional symptoms. Pain on ambulation in affected weight-bearing joints is common, but nonspecific. Spinal disease may be associated with neurologic deficits caused by impingement of the spinal cord, nerve roots, or nerves. Patients with thoracic spine disease are at particular risk for paraparesis or paraplegia.

In the authors' experience, a significant number of patients have had local symptoms for greater than a year and have been treated unsuccessfully for osteoarthritis, the diagnosis only being considered when fistulae develop, or on referral to an orthopedic surgeon. The clinical presentation of NTM bone and joint disease is similar to that of tuberculosis. In these cases, a history of trauma, surgery, or immune compromise are clues that an NTM infection may be present.

Diagnosis

Tuberculin skin testing

The most significant step toward diagnosing tuberculous bone and joint infections is to consider the possibility of the diagnosis in the appropriate clinical setting. Often, a tuberculin skin test is performed. This test is of limited use in determining active disease, however, and is best used for screening for latent infection in high-risk populations. Although skin test positivity has been reported to be as high as 90% in immunocompetent patients with bone and joint tuberculosis [35], positivity neither confirms nor excludes the diagnosis. In debilitated or immunocompromised patients, the sensitivity of the test decreases substantially, making it largely irrelevant in making the diagnosis of tuberculosis disease in this population. Tuberculin skin testing is not useful in diagnosing disease caused by NTM.

Mycobacterial culture

Once considered, a clinical diagnosis should be supported by mycobacterial culture from the affected area. Culture is also crucial to provide antibiotic sensitivities to guide therapy. It is important to culture material from deep structures, such as bone, abscesses, synovial fluid, or synovial tissue rather than culturing drainage fluid, because these specimens may grow colonizing organisms, such as bacteria or fungi, which may cloud the diagnosis. An older review of the use of synovial fluid culture for *M tuberculosis* reported a sensitivity of 79%, whereas synovial tissue culture had a sensitivity of 94% [36]. Acid-fast smears are positive in a minority of patients. The use of molecular diagnostic tests in the assessment of smear-negative or culture-negative patients with suspected extrapulmonary tuberculosis remains unclear [37,38].

Histology

In cases where a biopsy was performed but material was not sent for mycobacterial culture, histology can be very useful in suggesting the diagnosis. Histologic evidence of mycobacterial infection has been reported in 94% of synovial biopsy specimens [36], although the presence of granulomatous inflammation is not specific for mycobacterial infection [39]. The detection of mycobacterial genetic material from pathology specimens may aid in diagnosis, although the positive and negative predictive value of these techniques is not well defined [40].

Cell counts and fluid biochemistry

The cell count and biochemistry findings from tuberculous joint fluids, although typical of inflammatory arthritis, are not specific for a mycobacterial infection [34]. Moderately elevated leukocyte counts with a neutrophilic predominance, low glucose, and increased protein are typical [36].

Radiology

Multiple imaging modalities, such as plain radiographs, CT, MRI, and ultrasound, may all play a role in suggesting the diagnosis and aiding in the recovery of culture material through directed biopsies (Figs. 1–3). Imaging of extraspinal bones may show soft tissue swelling, evidence of bone destruction with relative preservation of the joint space, and osteopenia [24]. Osteomyelitis without involvement of the adjacent joint is unusual. In advanced stages, gross bone destruction and soft tissue calcification may be evident (see Figs. 1 and 2). These changes, however, can be seen with other causes of chronic osteomyelitis.

Spinal imaging may reveal findings that favor tuberculosis over other causes of bone destruction, such as malignancy (see Fig. 3). Typically, infection starts at the anteroinferior aspect of the vertebral body, and spreads to contiguous vertebrae along the anterior longitudinal ligament of the spine. The infection, however, may also track down the posterior aspect of the spine [24]. The infection may also "skip" vertebrae. The disks and posterior elements are typically spared, at least early in the course of disease

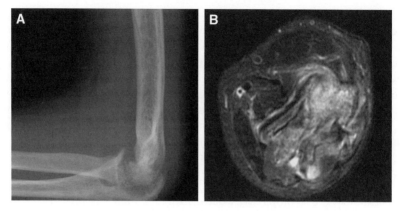

Fig. 1. Plain radiograph (*A*) and MRI (*B*) of the left elbow of a 49-year-old man of Chinese origin with a 1-year history of progressive elbow swelling, immobilization, and pain. The plain film reveals a large joint effusion and periosteal reaction of the radius and ulna. The MRI reveals a complicated effusion with partial destruction and erosion of the joint. Extensive edema of the surrounding musculature was noted. Cultures from the joint effusion grew drug-sensitive *M tuberculosis*. The patient's pain and swelling significantly worsened after several weeks of appropriate antituberculous therapy and were unrelieved by nonsteroidal anti-inflammatory drugs. He was subsequently treated with prednisone for 4 weeks, which dramatically decreased his symptoms.

[41]. As the disease progresses, collapse of the anterior portion of the vertebrae can lead to a kyphotic wedging deformity of the spine, the gibbus of Pott's disease. Fusiform cold paraspinal abscesses, with or without calcification, occur in roughly 70% of cases [20].

Treatment

Medical therapy

Antituberculous chemotherapy for bone and joint tuberculosis does not differ significantly from that recommended for most other forms of the disease. Large clinical trials have confirmed that standard short-course therapy for drug-sensitive disease consisting of 6 months of isoniazid and rifampin, and 2 months of pyrazinamide, is effective [42–44]. Concerns regarding tissue penetration and difficulty in measuring a microbiologic response to treatment have led some experts to recommend prolonging therapy to 9 months; however, there are little clinical data to support this. The American Thoracic Society recommends 6- to 9-month duration of therapy for patients with drug-sensitive disease [45]. Prolonged therapy should be considered for patients slow to respond to otherwise adequate treatment. The treatment of drug-resistant disease follows the same principles for treatment of other sites.

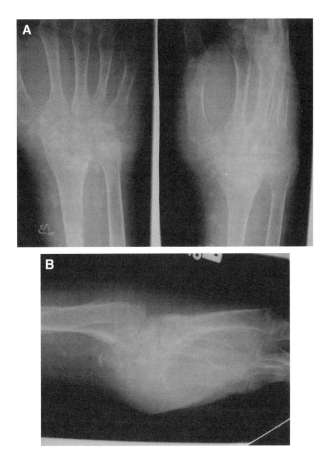

Fig. 2. (*A, B*) Plain radiographs of a 37-year-old man of Indian origin who presented to the hand clinic with a several year history of pain and swelling of the right wrist. Cultures obtained at the time of bone debridement grew *M tuberculosis*. Imaging reveals extensive destruction of the wrist with pancarpal erosive changes. Erosion is also noted at the distal radius and ulna, and at the metacarpal bases. There is a significant amount of soft tissue calcification, typical of long-standing tuberculous infection. The patient's treatment course was complicated by the development of worsening swelling and fistulae while on therapy. The degree of drainage required several episodes of surgical debridement.

Adjunctive corticosteroids

The use of corticosteroids in tuberculous osteomyelitis and arthritis is generally not recommended [45]. The authors have occasionally used steroids (40–60 mg prednisone per day followed by tapering doses) in situations where significant swelling has developed, resulting in severe pain and immobilization of the joint. This situation may infrequently occur several weeks after the start of appropriate therapy, and is typically considered a paradoxical reaction resulting from effective therapy, rather than an indication that treatment is ineffective.

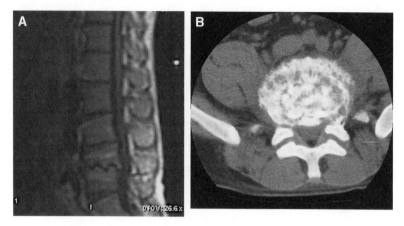

Fig. 3. MRI and CT scan of a 47-year-old man of Jamaican origin who presented with a several month history of lower back pain. (*A*) The MRI reveals marked destruction of the L4-L5 disk, with marked irregularity of the end plates. No impingement on nervous structures was noted. (*B*) The CT revealed partial anterior collapse of the L4 vertebrae, and destruction of the L4-L5 end plate. A CT-guided biopsy revealed chronic inflammation, but mycobacterial cultures were negative. A clinical decision was made to treat the patient for vertebral tuberculosis, and he rapidly recovered.

Surgery

The role of surgery for bone and joint tuberculosis, for sites other than the spine, is relatively straightforward. Surgery is not necessary for cure, but can play a supportive role in draining abscesses and decompressing vital structures, such as nerves. Joints that are significantly damaged may require debridement and possible fusion or replacement. Placement of a prosthetic joint into a previously infected space is possible, provided the patient has received adequate therapy before the replacement [14,34].

Spinal tuberculosis can also be cured by medical therapy [44]. Patients treated medically, however, have a tendency to develop late neurologic and musculoskeletal complications from progressive kyphosis and spinal instability. Given the close proximity of vital structures, such as the spinal cord and nerve roots, it has been argued that aggressive surgical treatment should be used to stabilize the spine and prevent kyphosis, unless only very mild disease is present [46]. There is evidence to suggest that radical debridement and bone grafting may be superior to simple debridement in improving kyphosis and preventing late deterioration [47–49].

Although there have been no large randomized trials studying the treatment of bone infections caused by NTM, a combination of surgery and antibiotics is usually advocated. Aggressive surgical intervention has been emphasized, particularly in the setting of abscess formation. In general, NTM are more resistant to antituberculous drugs than *M tuberculosis*, and in vitro resistance testing may not correlate with clinical response [25].

Although the combination of agents used is based on the particular mycobacterium species or group isolated, agents used for treating NTM infections have included macrolides (clarithromycin, azithromycin); rifampin or rifabutin; ethambutol; doxycycline; minocycline; quinolones (ciprofloxacin, moxifloxacin, gatifloxacin); sulfonamides; amikacin; streptomycin; isoniazid; ethionamide; cefmetazole; and imipenem [50]. The number of agents required for effective treatment is not clear, although three-drug regimens are often adopted. Furthermore, the optimal duration of therapy is unknown, although courses of 6 to 12 months are generally used. Severely immunocompromised patients may require treatment for years [51].

Follow-up during treatment

As per any type of tuberculosis, regularly scheduled follow-up, at least monthly, is essential. Patients must be warned of the possible side effects of therapy and questioned regarding suspicious symptoms at each visit. The authors perform liver function tests at the initial visit, repeated monthly for the first 3 months, and then as needed based on patient symptoms, until therapy is completed. Baseline measurement of visual acuity and color vision, followed by regular assessments thereafter, is necessary for patients receiving prolonged ethambutol therapy, especially at doses >15 mg/kg.

Similarly, the prolonged duration of therapy and use of toxic agents demands that patients with NTM bone infections be followed closely for adverse drug events. Although little evidence exists on the management of these patients, clinical and radiologic improvement on therapy can direct the frequency of follow-up and intervention.

Proof of cure is not easily available for mycobacterial bone and joint disease, unlike pulmonary disease. Repeat cultures of the affected area are typically difficult to obtain and generally not required, unless there is a suspicion that the patient is not responding to therapy. Repeat imaging is helpful to show resolution of symptoms; however, the patient's ongoing history and physical examination findings are likely the most relevant.

Summary

Physicians can expect to see more mycobacterial bone and joint disease in North America as a result of increased travel, immigration, and use of immunosuppressive medications. The first step in treating infections caused by these organisms is to consider the diagnosis early in the course of illness. Long-standing untreated mycobacterial infections typically cause significant bone destruction and loss of function. The treatment of mycobacterial bone and joint infection requires prolonged antibiotic therapy, often in conjunction with surgical intervention, particularly for spinal tuberculosis.

References

[1] Good RC, Snider DE Jr. Isolation of nontuberculous mycobacteria in the United States, 1980. J Infect Dis 1982;146:829–33.

[2] Chastel C. When the Egyptian mummies are speaking about the infections that have made them ill. Hist Sci Med 2004;38:147–55.

[3] Zink A, Haas CJ, Reischl U, et al. Molecular analysis of skeletal tuberculosis in an ancient Egyptian population. J Med Microbiol 2001;50:355–66.

[4] Zink AR, Grabner W, Reischl U, et al. Molecular study on human tuberculosis in three geographically distinct and time delineated populations from ancient Egypt. Epidemiol Infect 2003;130:239–49.

[5] Tayles N, Buckley HR. Leprosy and tuberculosis in Iron Age Southeast Asia? Am J Phys Anthropol 2004;125:239–56.

[6] Zink AR, Grabner W, Nerlich AG. Molecular identification of human tuberculosis in recent and historic bone tissue samples: the role of molecular techniques for the study of historic tuberculosis. Am J Phys Anthropol 2005;126:32–47.

[7] Haas CJ, Zink A, Molnar E, et al. Molecular evidence for different stages of tuberculosis in ancient bone samples from Hungary. Am J Phys Anthropol 2000;113:293–304.

[8] Kapur V, Whittam TS, Musser JM. Is *Mycobacterium tuberculosis* 15,000 years old? J Infect Dis 1994;170:1348–9.

[9] Falkinham JO III. Epidemiology of infection by nontuberculous mycobacteria. Clin Microbiol Rev 1996;9:177–215.

[10] O'Brien RJ, Geiter LJ, Snider DE Jr. The epidemiology of nontuberculous mycobacterial diseases in the United States: results from a national survey. Am Rev Respir Dis 1987;135: 1007–14.

[11] Heathcock R, Dave J, Yates MD. *Mycobacterium chelonae* hip infection. J Infect 1994;28: 104–5.

[12] Oz O, Lee DH, Smetana SM, et al. A case of infected scleral buckle with *Mycobacterium chelonae* associated with chronic intraocular inflammation. Ocul Immunol Inflamm 2004;12: 65–7.

[13] Pring M, Eckhoff DG. *Mycobacterium chelonae* infection following a total knee arthroplasty. J Arthroplasty 1996;11:115–6.

[14] Spinner RJ, Sexton DJ, Goldner RD, et al. Periprosthetic infections due to *Mycobacterium tuberculosis* in patients with no prior history of tuberculosis. J Arthroplasty 1996;11:217–22.

[15] Nightingale SD, Byrd LT, Southern PM, et al. Incidence of *Mycobacterium avium-intracellulare* complex bacteremia in human immunodeficiency virus-positive patients. J Infect Dis 1992;165:1082–5.

[16] Farer LS, Lowell AM, Meador MP. Extrapulmonary tuberculosis in the United States. Am J Epidemiol 1979;109:205–17.

[17] Davies PD, Humphries MJ, Byfield SP, et al. Bone and joint tuberculosis: a survey of notifications in England and Wales. J Bone Joint Surg Br 1984;66:326–30.

[18] Jutte PC, van Loenhout-Rooyackers JH, Borgdorff MW, et al. Increase of bone and joint tuberculosis in The Netherlands. J Bone Joint Surg Br 2004;86:901–4.

[19] Houshian S, Poulsen S, Riegels-Nielsen P. Bone and joint tuberculosis in Denmark: increase due to immigration. Acta Orthop Scand 2000;71:312–5.

[20] Hoffman EB, Crosier JH, Cremin BJ. Imaging in children with spinal tuberculosis: a comparison of radiography, computed tomography and magnetic resonance imaging. J Bone Joint Surg Br 1993;75:233–9.

[21] Weaver P, Lifeso RM. The radiological diagnosis of tuberculosis of the adult spine. Skeletal Radiol 1984;12:178–86.

[22] Omari B, Robertson JM, Nelson RJ, et al. Pott's disease: a resurgent challenge to the thoracic surgeon. Chest 1989;95:145–50.

[23] Kumar K, Saxena MB. Multifocal osteoarticular tuberculosis. Int Orthop 1988;12:135–8.

[24] Griffith JF, Kumta SM, Leung PC, et al. Imaging of musculoskeletal tuberculosis: a new look at an old disease. Clin Orthop Relat Res 2002;398:32–9.

[25] Petitjean G, Fluckiger U, Scharen S, et al. Vertebral osteomyelitis caused by non-tuberculous mycobacteria. Clin Microbiol Infect 2004;10:951–3.

[26] Rieder HL, Snider DE Jr, Cauthen GM. Extrapulmonary tuberculosis in the United States. Am Rev Respir Dis 1990;141:347–51.

[27] Crow HE, King CT, Smith CE, et al. A limited clinical, pathologic, and epidemiologic study of patients with pulmonary lesions associated with atypical acid-fast bacilli in the sputum. Am Rev Tuberc 1957;75:199–222.

[28] Lewis AG Jr, Lasche EM, Armstrong AL, et al. A clinical study of the chronic lung disease due to nonphotochromogenic acid-fast bacilli. Ann Intern Med 1960;53:273–85.

[29] Timpe A, Runyon EH. The relationship of atypical acid-fast bacteria to human disease: a preliminary report. J Lab Clin Med 1954;44:202–9.

[30] Collins CH, Grange JM, Yates MD. Mycobacteria in water. J Appl Bacteriol 1984;57: 193–211.

[31] Reznikov M, Leggo JH. Examination of soil in the Brisbane area for organisms of the *Mycobacterium avium-intracellulare-scrofulaceum* complex. Pathology 1974;6:269–73.

[32] Christianson LC, Dewlett HJ. Pulmonary disease in adults associated with unclassified mycobacteria. Am J Med 1960;29:980–91.

[33] Hodgson SP, Ormerod LP. Ten-year experience of bone and joint tuberculosis in Blackburn 1978–1987. J R Coll Surg Edinb 1990;35:259–62.

[34] Iseman MD. A clinician's guide to tuberculosis. 1st edition. Philadelphia: Lippincott, Williams, and Wilkins; 2000.

[35] Berney S, Goldstein M, Bishko F. Clinical and diagnostic features of tuberculous arthritis. Am J Med 1972;53:36–42.

[36] Wallace R, Cohen AS. Tuberculous arthritis: a report of two cases with review of biopsy and synovial fluid findings. Am J Med 1976;61:277–82.

[37] Coll P, Garrigo M, Moreno C, et al. Routine use of Gen-Probe Amplified Mycobacterium Tuberculosis Direct (MTD) test for detection of *Mycobacterium tuberculosis* with smear-positive and smear-negative specimens. Int J Tuberc Lung Dis 2003;7:886–91.

[38] Honore-Bouakline S, Vincensini JP, Giacuzzo V, et al. Rapid diagnosis of extrapulmonary tuberculosis by PCR: impact of sample preparation and DNA extraction. J Clin Microbiol 2003;41:2323–9.

[39] Kostman JR, Rush P, Reginato AJ. Granulomatous tophaceous gout mimicking tuberculous tenosynovitis: report of two cases. Clin Infect Dis 1995;21:217–9.

[40] Schulz S, Cabras AD, Kremer M, et al. Species identification of mycobacteria in paraffin-embedded tissues: frequent detection of nontuberculous mycobacteria. Mod Pathol 2005;18: 274–82.

[41] Pertuiset E, Beaudreuil J, Horusitzky A, et al. Epidemiological aspects of osteoarticular tuberculosis in adults: retrospective study of 206 cases diagnosed in the Paris area from 1980 to 1994. Presse Med 1997;26:311–5.

[42] Medical Research Council Working Party on Tuberculosis of the Spine. Five-year assessment of controlled trials of short-course chemotherapy regimens of 6, 9 or 18 months' duration for spinal tuberculosis in patients ambulatory from the start or undergoing radical surgery. Fourteenth report of the Medical Research Council Working Party on Tuberculosis of the Spine. Int Orthop 1999;23:73–81.

[43] Medical Research Council Working Party on Tuberculosis of the Spine. A controlled trial of six-month and nine-month regimens of chemotherapy in patients undergoing radical surgery for tuberculosis of the spine in Hong Kong. Tenth report of the Medical Research Council Working Party on Tuberculosis of the Spine. Tubercle 1986;67:243–59.

[44] Medical Research Council Working Party on Tuberculosis of the Spine. Controlled trial of short-course regimens of chemotherapy in the ambulatory treatment of spinal tuberculosis:

results at three years of a study in Korea. Twelfth report of the Medical Research Council
Working Party on Tuberculosis of the Spine. J Bone Joint Surg Br 1993;75:240–8.

[45] American Thoracic Society, Centers for Disease Control and Prevention, Infectious Diseases
Society of America. Treatment of tuberculosis. Am J Respir Crit Care Med 2003;167:603–62.

[46] Leong JC. Tuberculosis of the spine. J Bone Joint Surg Br 1993;75:173–5.

[47] Upadhyay SS, Sell P, Saji MJ, et al. Surgical management of spinal tuberculosis in adults:
Hong Kong operation compared with debridement surgery for short and long term outcome
of deformity. Clin Orthop 1994;302:173–82.

[48] Upadhyay SS, Saji MJ, Sell P, et al. Longitudinal changes in spinal deformity after anterior
spinal surgery for tuberculosis of the spine in adults: a comparative analysis between radical
and debridement surgery. Spine 1994;19:542–9.

[49] Upadhyay SS, Saji MJ, Sell P, et al. Spinal deformity after childhood surgery for tuberculosis
of the spine: a comparison of radical surgery and debridement. J Bone Joint Surg Br 1994;76:
91–8.

[50] Medical Section of the American Lung Association. Diagnosis and treatment of disease
caused by nontuberculous mycobacteria. Am J Respir Crit Care Med 1997;156(2 Pt 2):
S1–25.

[51] Ingram CW, Tanner DC, Durack DT, et al. Disseminated infection with rapidly growing
mycobacteria. Clin Infect Dis 1993;16:463–71.

ELSEVIER
SAUNDERS

INFECTIOUS
DISEASE CLINICS
OF NORTH AMERICA

Infect Dis Clin N Am 19 (2005) 831–851

Fungal Arthritis and Osteomyelitis

Rakhi Kohli, MD, MS, Susan Hadley, MD*

*Tufts University School of Medicine, Division of Geographic Medicine and Infectious Disease,
Tufts-New England Medical Center, 750 Washington Street, Boston, MA 02111, USA*

Fungal osteomyelitis and arthritis are uncommon diseases, often presenting in an indolent fashion. Alterations of human flora, disruption of mucocutaneous membranes, and impaired immune function may predispose to fungal infection [1–3]. There is frequently a long period between onset of symptoms and diagnosis.

Fungal osteomyelitis and arthritis arise as a result of hematogenous dissemination, direct inoculation from an exogenous source, such as trauma, surgery, joint injection, or aspiration [1,4,5], or direct extension from an adjacent focus [4,6]. Most cases of septic arthritis occur following hematogenous spread, owing to the vascularity of synovial tissue [7]. With disseminated infection, organisms traverse the bloodstream by direct spread from the primary site, seeding distant sites. The specific metastatic site likely depends on factors pertaining to the pathogen and host [4].

Much of the current understanding of the pathophysiology of bone and joint infection stems from studies of *Staphylococcus aureus* [4]. Blood vessel occlusion by bacteria and inflammatory cells results in tissue necrosis. Bacteria adhere to avascular bone and form a glycocalyx. Following infection of the synovial membrane, polymorphonuclear leukocytes release enzymes that destroy the articular surface [7]. Release of cytokines leads to bone lysis, with destruction of bony trabeculae and matrix and inhibition of collagen synthesis. Segments of avascular bone form sequestra; however, this process occurs less commonly in fungal osteomyelitis. In contrast to bacterial osteomyelitis, reactive new bone formation occurs later in the disease process [4].

Fungal osteomyelitis may occur as part of a multisystem process or in isolation. The most common chief complaint is localized pain. Although virtually any joint can be affected, large, weight-bearing joints such as the knees are most commonly involved [4,8,9]. On physical examination,

---

* Corresponding author.
E-mail address: shadley@tufts-nemc.org (S. Hadley).

common findings associated with arthritis may be present, including decreased range of motion, tenderness, swelling, erythema, and joint effusion. Chronic infection may lead to cold soft tissue abscesses and sinus tract formation [4]. Diagnosis may be delayed because of slow progression of disease, absence of characteristic laboratory findings, and failure to recognize fungi as potential pathogens. Patients may have other factors that mask physical signs of inflammation. Initial imaging may reveal lytic lesions with little new bone formation. Adjacent osteoporosis and osteomyelitis and cortical erosion may also be seen [4]. The differential diagnosis based on clinical and radiographic findings includes bacterial osteomyelitis, tuberculosis, sarcoidosis, osteogenic sarcoma, Ewing sarcoma, Langerhans cell histiocytosis, and malignant metastasis. The absence of new bone formation or a periosteal reaction may suggest fungal osteomyelitis [4]. Direct examination of potassium hydroxide–treated or Gram stain smears of synovial fluid usually fail to allow visualization of the organism. Synovial fluid leukocyte counts often resemble noninfectious inflammatory arthritis, and routine cultures are frequently nondiagnostic. Synovial fluid protein concentration is usually greater than 3 g/dL, and the glucose concentration varies from low to normal [4]. On pathologic examination, necrotizing granulomas may suggest the presence of a fungal infection, but do not exclude tuberculosis. Aggressive management and bone or synovial biopsy and culture are often necessary to confirm a diagnosis [3,10,11].

Clinical presentation and outcome differ according to the specific fungal pathogen and host factors [4]. This article discusses each fungal pathogen separately, and addresses special populations, namely neonates and intravenous drug abusers.

Candida

Overview

Candida spp are commensals commonly found in the gastrointestinal tract, female genital tract, skin, sputum, and urine. These organisms are the most common fungi associated with opportunistic infections. When the dermal integrity is impaired, Candida spp easily gain entry into underlying tissues [1,13]. Several Candida spp have been reported to cause bone and joint disease, including C albicans, C glabrata, C guilliermondii, C lambica, C krusei, C parapsilosis, C tropicalis, C stellatoidea, and C zeylanoides [4–6,11,14]. Candida osteomyelitis involving the femur, calcaneus, phalanges, metacarpals, metatarsals, mandible, zygoma, and talus, and arthritis of the knee, hip, ankle, costochondral, and clavicular joints have been described [1,5,13,15].

Bone and joint infections involving Candida spp most often occur in the setting of disseminated disease, but may also result from direct inoculation during surgery or trauma, or direct extension from a contiguous focus such as diabetic foot ulcers [1,4,5]. Candida osteomyelitis can also follow direct extension from a joint infection [6]. Factors predisposing to candidemia include immunosuppression, parenteral hyperalimentation, indwelling catheters, intravenous drug use, diabetes, HIV infection, multiple surgeries, malignancy, cirrhosis, malnutrition, steroids, and broad-spectrum antibiotics [1–3]. Candida bone infections can occur simultaneously or several months after an episode of fungemia, despite adequate antifungal treatment of the initial bloodstream infection [5].

Osteomyelitis

Reports of *Candida* osteomyelitis did not begin to rise until the 1970s. It is a rare disease, but with the increased prevalence of factors predisposing to invasive candidiasis, *Candida* osteomyelitis is emerging more frequently in select populations. This condition is associated with significant morbidity, particularly when diagnosis is delayed because of late recognition of *Candida* spp as potential bone pathogens [1]. *Candida* osteomyelitis in a patient who does not have predisposing factors, particularly a child, should raise concern for polymorphonuclear leukocyte dysfunction [4].

The most common presenting complaint is localized pain. Pain frequently occurs without constitutional symptoms; less than half of reported cases demonstrated fever or elevated sedimentation rates [5,13].

The vertebrae [5,11,16], followed by the sternum [1,5], are the sites most commonly affected after an episode of candidemia. When the sternum is involved, draining sinus tracts are commonly seen [5]. One such case of *C albicans* sternal osteomyelitis in a patient who had undergone coronary artery bypass graft surgery 1 year prior was characterized by multiple draining sinus tracts along the midline incision extending to the anterior mediastinum and destroying the manubrium and upper sternum [5].

In addition to hematogenous spread, osteomyelitis may occur because of contiguous spread or inoculation during surgery. The frequent occurrence of vertebral osteomyelitis in patients who have intra-abdominal infection suggests that contiguous spread through the retroperitoneum may be a source of infection [11]. Gathe and colleagues [5] described a case of *C parapsilosis* osteomyelitis of the lumbar spine in a patient who had undergone lumbar laminectomy 3 months prior. Given the absence of a central venous catheter, prior antibiotic use, and immunosuppression, the osteomyelitis was attributed to inoculation of *Candida* during surgery.

Arthritis

When hematogenous dissemination of *Candida* spp involves joints, it most commonly results in a monoarticular arthritis affecting normal joints [12,17]. Persons who have candida arthritis as a result of disseminated infection are often febrile, with either leukopenia or leukocytosis [18].

Conversely, septic arthritis has been reported as the first presenting sign in an immunocompromised patient who has candidemia [19]. A long latent period between an episode of fungemia and disseminated disease is not uncommon; in one report, a patient developed *C glabrata* arthritis of the hip 31 months after an episode of *C glabrata* fungemia, appropriately treated with amphotericin B [20].

Candida arthritis has also been associated with intra-articular administration of steroids, highlighting the importance of aseptic technique and the ability of cortisone to impair local defenses [12,18]. Patients who have localized candida arthritis as a result of an exogenous source are generally over 60 years of age and have a history of chronic arthritis. They typically present with a monoarticular arthritis and normal white blood cell count and body temperature [12,17]. The use of systemic or local corticosteroids may mask an inflammatory reaction and lead to a more indolent course and delayed presentation and diagnosis.

Candida typically affects large weight-bearing joints [8]. Knee involvement has been reported most frequently, although the hip, shoulder, ankle, cuneiform bone, and costochondral joint have also been described [1,3,5,15,17]. In contrast to bacterial arthritis, candida arthritis begins as a synovitis and can eventually involve adjacent bone, resulting in osteomyelitis [3]. Clinical findings may include pain, restriction of motion, and inability to bear weight [8]. The affected joints are generally tender, swollen, and mildly warm.

Diagnosis

The diagnosis of candida osteomyelitis or septic arthritis is not easy to establish. Blood cultures are frequently negative, as only 30% to 50% of persons who have disseminated candidiasis have positive blood cultures [17,21]. There are few characteristic clinical or radiologic features to suggest a fungal origin of bone destruction or joint invasion [5]. A high index of suspicion must be maintained in the appropriate host or in those who have bone or joint infections unresponsive to antibiotic therapy. Appropriate cultures may yield results in a timely fashion.

Radiographic findings associated with candida vertebral osteomyelitis are indistinguishable from those found with bacterial infection. They include destruction of the superior plate of one vertebral body and the inferior plate of the adjoining body, along with narrowing of the respective disc space [5]. CT and MRI may be useful to delineate cord compression, paraspinal abscess, and the degree of disc space or vertebral body involvement [16]. Bone or gallium scans may be helpful in diagnosing the presence of spinal osteomyelitis, but culture of biopsy tissue is needed to identify the causative microorganisms. In cases of sternal osteomyelitis, percutaneous needle biopsy has been efficacious in establishing the diagnosis [5]. Osteomyelitis of the long bones may reveal demineralization and a mottled trabecular pattern [5].

In cases of arthritis, synovial effusions are commonly visualized on plain radiographs, and radiographic evidence of adjacent osteomyelitis may also be seen. The synovial fluid is commonly purulent, distinguishing *Candida* from other fungal pathogens. The white blood cell count ranges from 15,000 to 100,000 cells/mm^3 with a predominance of neutrophils [3,4]. The synovial fluid glucose is usually either low or normal, whereas the protein concentration is most often high. Biopsy of the synovium may reveal a mononuclear cell infiltration, but granulomas are typically absent [4]. Direct examination of synovial fluid by Gram stain results in visualization of the organism in only 20% of cases, whereas better results are achieved with culture of synovial fluid or tissue [4]. The presence of *Candida* spp in synovial fluid should not be attributed to contamination caused by lack of predisposing factors for invasive candidiasis, as there are reports of candida arthritis in persons who are immunocompetent [15,22]. Surgical findings in the setting of fungal arthritis include a thickened and hyperemic synovium with fibrosis and scarring, erosion of cartilage, and purulent pyoarthrosis [3].

Polymerase chain reaction analysis has been reported to confirm an identical isolate in the setting of candida monoarthritis with antecedent fungemia [18]. Early diagnosis of candida bone infection may be achieved by measuring the serum level of β–D-glucan, a constituent of fungi that is elevated in the plasma in the setting of invasive mycosis or fungemia [15]. However, it does not distinguish between types of fungi. The specific *Candida* sp should be identified to guide therapy owing to the rise in non–*albicans* spp. This practice is particularly important because susceptibilities of *C albicans* and non–*albicans* spp are variable [1].

Treatment

Treatment of candida bone and joint infections is not well established, but almost always includes antifungal chemotherapy, with or without surgical debridement. Most successfully treated cases of candida arthritis and osteomyelitis described in the literature have reported the use of intravenous amphotericin B [3,5,9,11,14,17]. Although the combined use of amphotericin B and flucytosine has resulted in favorable outcomes [18], there is no evidence that flucytosine in combination with amphotericin B is more efficacious than amphotericin B alone [1,5,23]. The use of flucytosine alone is not recommended because resistance and significant bone marrow suppression may develop [1,5,12]. A major difficulty with the use of amphotericin B is the selection of an appropriate dose and duration of treatment, given the significant toxicity associated with the drug [11]. In case reports of candida arthritis and osteomyelitis, amphotericin B doses of 900 mg to 3.5 g over 4 to 12 weeks have been described [5,6,8,11]. Liposomal amphotericin B is less toxic, and has been reported to be as effective as conventional amphotericin B [9,24]. A patient who has *C albicans* arthritis of the knee was successfully treated with liposomal amphotericin B at a dose of 1 mg/kg/d [9]. Eradication of *Candida* spp may require several months of antifungal treatment [6].

If standard antifungal treatment with intravenous amphotericin B cannot be followed or fails, the choice of other drugs (eg, azoles) should be based on susceptibility testing, although clinical correlation data are lacking [9]. Successful treatment of candida infections has been noted with drugs that were observed to be resistant in vitro [14]. The newer azoles such as fluconazole, itraconazole, voriconazole, and posaconazole may be potential alternative agents and are associated with less toxicity [24,25]. In one report, *C albicans* knee arthritis in a person who was immunocompetent was successfully treated with joint aspiration and lavage and 200 to 400 mg of fluconazole daily for 3 months [22]. Prolonged maintenance treatment with fluconazole for up to 2 years has been reported [6]. There are limited data on the use of caspofungin in the treatment of candida arthritis and osteomyelitis.

Investigators have measured serum and joint fluid levels of amphotericin B in patients who have candida arthritis, and have found that levels vary from 20% to more than 100% of the serum concentration. These variations notwithstanding, the joint-fluid drug levels are felt to be sufficient to inhibit fungal growth [12,18]. Joint-fluid drug levels of fluconazole have been reported to approximate those in plasma [12].

There is controversy over the usefulness of intra-articular amphotericin as an adjunct in infections limited to the joint capsule [3,12,17]. Surgery, including synovectomy combined with arthrodesis, has been required for successful management in some joint infection cases [17]. Vertebral osteomyelitis may require surgical stabilization and decompression, but in cases without neurologic compromise, medical treatment alone has been successful [5].

Outcome of candida bone and joint infection is assessed by radiologic findings and improvement in clinical symptoms. Successful eradication is best confirmed by posttreatment biopsy [11]. Clinically significant treatment failure of *C albicans* septic arthritis, as defined by failure to clear *Candida* from synovial fluid, has been reported with the use of fluconazole despite in vitro susceptibility [8,9]. Failure of ketoconazole in the treatment of isolated candida arthritis has also been reported [20].

Prosthetic joint infections

Fungal prosthetic joint infections account for less than 1% of all such infections, and most are caused by *Candida* spp [23,26,27]. Prosthetic joint infections caused by *C albicans*, *C parapsilosis*, *C tropicalis*, and *C glabrata* have been reported [26,28], with *C albicans* being the most common isolate [2,27]. Given the paucity of cases, clinical features are not well understood and treatment recommendations are often based on anecdotal reports [26,28].

The hip and knee are most commonly involved, although the shoulder has also been affected [26,28–31]. Hip and knee prostheses are associated with a higher risk for infection given the long duration of surgery, large size of the foreign device, and low blood flow to cortical bone. Hematomas may form around a prosthesis, which can devascularize surrounding tissue and inhibit penetration of antibiotics [26].

Risk factors for prosthetic joint infection include surgical site infection, history of prior total joint arthroplasty, malignancy, advanced age, and obesity [26]. Bacterial infection of the prosthesis may precede fungal infection [2,32,33]. Patients who have candida prosthetic joint infections often do not have an underlying predisposing condition [27], in contrast to candida native joint infections, which typically occur in association with immunosuppression, prolonged intravenous antibiotics, or drug abuse [34].

Cellular and mechanical factors may contribute to the development of candida prosthetic joint infections. *Candida* spp have a mannoprotein coat that facilitates adherence to plastic surfaces and fibrin platelet matrices. Fibronectin, a glycoprotein produced by mammalian cells, is deposited on the surface of implanted foreign bodies. *C albicans* and *C tropicalis* adhere avidly to fibronectin, more so than less-virulent *Candida* spp such as *C pseudotropicalis* and *C krusei*. Bone cement may extend to surrounding tissues after implantation, and has been described to inhibit neutrophil chemotaxis [23].

Early prosthetic joint infection, defined as occurring less than 3 months after surgery, is characterized by pain, erythema, edema, poor would healing, and fever [26,28]. Early infection often arises as a result of an infected hematoma or superficial wound [28]. Candida prosthetic joint infection occurs later than typical early bacterial infections. It most commonly occurs between 3 months and 2 years after surgery, and presents in an indolent fashion [2,23,28–30,32]. It most likely occurs as a result of intraoperative contamination from organisms residing on the skin [2,28,30]. However, hematogenous spread and direct extension from an adjacent focus of infection may also play a role [30]. In particular, the long latency between surgery and clinical presentation suggests hematogenous dissemination may be important in the pathogenesis [2].

Diagnosis of prosthetic joint infection often proves difficult given the indolent presentation, difficulty detecting fungi, and false interpretation of positive fungal cultures as contaminants [28,29]. Patients may complain of pain caused by loosening of the joint, but commonly lack signs of inflammation, including fever [28]. Prosthetic loosening and radiolucency may be evident radiographically, but interpreted as mechanical failure [28]. Periosteal bone formation is suggestive of a deep periprosthetic infection [35]. Sedimentation rates may be normal early in the course of infection [28], and total leukocyte count is infrequently elevated. C-reactive protein may be useful for evaluating and monitoring treatment response [35]. Blood and urine cultures are most often sterile [23]. Diagnosis is facilitated by joint aspiration and culture. A neutrophilic predominance suggests infection, whereas lymphocytes and histiocytes are predominant in the setting of mechanical failure [28]. A microbiologic diagnosis is generally achieved by culturing the joint fluid. Additionally, culture of periprosthetic tissue has been helpful in problematic cases [23]. Organisms are visualized microscopically in less than 20% of cases with culture-positive joint fluid [23]. In one patient, microbiologic diagnosis required culture of a knee implant biofilm [29]. Given that *Candida* spp can be nonpathogenic colonizers of hospitalized persons, it is not uncommon for their identification in synovial fluid to be disregarded [2]. However, the appropriate clinical setting and repeated identification of the organism highly suggests the diagnosis [2]. Ultimately, culture from intraoperative tissue specimens may confirm the diagnosis [2].

Successful treatment of candida prosthetic joint infection most often requires removal of the prosthesis in combination with antifungal therapy [27], although medical treatment without prosthetic removal has been described in a few cases [31,36–38]. Initial surgical resection should include removal of the prosthesis and all foreign bodies, including cement fragments, and debridement of involved tissues [28].

Delayed reimplantation offers the best chance of good functional outcome [27]. A recent review of candida prosthetic joint infection identified 46 cases between 1969 and 1999, 10 of which were treated with delayed reimplantation [27,34]. Of the 10 patients, 8 received amphotericin B, with or without concurrent 5-fluorocytosine, fluconazole, or ketoconazole [27,34]. One patient received fluconazole alone, but in combination with a fluconazole-impregnated spacer. Another patient was treated with surgery alone, and underwent reimplantation 8 days after resection. These 10 patients were followed for a median of 50.7 months after reimplantation and 8 did not have evidence of recurrent infection. The two failures occurred in one person who was HIV-infected and treated with amphotericin B followed by ketoconazole before reimplantation, and the second in a patient who underwent reimplantation 18 days after resection arthroplasty and treatment with amphotericin B [27].

The optimal time to reimplantation is unclear [27]. It has been advised that an infection-free interval of at least 3 months after completion of intravenous antifungal therapy, as confirmed by culture of aspirated fluid, occur before reimplantation [34]. In the previously described ten cases of candida prosthetic joint infection treated with delayed reimplantation, median time from initial resection to reimplantation was 8.6 and 2.3 months for total hip and knee arthroplasties, respectively [27]. The use of antifungal beads or spacers may be effective adjunctive therapy, but requires further study [27].

The choice of antifungal agents and duration of treatment has varied considerably. Amphotericin B has been used most commonly, but successful treatment with fluconazole as the sole antifungal agent has been described [27,31,36,37]. Although data are limited, fluconazole appears to be as effective as amphotericin B for susceptible strains when combined with surgical drainage. Clinical and in vitro data demonstrate good synovial penetration with fluconazole [27]. No studies have documented the equivalence of lipid formulations of amphotericin B to conventional amphotericin B in the treatment of candida osteomyelitis and prosthetic joint infection [27]. Moreover, the efficacy of newer antifungal agents, such as voriconazole and caspofungin, is unknown. The total duration of antifungal therapy needed for eradication of infection is unknown, but in one series, amphotericin B was used for a median of 6 weeks and fluconazole for a median of 17 weeks [27]. It is not clear if supplemental treatment with an azole or 5-fluorocytosine is beneficial [34]. Doses of amphotericin B ranging from 0.5 to 1 mg/kg/d for 6 weeks have been described [2,34,39]. Initial doses of fluconazole ranging from 200 to 800 mg/d have been reported [31,36,37,40]. Early removal of the prosthesis may reduce the dose and duration of antifungal treatment [17].

Aspergillus

Aspergillus spp are ubiquitous in the environment, but only a few species, including *A fumigatus*, *A flavus*, *A niger*, and *A terreus*, are pathogenic in humans [41]. Aspergillosis occurs primarily in immunocompromised hosts at high risk for infection from neutropenia or organ transplantation [41–43]. Infection is most commonly acquired through inhalation of *Aspergillus* spores. Dissemination from a primary pulmonary focus can occur through hematogenous spread [44]. Aspergillus musculoskeletal disease is rare. Like other fungal bone and joint infections, it can occur in association with invasive aspergillosis or in isolation [45–47]. Vertebral, skull, sternal, shoulder, pelvic, tibia, knee, ankle, wrist, and rib involvement have been described [41–50]. The axial skeleton is the most common site of hematogenous spread to bone, and most frequently involves the lumbar spine [43].

Most cases of aspergillus bone and joint disease occur in association with immunosuppression, chronic granulomatous disease, surgery, or trauma [44,48], although there are a few reports of disease in persons who are immunocompetent [41,48–50]. Aspergillus sternal osteomyelitis in persons who are immunocompetent has been described after sternal trauma or surgery [46]. Direct inoculation is thought to be responsible for some cases of intra-articular aspergillus infection [48,50]. Septic arthritis can also arise from direct extension of infected bone [7]. *A fumigatus* septic arthritis and adjacent osteomyelitis of the shoulder have been described in persons who were immunocompetent and receiving intra-articular corticosteroid injections [48]. *A fumigatus* septic arthritis of the knee occurring months after vascular surgery likely results from contamination during surgery [41].

Diagnosis of aspergillus bone and joint infection is achieved by culture of synovial fluid, tissue, or bone [44,45,49]. Silver staining may show the presence of fungal hyphae. The recovery of *Aspergillus* spp in synovial fluid should not be casually attributed to colonization, especially in immunocompromised hosts [41]. An elevated erythrocyte sedimentation rate and radiologic evidence of bone and joint destruction are frequently observed [41,49].

Optimal treatment of aspergillus bone and joint infections has generally required a combination of medical and surgical modalities. Successful treatment has included surgical debridement, long or short courses of amphotericin B, and suppressive therapy with oral itraconazole [43,49,50]. There have been reports of patients who had aspergillus bone and joint infections successfully treated with surgical debridement and itraconazole alone at a dose of 400 mg/d [41,46]. It should be noted that itraconazole exhibits poor penetration into the central nervous system, and thus should not be used as the sole antifungal agent in patients who have disseminated aspergillus bone and joint infection and evidence of central nervous system disease [44,47]. One report described a renal transplant recipient who had *A fumigatus* arthritis of the shoulder who was treated with itraconazole and expired 9 months later because of an *A fumigatus* cranial abscess [47].

Although amphotericin B has long been the drug of choice, newer azole agents are being employed given excellent in vitro activity against *Aspergillus*, less toxicity, and good bone penetration [24,25,48]. A lung transplant recipient with *A fumigatus* pleuropulmonary disease that disseminated to the ankle was successfully treated with posaconazole after failing treatment with itraconazole and liposomal amphotericin B lipid complex in combination with surgical management [42]. Another patient who had *A fumigatus* septic arthritis was successfully treated with surgical debridement and voriconazole 200 mg by mouth twice daily for 9 months [48]. Caspofungin has been successful in the management of invasive aspergillosis in patients who are refractory or intolerant of other antifungal agents; however, its role in treatment of osteoarticular disease has not been well studied [24].

Endemic and community-acquired mycoses

Fungal arthritis or osteomyelitis caused by endemic dimorphic fungi, including *Histoplasma capsulatum*, *Blastomyces dermatitidis*, and *Coccidioides immitis* often occur secondary to hematogenous dissemination in persons who are immunocompetent [4,51,52].

Coccidioides immitis

C immitis is a fungus that exists in the mycelial phase in nature and as a spherule containing endospores in the tissues. It is endemic in the arid conditions of the southwestern United States. Infection usually occurs by inhalation of arthrospores. In persons who are immunocompetent, approximately 60% of primary infections are clinically silent and are recognized by a positive skin test with coccidioidal antigen [53]. Less than 1% of pulmonary infections progress to disseminated disease, and approximately 20% of disseminated cases involve the bone or joints [54]. Disseminated disease can arise in nonendemic regions several years after primary infection [54]. Reactivation of pre-existing infection can occur in persons who are immunosuppressed [55]. Epidemiologic reviews have observed that nonwhite ethnic groups have an increased propensity toward disseminated disease [51,53]. Many patients do not have an underlying systemic disease, and there is rarely a history of antecedent trauma.

C immitis has been associated with a sterile, immune-complex arthritis that occurs in the setting of primary pulmonary coccidioidomycosis. This arthritis is typically part of a self-limited hypersensitivity syndrome that includes fever, rash, eosinophilia, and hilar adenopathy [4,51]. Bone and joint infection can occur in isolation or in the setting of disseminated disease. Large weight-bearing joints, such as the knee, are most commonly involved. Symptoms may include fever, pain, restricted range of motion, joint effusion, warmth, and tenderness of the affected area [51,54,55]. Coccidioidal arthritis can be slowly progressive, or rapidly destructive and serving as a nidus for further hematogenous dissemination [51]. Untreated infection can result in pannus formation with infiltration into surrounding joint structures, bony invasion, and sinus tract formation [51].

Radiologic findings reflect the duration of infection. Cysts, cartilage erosion, and lytic lesions are seen in the setting of advanced disease (Fig. 1) [51]. The coccidioidin skin test is reactive in most cases. Serum coccidioidal complement fixation titers are usually elevated. A titer of 1:32 or more is generally indicative of disseminated disease [51]. Peripheral eosinophilia may be present [53,55]. Synovial fluid analysis may reveal a leukocytosis with

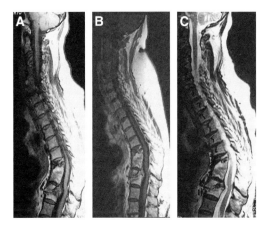

Fig. 1. Sagittal thoracic spine MRI of patient 4 years after diagnosis of disseminated coccidioidomycosis with multiple bone and joint involvement. Enhancing lesions at T 7-8 showing severe bone destruction extending into the paraspinal soft tissues, neural foramen, and epidural space, deforming spinal cord. Less-severe enhancing lesion noted at T-5 level. (*A*) T1 weighted MRI image pregadolinium. (*B*) Postgadolinium. (*C*) T2 weighted MRI image.

lymphocytic predominance [51]. Diagnosis may be confirmed by synovial fluid culture, but most often requires culture of surgical or biopsy tissue [51,54]. The diagnosis is highly suspected in the presence of characteristic endospores or chronic granulomatous inflammation on histopathology.

Treatment generally consists of aggressive debridement and long courses of amphotericin B. Management should be individualized based on the severity and progression of disease and the patient's underlying immune status [51]. It can be exceedingly difficult to eradicate C immitis from the bone or joint once chronic infection has occurred. Intra-articular amphotericin B has been used, but its efficacy is unclear [54]. Therapy can be initiated with azole antifungal agents, but amphotericin B may be preferable with vertebral column involvement and rapidly progressive lesions [54–56]. Isolated, early infections have been successfully treated with fluconazole and itraconazole. The newer agent, posaconazole, may also have a role in treatment [55]. Long-term fluconazole prophylaxis should be given in patients who are immunosuppressed (eg, transplant recipients) to minimize the risk for reactivation [55].

Histoplasma capsulatum

H capsulatum, a spore-producing dimorphic fungus, is found worldwide but is heavily endemic in the Midwestern United States [57,58]. Like coccidioidomycosis, infection occurs through inhalation of spores and can result in primary pulmonary, chronic pulmonary, and disseminated manifestations [59]. Primary pulmonary histoplasmosis is associated with a self-limited, sterile, migratory polyarthritis as part of a hypersensitivity syndrome [59]. Disseminated histoplasmosis is most frequently seen in persons who are HIV-infected. Although H capsulatum frequently infects the bone marrow in disseminated cases, bone and joint infection is rare [4,59]. A few cases of septic arthritis involving the knee, hip, and wrist have been described [57,60,61]. Infectious arthritis can occur in the setting of disseminated histoplasmosis or as a solitary monoarthritis [57,59,61]. C immitis and H capsulatum are the two fungi most commonly associated with immune complex arthritis, often manifested by symmetrical joint involvement [4]. In these cases, joint swelling is largely caused by synovial proliferation rather than accumulation of fluid [4].

Given the paucity of cases, there are little data to support diagnostic or therapeutic guidelines. Bone or joint involvement may be associated with normal radiographs or atrophy of articular surfaces with secondary changes of surrounding bone. Positive synovial fluid or surgical tissue culture confirms the diagnosis [57,60,61]. Histopathology of infected bone may reveal caseating or noncaseating granulomas [59,61]. Treatment has consisted of surgical debridement combined with amphotericin B, amphotericin B alone, and oral azoles. Although fluconazole has poor in vitro activity against H capsulatum, it has good in vivo efficacy in a limited number of patients [57]. One reported case of a prosthetic hip joint infection caused by

H capsulatum was treated with surgical debridement and itraconazole 200 mg daily as lifelong suppressive therapy [60].

African histoplasmosis, caused by *H capsulatum* subsp *duboisii*, is endemic in Central and West Africa. Unlike *H capsulatum*, approximately 50% of African histoplasmosis cases develop osteomyelitis [58]. Histology of infected tissue reveals giant cell granulomas and large yeast cells [58].

Blastomyces dermatitidis

B dermatitidis is found in soil in the mycelial form and in yeast form in host tissue. It is endemic in the south-central, southeastern, and Midwestern United States, and several regions of Canada. It is more common in men between 20 and 50 years of age and is associated with outdoor occupations [52,62]. Unlike other invasive fungal infections, such as candidiasis, it is infrequently associated with severe underlying illness [52,63].

The organism is inhaled as spores, and once ingested by alveolar macrophages is either contained by the host immune system or disseminated hematogenously to distant sites, including the skin, bone, kidney, and central nervous system. The disease has a predilection for the lungs, skin, soft tissue, and bone [52,62]. Isolated bone and skin involvement has been reported, and is attributed to direct inoculation [64].

Constitutional symptoms, including fever, chills, malaise, and weight loss, are common during the initial presentation. Blastomycosis bone and joint disease commonly presents with pain and swelling in the affected area, and may be accompanied by nodular and ulcerative skin lesions [52]. The most commonly involved bones are the vertebrae, pelvis, sacrum, skull, face, ribs, and long bones [62]. Joint involvement is uncommon and usually occurs as a result of local spread from an osteomyelitic focus [7]. The most commonly affected joints are those of the knee, ankle, elbow, wrist, and hand [52,63]. The arthritis is usually monoarticular, although oligoarticular cases have been reported [63]. Once bone and joint involvement occurs, the disease rapidly progresses without antifungal treatment [52].

Given the systemic toxicity associated with disseminated blastomycosis, leukocytosis and an elevated erythrocyte sedimentation rate are frequently seen [52]. The most frequent radiographic findings include osteolytic, "punched out" lesions and synovial effusions (Fig. 2) [52]. The synovial fluid is usually purulent [52,63]. Of all fungal arthritides, blastomycosis is the only one associated with positive wet mount microscopy of synovial fluid [52,62]. Definitive diagnosis can be made by identifying the characteristic round and broad-based budding yeast of *B dermatitidis* on histologic examination of synovial or bone tissue or culture of joint fluid or tissue [62].

Itraconazole at 200 to 400 mg/d for 1 year has been recommended for the treatment of osteomyelitis secondary to blastomycosis [62]. Amphotericin B is recommended for disseminated, life-threatening disease [62]. Medical

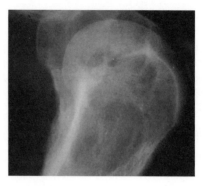

Fig. 2. Large osteolytic, punched-out tibial lesions in a patient who has *Blastomyces dermatitidis* osteomyelitis. (Courtesy of Michael Barza, MD, Boston, MA.)

treatment alone is usually sufficient to clear infection, although arthroscopic drainage has been needed in recalcitrant cases [63].

Cryptococcus neoformans

Cryptococcus neoformans is a ubiquitous, encapsulated, budding yeast. Cryptococcosis can have acute, subacute, or chronic manifestations. Persons receiving corticosteroids and who have hematologic malignancies have an increased predisposition to cryptococcosis. Primary infection typically results in pulmonary disease. In persons who are immunocompetent, respiratory disease is usually mild and self-limited. In persons who have impaired cell-mediated immunity, hematogenous dissemination can occur and involve many extrapulmonary sites, including the meninges, kidneys, skin, subcutaneous tissues, and bone. Bony involvement caused by hematologic spread occurs in 10% of cases of systemic cryptococcosis [59,65]. Cryptococcal vertebral osteomyelitis is well described and has been reported in normal hosts [58]. Cryptococcal arthritis most often results from local invasion of infected bone into the adjacent synovial space [59]. It most commonly affects the knee, although there are also reports of infection of the elbow, ankle, wrist, sacroiliac, metacarpophalangeal, and sternoclavicular joints [59,65,66]. Radiographic findings include soft tissue swelling, synovial effusion, and lytic lesions of contiguous bone [59,65].

Disease onset is typically subacute, with swelling and pain as the most common symptoms. Testing for cryptococcal antigen in the serum or cerebrospinal fluid may be helpful in diagnosis, although there are reports of cryptococcal bone and joint disease in the setting of negative antigen tests [66]. Diagnosis is confirmed by positive culture of synovial fluid, tissue, or draining sinus tracts [65]. Histopathology of biopsy or surgical specimens reveals multinucleated giant cells and granuloma formation. Special stains of bone and synovial tissue, including methenamine silver and periodic acid-Schiff stains, may demonstrate characteristic budding cryptococci.

Treatment generally involves surgical drainage and antifungal therapy. Two cases of cryptococcal arthritis were successfully treated with a combination of intravenous amphotericin B and 5-fluorocytosine [59]. A case of cryptococcal arthritis of the ankle was successfully treated with surgical drainage and fluconazole [65]. Current limited data suggest that, in immuno-compromised hosts, cryptococcal joint infection is best treated with amphotericin B and 5-fluorocytosine initially, followed by fluconazole [66].

Sporothrix schenckii

Sporothrix schenckii is a ubiquitous dimorphic fungus commonly found in soil, on animals, and on vegetation [58,67,68]. Persons who have an outdoor occupation are at increased risk for infection [67,68]. Alcoholism and myeloproliferative disorders have also been associated with sporotrichosis [67–69]. The most common mode of entry is through a minor skin wound, although the respiratory tract may also play a role [67,68]. Sporotrichal infections are usually either lymphocutaneous or extracutaneous. The lymphocutaneous form is the most common, and manifests as skin ulcerations and subcutaneous nodules. The extracutaneous form occurs in isolation or after dissemination, resulting in pneumonitis, arthritis, or osteomyelitis [67–69]. A history of direct penetrating trauma is often absent. Osteoarticular sporotrichosis comprises approximately 80% of extracutaneous cases and most commonly affects the knee, followed by the wrist, hand, elbow, and ankle [67,69,70]. One joint or several may be involved [68].

Sporothrix bone and joint disease is extremely rare; the incidence of *S schenckii* knee arthritis ranges from 0.03% to 0.04% [67]. Sporotrichal arthritis usually presents with pain, swelling, and decreased range of motion of the affected joint [67,70]. Symptoms are typically chronic and progressively worsen. Sporotrichal arthritis that remains unchecked may extend to contiguous subcutaneous or cutaneous tissues, resulting in parasynovial abscesses, cutaneous fistulae, and draining sinuses [68,70].

Diagnosis is often difficult because of the insidious onset, slow progression of joint disease, rarity of the disease, and difficulty in culturing the organism from synovial fluid or tissue. A review of 44 cases of sporotrichal arthritis noted that the interval between onset of symptoms and diagnosis ranged from 2 months to 8 years [68]. Patients infrequently have constitutional symptoms [68]. The erythrocyte sedimentation rate may be elevated, and the white blood cell count may be normal or slightly elevated [67,68]. Synovial fluid leukocytosis is generally moderate, ranging from 8,000 to 23,600 cells/mm^3 in one series [68]. Neutrophilic and lymphocytic predominances were noted [68]. In contrast to cases of histoplasmosis and coccidioidomycosis, serology has not been well studied in the diagnosis of sporotrichosis [71].

Radiographic findings include joint-space narrowing, joint effusions, erosion of articular surfaces, soft-tissue swelling, and periarticular osteopenia [67–69]. Surgical findings include a thickened synovial lining with pannus formation [68]. Diagnosis generally requires mycologic culture at the site of infection. Synovial tissue generally has a higher yield than synovial fluid [67,71]. Visualization of the organism using fungal stains is difficult [7]. Histopathology commonly reveals chronic granulomatous infection; multinucleated giant cells and caseating or noncaseating granulomas may be seen [67].

Itraconazole at a dosage of 200 mg twice per day is the initial treatment of choice [72]. Amphotericin B should be used in patients who have extensive disease or in those who fail itraconazole. Success rates with the use of itraconazole or amphotericin B are approximately 60% to 80% [72]. Itraconazole may be useful for long-term suppressive treatment in cases initially treated with amphotericin B [70]. A prosthetic knee joint infection caused by *S schenckii* successfully treated with a combination of surgical debridement, amphotericin B at a total dose of 2.4 g, and maintenance treatment with 200 mg of itraconazole daily for 2 years has been described [70]. Another case of sporotrichal arthritis involving a native knee was successfully treated with 11 months of itraconazole in combination with arthroscopic irrigation and debridement [67]. Surgical therapy alone has been largely unsuccessful [68].

Special populations

Neonates

The first case of neonatal candida arthritis and osteomyelitis was first described in 1972 in premature infants who had an umbilical catheter–related candidemia. Infants younger than 6 months of age now represent approximately 85% of cases of pediatric fungal arthritis, and most of these cases occur in neonates [12,73]. *Candida* sp is the causative organism in almost one out of five cases of neonatal nosocomial bone and joint disease [4,73]. Given the extensive blood supply in growing bones and joints, hematogenous candida arthritis is common in infants who have invasive candidiasis [12]. Fungal bone and joint disease is generally seen concomitant with or shortly after fungemia, although candida arthritis occurring 1 year after an initial episode of candidemia appropriately treated with amphotericin B has been described [73].

Neonatal candida arthritis is predominantly a nosocomial infection of low birth weight infants with underlying diseases, such as respiratory distress syndrome, aspiration pneumonia, and gastrointestinal defects [12,17]. These conditions are associated with many predisposing factors for candidemia, including prematurity, broad-spectrum antibiotics, hyperalimentation, abdominal surgery, intravenous or arterial catheters, and malnutrition [4,12,73]. Maternal vaginal candidiasis before or during delivery may also increase the risk for neonatal invasive candidiasis [73,74].

Patients commonly present with fever and a swollen, tender joint. Infants may demonstrate abnormal positioning of the affected limb. Polyarticular involvement occurs in one third of cases, and the knee is most commonly affected [12,74]. Neonatal candida arthritis may also be one manifestation of disseminated disease. The organism is frequently recovered from blood, urine, cerebrospinal fluid, and joint fluid [4,74]. Neonatal candida arthritis frequently occurs in association with metaphyseal osteomyelitis [14,73]. Bone infection may occur through contiguous spread from infected synovium, or the bone and joint may be simultaneously infected through the metaphyseal vessels [3,12]. Radiographs may reveal a joint effusion, dislocation of the joint, or irregularities at the metaphysis [3,12].

Candida arthritis in neonates is generally treated with intravenous amphotericin B at a dose of 0.5 to 1.0 mg/kg/d for 2 to 10 weeks [73,74]. Fluconazole at a dose of 7.5 mg/kg/d for 6 weeks has also been used with success [75]. Surgical debridement is generally not needed for successful treatment [73].

HIV and intravenous drug users

Candida sp is the most frequent fungal pathogen seen in intravenous drug abusers [76–78]. Intravenous drug users, regardless of HIV status, are at increased risk for musculoskeletal infection, and the clinical outcome does not appear to be affected by HIV status [77]. Approximately one third of heroin abusers with systemic candidiasis have osteoarticular involvement [12].

In a retrospective review of musculoskeletal infections in intravenous drug addicts, septic arthritis was seen in almost 80% of cases and *C albicans* was the most common fungal pathogen [77]. The axial skeleton is most commonly involved, with the sternoclavicular joint, costochondral joint, sacroiliac joint, hip, and vertebral body most commonly affected [14,77,78]. In addition to *C albicans*, aspergillus sternal osteomyelitis in intravenous drug users has been described [46]. Drug abusers are also at increased risk for infection with non-*albicans Candida* spp [5].

Persons who have HIV infection infrequently develop septic arthritis despite their immunosuppressed state. Furthermore, among those who have septic arthritis, candida arthritis is rare [12,17]. The presence of candida arthritis in persons who are HIV-infected appears to be associated with intravenous drug abuse rather than HIV itself [12].

Disseminated candidiasis, followed by cutaneous, ocular, and osteoarticular manifestations, has been described in intravenous drug users who use brown heroin diluted in lemon juice [12,17,76,79]. This clinical syndrome presents with fever during the candidemic phase, followed days to weeks later by painful cutaneous nodules over the scalp or bearded areas; chorioretinitis or endophthalmitis; and osteoarticular lesions. Osteoarticular involvement is characterized by multiple costochondral tumors, although large joint involvement has also been described. The costochondral lesions are usually painful and most commonly occur in the anterior thorax at the costochondral junction, and occasionally pus can be expressed. They can occur in isolation or simultaneously with cutaneous or ocular lesions.

The source of disseminated candidiasis in brown heroin users is likely contamination with *C albicans* on the skin. Lemon juice is an excellent growth medium for *C albicans*. Fluconazole or amphotericin B has been used in the treatment of this syndrome, although amphotericin B is the drug of choice in the setting of ocular involvement [76].

Summary

Fungal arthritis and osteomyelitis are uncommon diseases and generally present in an indolent fashion. The incidence of fungal bone and joint disease is increasing with an increase in the prevalence of factors predisposing to invasive fungal disease, such as the use of central venous catheters, broad spectrum antibiotics, immunosuppression, and abdominal surgery. Definitive diagnosis relies on bone or synovial culture or biopsy. Successful management has traditionally consisted of amphotericin B in combination with surgical debridement. Given the rarity of this disease, treatment is not well defined, but reports of success with the use of azole antifungal agents, including itraconazole, fluconazole, voriconazole, and posaconazole, are promising.

References

[1] Arias F, Mata-Essayag S, Landaeta ME, et al. Candida albicans osteomyelitis: case report and literature review. Int J Infect Dis 2004;8(5):307–14.
[2] Cardinal E, Braunstein EM, Capello WN, et al. Candida albicans infection of prosthetic joints. Orthopedics 1996;19(3):247–51.
[3] Bayer AS, Guze LB. Fungal arthritis. I. Candida arthritis: diagnostic and prognostic implications and therapeutic considerations. Semin Arthritis Rheum 1978;8(2):142–50.
[4] Kemper CA, Deresinski SC. Fungal disease of bone and joint. In: Kibbler CC, Mackenzie DWR, Odds FC, editors. Principles and practice of clinical mycology. Chichester: John Wiley & Sons; 1996. p. 49–68.
[5] Gathe JC Jr, Harris RL, Garland B, et al. Candida osteomyelitis. Report of five cases and review of the literature. Am J Med 1987;82(5):927–37.
[6] Trowbridge J, Ludmer LM, Riddle VD, et al. Candida lambica polyarthritis in a patient with chronic alcoholism. J Rheumatol 1999;26(8):1846–8.
[7] Smith JW, Piercy EA. Infectious arthritis. Clin Infect Dis 1995;20(2):225–30.
[8] Choi IS, Kim SJ, Kim BY, et al. Candida polyarthritis in a renal transplant patient: case report of a patient successfully treated with amphotericin B. Transplant Proc 2000;32(7): 1963–4.
[9] Turgut B, Vural O, Demir M, et al. Candida arthritis in a patient with chronic myelogenous leukemia (CML) in blastic transformation, unresponsive to fluconazole, but treated effectively with liposomal amphotericin B. Ann Hematol 2002;81(9):529–31.
[10] Harrington JT. Mycobacterial and fungal arthritis. Curr Opin Rheumatol 1998;10(4): 335–8.

[11] Friedman BC, Simon GL. Candida vertebral osteomyelitis: report of three cases and a review of the literature. Diagn Microbiol Infect Dis 1987;8(1):31–6.

[12] Silveira LH, Cuellar ML, Citera G, et al. Candida arthritis. Rheum Dis Clin North Am 1993; 19(2):427–37.

[13] Lasday SD, Jay RM. Candida osteomyelitis. J Foot Ankle Surg 1994;33(2):173–6.

[14] Zmierczak H, Goemaere S, Mielants H, et al. Candida glabrata arthritis: case report and review of the literature of Candida arthritis. Clin Rheumatol 1999;18(5):406–9.

[15] Kawanabe K, Hayashi H, Miyamoto M, et al. Candida septic arthritis of the hip in a young patient without predisposing factors. J Bone Joint Surg Br 2003;85(5):734–5.

[16] Frazier DD, Campbell DR, Garvey TA, et al. Fungal infections of the spine. Report of eleven patients with long-term follow-up. J Bone Joint Surg Am 2001;83-A(4):560–5.

[17] Cuende E, Barbadillo C, Mazzucchelli R, et al. Candida arthritis in adult patients who are not intravenous drug addicts: report of three cases and review of the literature. Semin Arthritis Rheum 1993;22(4):224–41.

[18] Katzenstein D. Isolated Candida arthritis: report of a case and definition of a distinct clinical syndrome. Arthritis Rheum 1985;28(12):1421–4.

[19] Vicari P, Feitosa PR, Chauffaille ML, et al. Septic arthritis as the first sign of Candida tropicalis fungaemia in an acute lymphoid leukemia patient. Braz J Infect Dis 2003;7(6):426–8.

[20] Gumbo T, Isada CM, Muschler GF, et al. Candida (Torulopsis) glabrata septic arthritis. Clin Infect Dis 1999;29(1):208–9.

[21] Jones JM. Laboratory diagnosis of invasive candidiasis. Clin Microbiol Rev 1990;3(1): 32–45.

[22] Calvo Romero JM, Alvarez Vega JL, Salazar Vallinas JM, et al. Candida arthritis in an immunocompetent patient without predisposing factors. Clin Rheumatol 1998;17(5):393–4.

[23] Darouiche RO, Hamill RJ, Musher DM, et al. Periprosthetic candidal infections following arthroplasty. Rev Infect Dis 1989;11(1):89–96.

[24] Maschmeyer G, Ruhnke M. Update on antifungal treatment of invasive Candida and Aspergillus infections. Mycoses 2004;47(7):263–76.

[25] Perez-Gomez A, Prieto A, Torresano M, et al. Role of the new azoles in the treatment of fungal osteoarticular infections. Semin Arthritis Rheum 1998;27(4):226–44.

[26] Kojic EM, Darouiche RO. Candida infections of medical devices. Clin Microbiol Rev 2004; 17(2):255–67.

[27] Phelan DM, Osmon DR, Keating MR, et al. Delayed reimplantation arthroplasty for candidal prosthetic joint infection: a report of 4 cases and review of the literature. Clin Infect Dis 2002;34(7):930–8.

[28] Lambertus M, Thordarson D, Goetz MB. Fungal prosthetic arthritis: presentation of two cases and review of the literature. Rev Infect Dis 1988;10(5):1038–43.

[29] Acikgoz ZC, Sayli U, Avci S, et al. An extremely uncommon infection: Candida glabrata arthritis after total knee arthroplasty. Scand J Infect Dis 2002;34(5):394–6.

[30] Lazzarini L, Manfrin V, De Lalla F. Candidal prosthetic hip infection in a patient with previous candidal septic arthritis. J Arthroplasty 2004;19(2):248–52.

[31] Tunkel AR, Thomas CY, Wispelwey B. Candida prosthetic arthritis: report of a case treated with fluconazole and review of the literature. Am J Med 1993;94(1):100–3.

[32] Brooks DH, Pupparo F. Successful salvage of a primary total knee arthroplasty infected with Candida parapsilosis. J Arthroplasty 1998;13(6):707–12.

[33] Koch AE. Candida albicans infection of a prosthetic knee replacement: a report and review of the literature. J Rheumatol 1988;15(2):362–5.

[34] Evans RP, Nelson CL. Staged reimplantation of a total hip prosthesis after infection with Candida albicans. A report of two cases. J Bone Joint Surg 1990;72(10):1551–3.

[35] Garvin KL, Hanssen AD. Infection after total hip arthroplasty. Past, present, and future. J Bone Joint Surg Am 1995;77(10):1576–88.

[36] Wada M, Baba H, Imura S. Prosthetic knee Candida parapsilosis infection. J Arthroplasty 1998;13(4):479–82.

[37] Merrer J, Dupont B, Nieszkowska A, et al. Candida albicans prosthetic arthritis treated with fluconazole alone. J Infect 2001;42(3):208–9.

[38] Simonian PT, Brause BD, Wickiewicz TL. Candida infection after total knee arthroplasty. Management without resection or amphotericin B. J Arthroplasty 1997;12(7):825–9.

[39] Pappas PG, Rex JH, Sobel JD, et al. Guidelines for treatment of candidiasis. Clin Infect Dis 2004;38(2):161–89.

[40] Lerch K, Kalteis T, Schubert T, et al. Prosthetic joint infections with osteomyelitis due to Candida albicans. Mycoses 2003;46(11–12):462–6.

[41] Steinfeld S, Durez P, Hauzeur JP, et al. Articular aspergillosis: two case reports and review of the literature. Br J Rheumatol 1997;36(12):1331–4.

[42] Lodge BA, Ashley ED, Steele MP, et al. *Aspergillus fumigatus* empyema, arthritis, and calcaneal osteomyelitis in a lung transplant patient successfully treated with posaconazole. J Clin Microbiol 2004;42(3):1376–8.

[43] Park KU, Lee HS, Kim CJ, et al. Fungal discitis due to Aspergillus terreus in a patient with acute lymphoblastic leukemia. J Korean Med Sci 2000;15(6):704–7.

[44] Gunsilius E, Lass-Florl C, Mur E, et al. Aspergillus osteoarthritis in acute lymphoblastic leukemia. Ann Hematol 1999;78(11):529–30.

[45] Panigrahi S, Nagler A, Or R, et al. Indolent aspergillus arthritis complicating fludarabine-based non-myeloablative stem cell transplantation. Bone Marrow Transplant 2001;27(6): 659–61.

[46] Allen D, Ng S, Beaton K, et al. Sternal osteomyelitis caused by Aspergillus fumigatus in a patient with previously treated Hodgkin's disease. J Clin Path 2002;55(8):616–8.

[47] Cassuto-Viguier E, Mondain JR, Van Elslande L, et al. Fatal outcome of Aspergillus fumigatus arthritis in a renal transplant recipient. Transplant Proc 1995;27(4):2461.

[48] Sohail MR, Smilack JD. Aspergillus fumigatus septic arthritis complicating intra-articular corticosteroid injection. Mayo Clin Proc 2004;79(4):578–9.

[49] McGregor A, McNicol D, Collignon P. Aspergillus-induced discitis. A role for itraconazole in therapy? Spine 1992;17(12):1512–4.

[50] Garcia-Porrua C, Blanco FJ, Atanes A, et al. Septic arthritis by Aspergillus fumigatus: a complication of corticosteroid infiltration. Br J Rheumatol 1997;36(5):610–1.

[51] Bayer AS, Guze LB. Fungal arthritis. II. Coccidioidal synovitis: clinical, diagnostic, therapeutic, and prognostic considerations. Semin Arthritis Rheum 1979;8(3):200–11.

[52] Bayer AS, Scott VJ, Guze LB. Fungal arthritis. IV. Blastomycotic arthritis. Semin Arthritis Rheum 1979;9(2):145–51.

[53] Pappagianis D, Zimmer BL. Serology of coccidioidomycosis. Clin Microbiol Rev 1990;3(3): 247–68.

[54] Lantz B, Selakovich WG, Collins DN, et al. Coccidioidomycosis of the knee with a 26-year follow-up evaluation. A case report. Clin Ortho Related Res 1988;(234):183–7.

[55] Blair JE. Coccidioidal pneumonia, arthritis, and soft-tissue infection after kidney transplantation. Transpl Infect Dis 2004;6(2):74–6.

[56] Galgiani JN, Ampel NM, Catanzaro A, et al. Practice guidelines for the treatment of Coccidioidomycosis. Clin Infect Dis 2000;30(4):658–61.

[57] Darouiche RO, Cadle RM, Zenon GJ, et al. Articular histoplasmosis. J Rheumatol 1992; 19(12):1991–3.

[58] McGill PE. Geographically specific infections and arthritis, including rheumatic syndromes associated with certain fungi and parasites, Brucella species and Mycobacterium leprae. Best Pract Res Clin Rheumatol 2003;17(2):289–307.

[59] Bayer AS, Choi C, Tillman DB, et al. Fungal arthritis. V. Cryptococcal and histoplasmal arthritis. Semin Arthritis Rheum 1980;9(3):218–27.

[60] Fowler VG Jr, Nacinovich FM, Alspaugh JA, et al. Prosthetic joint infection due to Histoplasma capsulatum: case report and review. Clin Infect Dis 1998;26(4):1017–22.

[61] Weinberg JM, Ali R, Badve S, et al. Musculoskeletal histoplasmosis. A case report and review of the literature. J Bone Joint Surg Am 2001;83-A(11):1718–22.

[62] Saiz P, Gitelis S, Virkus W, et al. Blastomycosis of long bones. Clin Orthop Relat Res 2004;(421):255–9.

[63] Abril A, Campbell MD, Cotten VR Jr, et al. Polyarticular blastomycotic arthritis. J Rheumatol 1998;25(5):1019–21.

[64] Marcellin-Little DJ, Sellon RK, Kyles AE, et al. Chronic localized osteomyelitis caused by atypical infection with Blastomyces dermatitidis in a dog. J Am Vet Med Assoc 1996;209(11): 1877–9.

[65] Agrawal A, Brown WS, McKenzie S. Cryptococcal arthritis in an immunocompetent host. J S C Med Assoc 2000;96(7):297–9.

[66] Bruno KM, Farhoomand L, Libman BS, et al. Cryptococcal arthritis, tendinitis, tenosynovitis, and carpal tunnel syndrome: report of a case and review of the literature. Arthritis Rheum 2002;47(1):104–8.

[67] Zacharias J, Crosby LA. Sporotrichal arthritis of the knee. Am J Knee Surg 1997;10(3): 171–4.

[68] Bayer AS, Scott VJ, Guze LB. Fungal arthritis. III. Sporotrichal arthritis. Semin Arthritis Rheum 1979;9(1):66–74.

[69] Gordhan A, Ramdial PK, Morar N, et al. Disseminated cutaneous sporotrichosis: a marker of osteoarticular sporotrichosis masquerading as gout. Int J Dermatol 2001;40(11):717–9.

[70] DeHart DJ. Use of itraconazole for treatment of sporotrichosis involving a knee prosthesis. Clin Infect Dis 1995;21(2):450.

[71] Kauffman CA. Sporotrichosis. Clin Infect Dis 1999;29(2):231–6.

[72] Kauffman CA, Hajjeh R, Chapman SW. Practice guidelines for the management of patients with sporotrichosis. Clin Infect Dis 2000;30(4):684–7.

[73] Swanson H, Hughes PA, Messer SA, et al. Candida albicans arthritis one year after successful treatment of fungemia in a healthy infant. J Pediatr 1996;129(5):688–94.

[74] Adler S, Randall J, Plotkin SA. Candidal osteomyelitis and arthritis in a neonate. Am J Dis Child 1972;123(6):595–6.

[75] Merchant RH, Sanghvi KP, Sridhar N, et al. Nursery outbreak of neonatal fungal arthritis treated with fluconazole. J Trop Pediatr 1997;43(2):106–8.

[76] Bisbe J, Miro JM, Latorre X, et al. Disseminated candidiasis in addicts who use brown heroin: report of 83 cases and review. Clin Infect Dis 1992;15(6):910–23.

[77] Belzunegui J, Rodriguez-Arrondo F, Gonzalez C, et al. Musculoskeletal infections in intravenous drug addicts: report of 34 cases with analysis of microbiological aspects and pathogenic mechanisms. Clin Exp Rheumatol 2000;18(3):383–6.

[78] Belzunegui J, Gonzalez C, Lopez L, et al. Osteoarticular and muscle infectious lesions in patients with the human immunodeficiency virus. Clin Rheumatol 1997;16(5):450–3.

[79] Collignon PJ, Sorrell TC. Disseminated candidiasis: evidence of a distinctive syndrome in heroin abusers. Br Med J (Clin Res Ed) 1983;287(6396):861–2.

ELSEVIER
SAUNDERS

Infect Dis Clin N Am 19 (2005) 853–861

INFECTIOUS
DISEASE CLINICS
OF NORTH AMERICA

Gonococcal Arthritis (Disseminated Gonococcal Infection)

Peter A. Rice, MD

Division of Infectious Diseases and Immunology, University of Massachusetts Medical School, Lazare Research Building (LRB), Room 321, 364 Plantation Street, Worcester, MA 01605, USA

Neisseria gonorrhoeae was once the most common cause of septic arthritis in the United States, but the prevalence of gonorrhea has plummeted in the United States since the onset of the AIDS epidemic. Gonorrhea may be poised to become more troublesome, because gonococcal resistance to fluoroquinolones and other antibiotics is increasing, and many contemporary physicians are unfamiliar with the musculoskeletal manifestations of gonococcal infection. Gonorrhea generally causes either a suppurative arthritis resembling septic arthritis caused by other bacteria, or a distinct syndrome of disseminated gonococcal infection, with tenosynovitis, skin lesions, and polyarthralgias, rather than frank arthritis.

Etiology and pathogenesis

Neisseria gonorrhoeae is the most common sexually transmitted bacterium causing infective arthritis. During the 1970s and 1980s, it was also the most common cause of infective arthritis in the United States [1–4]. Septic arthritis caused by *N gonorrhoeae* is usually monoarticular or pauciarticular, and is often associated with positive synovial fluid cultures. By contrast, in the overtly bacteremic form of the disease, suppurative arthritis almost never occurs. Instead, gonococcemia is usually associated with polyarthralgias and skin lesions, and may be more deserving of the term "disseminated gonococcal infection" (DGI).

An immunologic basis has been postulated for the polyarthralgias and skin lesions of DGI [5,6], but DGI may result directly from synovial and periarticular infection. Gonococcal bacteremia is commonly documented in

This work was supported by grant No. AI 032725 from the National Institutes of Health.
E-mail address: peter.rice@umassmed.edu

id.theclinics.com

this form of the disease with positive blood cultures in up to 50% of DGI patients with tenosynovitis and polyarthralgias, suggesting that the synovium and periarticular tissues are seeded early in the disease [1,4,7–10]. The skin and visceral lesions of DGI may also represent localized infection [4,5,10–13]. *N gonorrhoeae* can sometimes be identified micro-scopically or by immunochemical methods in apparently sterile joint fluids, periarticular tissues, or in skin lesions of patients with DGI [12,13]. The rapid improvement of polyarthralgias with appropriate antimicrobial therapy, usually within 48 hours, is consistent with a direct therapeutic effect against *N gonorrhoeae*, and is indirect diagnostic evidence of DGI [4,7,8,10,14–17].

Other evidence militates against an immunologic basis for most cases of DGI. Attempts to identify circulating immune complexes in patients with DGI have yielded conflicting results. Reduction of complement to abnormal levels is uncommon, although mild falls in complement often occur, presumably caused by consumption [4,18,19]. Nonetheless, the question of pathogenesis is still not resolved, and immune complex deposition or other immunologic mechanisms may play a role in individual patients. For example, the later entry of circulating gonococci into the joint space later may be facilitated by immune complex synovitis early in the course of DGI [20]. It is also possible that gonococcal cell wall constituents, such as lipo-oligosaccharide or peptidoglycan fragments, circulate from the site of mucosal infection to initiate arthritis in the absence of viable gonococci [21].

The lower incidence of DGI is caused by a lower prevalence of gonococcal strains able to enter the bloodstream and survive, going on to seed joint, tendon sheath, skin, and other tissues. DGI strains may have special growth requirements, particularly the arginine, hypoxanthine, and uracil auxotype, that make them fastidious and more difficult to isolate [22]. These strains often belong to the porin 1A serotype [23]. Porin is the most abundant gonococcal surface protein, accounting for more than 50% of outer membrane protein. Porins are aqueous anion channels penetrating an otherwise hydrophobic outer membrane. DGI strains resist the bactericidal action of human serum [24], and generally do not cause genital in-flammation, probably because of limited generation of chemotactic factors. These characteristics are related to the ability of porin 1A strains to bind to complement down-regulatory molecules, such as factor H and C4 binding protein [25,26], diminishing the local inflammatory response. Porin is an immunologic target of bactericidal and opsonophagocytic antibodies that arise after infection, or immunization with porin-containing vaccine candidates [27,28]. The critical role of humoral immunity is illustrated by the high rate of recurrent bacteremic gonococcal infection in patients with deficiencies of terminal complement components (C5-9) [29–31]. Up to 13% of patients with DGI have complement deficiencies [4], and persons with more than one episode of DGI should be screened with an assay for total hemolytic complement activity.

Epidemiology

The risk of DGI with gonorrhea infection was 0.5% to 3% in the 1970s, depending largely on the regional prevalence of specific strains of *N gonorrhoeae* [4,10,11]. These strains were then endemic in the Northwestern United States, where DGI occurred in up to 3% of patients with gonorrhea [32]. Current rates of DGI are low because of declines in the prevalence of these strains, and an overall drop in gonorrhea prevalence since the early 1980s. In the preantibiotic era, DGI was reported primarily in men [33], but studies in the 1960s and 1970s reported a female predominance of 78% to 97% [1,4,7–10,32,34]. Menstruation is a major risk factor for dissemination. In about half of affected women, symptoms of DGI begin within 7 days after the onset of menses. Hormonal factors and the more alkaline pH of genital secretions during menses may facilitate growth of *N gonorrhoeae*. The phenotypes of gonococci expressed during menses may be more likely to disseminate. Dissemination of *N gonorrhoeae* from a rectal source is uncommon in homosexual men, because these strains express phenotypes that are unlikely to disseminate [35].

Clinical and laboratory features

The clinical manifestations of DGI and gonococcal arthritis have sometimes been classified into two stages: a bacteremic stage, or a joint-localized stage with suppurative arthritis. An obvious progression from the bacteremic to the joint-localized stage usually is not evident [4]. Patients in the bacteremic stage have higher fever, often accompanied by rigors. Polyarthralgias are common during gonococcal bacteremia, and may occur in conjunction with tenosynovitis and skin lesions. Painful joints often include the knees, elbows, and the more distal joints; the axial skeleton is generally spared. Skin lesions are seen in about 75% of patients with bacteremia, although they usually are painless and patients may be unaware of their presence. They typically number between 5 and 40, appearing on the extremities and sometimes on the trunk, but rarely on the face. Papules or small macules are the most common lesions, followed by pustules, often with a hemorrhagic component. A wide variety of skin lesions are associated with DGI (Fig. 1), including vesicles and bullae, and immunologic lesions, such as erythema nodosum, erythema multiforme, and urticaria. *N gonorrhoeae* usually cannot be cultured from skin lesions by culture, and lesions may sometimes appear after appropriate antibiotic therapy has been started.

In the preantibiotic era, overt arthritis, confirmed by joint aspiration, was often reported; tenosynovitis was reported less frequently [32]. In more recent series of DGI, however, tenosynovitis was present in 67% to 68%, polyarthralgias in 52%, and monoarthritis in 42% to 48% [4,32]. The variable descriptions of these musculoskeletal manifestations may relate to

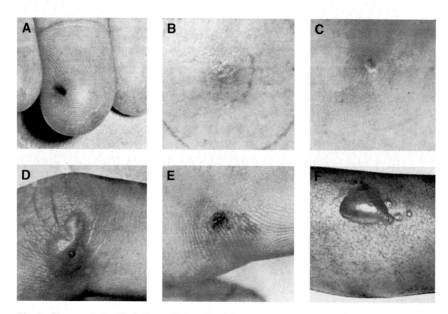

Fig. 1. Characteristic skin lesions of gonococcal bacteremia in various stages of evolution, from patients with proved gonococcal bacteremia. (*A*) Very early petechia on finger. (*B*) Early papular lesion, 7 mm in diameter, on lower leg. (*C*) Pustule with central eschar resulting from early petechial lesion. (*D*) Pustular lesion on finger. (*E*) Mature lesion with central necrosis (*black*) on hemorrhagic base. (*F*) Bullae on anterior tibial surface. (*From* Holmes KK, Counts GW, Beaty HN. Disseminated gonococcal infection. Ann Intern Med 1971;74:979–93; with permission.)

different definitions of arthritis and tenosynovitis in different series. For example, a common criterion for arthritis requires the demonstration of purulent synovial fluid having greater than 25,000 leukocytes/mm^3. Using this definition, frank arthritis may be less common than tenosynovitis accompanied by arthralgias [4]. It is unclear whether the increased reporting of tenosynovitis is related to a true change in the clinical manifestations, or whether it is simply resulting from increased recognition of tenosynovitis, instead of classifying all periarticular inflammation as arthritis. Tenosynovitis usually involves multiple sites, especially wrists, fingers, toes, and ankles. The differential diagnosis of the bacteremic stage of DGI includes reactive arthritis; acute rheumatoid arthritis; sarcoidosis; erythema nodosum; drug-induced arthritis; and viral infections (eg, hepatitis B and acute HIV infection). The distribution of joint symptoms in reactive arthritis, perhaps the most common differential diagnosis, differs from DGI (Fig. 2), as do the skin and genital manifestations [36,37].

Suppurative gonococcal arthritis usually involves one or two joints. The knees, wrists, ankles, and elbows are involved in decreasing order of frequency. The occurrence of arthritis in the absence of signs and symptoms of the bacteremic stage has led to the suggestion that these are separate

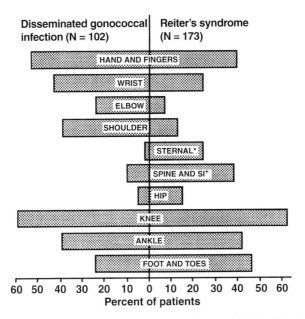

Fig. 2. Distribution of joints with arthritis in 102 patients with disseminated gonococcal infection and 173 patients with Reiter's syndrome. *Sternal includes the sternoclavicular joints. ⁺SI denotes the sacroiliac joint. (*From* Kousa M, Saikku P, Richmond S, et al. Frequent association of chlamydial infection with Reiter's syndrome. Sex Transm Dis 1978;5:57–61; with permission.)

syndromes. Most patients who develop gonococcal suppurative arthritis do so without prior polyarthralgias or skin lesions. In the absence of symptomatic genital infection, this disease cannot be distinguished from septic arthritis caused by other pathogens. Other joints, such as the sternoclavicular and temporomandibular joints, and the small joints of the feet are occasionally involved. Rarely, direct extension of an infection from the small joints of the hand to adjacent phalanges results in osteomyelitis [14]. The synovial fluid leukocyte count in suppurative arthritis ranges between 40,000 and 60,000 cells/mm^3 (with greater than 80% poly-morphonuclear leukocytes) in most series reporting synovial fluid analyses. Mean synovial fluid leukocyte counts in gonococcal suppurative arthritis are similar to those in staphylococcal and other types of nongonococcal bacterial arthritis [38]. Synovial fluid analysis and tests for *N gonorrhoeae* (ideally, both culture and DNA amplification) are important in identifying patients with crystal-induced arthritis and gonococcal septic arthritis. Other forms of septic arthritis should also be sought routinely with specific tests for pyogenic and other bacteria. Synovial fluid leukocyte counts are useful in establishing the presence of inflammation, but not in establishing its cause. Protein, glucose, and complement levels provide nonspecific but sometimes useful information.

Gonococcal endocarditis, although rare today [39,40], was relatively common in the preantibiotic era, causing about one quarter of reported cases of endocarditis [41,42]. Central nervous system infections including meningitis [43] and epidural abscess [44] occur rarely.

Although most patients with DGI have fever and many have shaking chills, up to 40% are afebrile [4]. Most DGI patients deny local genitourinary, rectal, or pharyngeal symptoms, despite the fact that genital, anorectal, or pharyngeal gonococcal infection can be identified in 70% to 80% of patients with DGI or in their sex partners. All potential mucosal sites of infection should be tested for gonococcal infection, regardless of the presence or absence of local symptoms. In a series from Seattle, N gonorrhoeae was identified by culture or by antigen detection using a direct fluorescent antibody test on blood, synovial fluid, or skin lesions in 52 (51%) of 102 subjects with DGI [1]; in Boston 23 (47%) of 49 patients were so identified [4]. Recent sex partners should also be examined. DGI is sometimes confirmed bacteriologically only by detection of gonorrhea in a partner [1,45]. Similarly, Chlamydia trachomatis should be sought in DGI patients and their sex partners.

Management

Hospitalization is indicated if the diagnosis of DGI is unclear, if the patient has frank suppurative arthritis, of if the patient cannot be relied on to comply with treatment. DGI may require higher dosages of antibiotics and longer durations of therapy. Ceftriaxone, 1 g intravenously given daily, is the mainstay of antibiotic therapy for DGI. Cefotaxime or ceftizoxime, 1 g intravenously every 8 hours, can be substituted as an initial regimen. A diagnostic test for C trachomatis should also be performed on genital secretions or urine. The initial regimens for DGI should be continued for 24 to 48 hours after clinical improvement begins. Thereafter, therapy may be switched to a fluoroquinolone (eg, levofloxacin, 500 mg orally daily), used as continuation therapy to complete a full week of antimicrobial therapy [46]. Levofloxacin also treats possible co-infection with C trachomatis. Because of developing resistance, fluoroquinolones are no longer recommended for the treatment of gonorrhea in men who have sex with men, or for gonorrhea acquired in California, Hawaii, Asia, and the Pacific Islands [47]. Clinicians in other areas need to monitor local resistance trends to fluoroquinolones. Cefixime, 400 mg orally twice a day, can also be used as continuation therapy. Cefixime is currently available in the United States as a suspension; the tablet form has been subject to availability problems. Because cefixime does not effectively treat the possibility of Chlamydia co-infection, patients should receive either a single oral dose of azithromycin, 1 g, or doxycycline, 100 mg, twice daily for 1 week.

Closed drainage of purulent effusions should be performed once or twice, which is all that is usually necessary. Nonsteroidal anti-inflammatory drugs may be indicated to alleviate pain, and are often useful to prevent recurrent joint effusions. Open drainage of suppurative joints is rarely necessary, but may be needed for joints that are difficult to drain percutaneously, such as the hip. All those who experience more than one episode of DGI should be evaluated for complement deficiency.

When the diagnosis is uncertain, a trial of antibiotic therapy may be warranted. Antibiotic-responsive, culture-negative acute arthritis in a sexually active young person often is caused by DGI. Blood cultures must be obtained before the therapeutic trial, not only to detect gonococcemia but also to help exclude other septic arthritides and infective endocarditis. Failure to respond to treatment necessitates evaluation either for other rheumatologic conditions, such as an acute presentation of a connective tissue disease, or another infection. If monoarticular suppurative arthritis persists during continued observation, synovial biopsy may be required to exclude tuberculosis, fungal infection, or a synovial tumor.

Summary

Septic arthritis caused by *N gonorrhoeae* is monoarticular or pauciarticular, and is more commonly associated with positive synovial fluid cultures and negative blood cultures. Gonococcal bacteremia is more likely to be associated with polyarthralgias and skin lesions. The diagnosis of gonococcal arthritis or DGI is also secure if a mucosal gonococcal infection is documented in the presence of a typical clinical syndrome that responds promptly to appropriate antimicrobial therapy. Hospitalization is indicated in patients with suppurative arthritis or when the diagnosis is in doubt. Initial treatment with ceftriaxone or another advanced-generation cephalosporin is warranted until signs and symptoms have improved; continuation of treatment for a total period of therapy of 1 week can be accomplished with a fluoroquinolone.

References

[1] Handsfield HH. Disseminated gonococcal infection. Clin Obstet Gynecol 1975;18:131–42.
[2] Calin A. Reiter's Syndrome. In: Kelly WN, Harris ED, Ruddy S, et al, editors. Textbook of rheumatology. Philadelphia: WB Saunders; 1985. p. 1007–9.
[3] Manshady BM, Thompson GR, Weiss JJ. Septic arthritis in a general hospital, 1966–1977. J Rheumatol 1980;7:523–30.
[4] O'Brien JP, Goldenberg DL, Rice PA. Disseminated gonococcal infection: a prospective analysis of 49 patients and a review of pathophysiology and immune mechanisms. Medicine 1983;62:395–406.
[5] Shapiro L, Teisch JA, Brownstein MH. Dermatohistopathology of chronic gonococcal sepsis. Arch Dermatol 1973;107:403–6.
[6] Williams RC. Immune complexes in clinical and experimental medicine. Cambridge (MA): Harvard University Press; 1980.
[7] Keiser H, Ruben FL, Wolinsky E, et al. Clinical forms of gonococcal arthritis. N Engl J Med 1968;279:234–40.

[8] Brandt KD, Cathcart ES, Cohen AS. Gonococcal arthritis: clinical features correlated with blood, synovial fluid and genitourinary cultures. Arthritis Rheum 1974;17:503–10.

[9] Gelfand SG, Masi AT, Garcia-Kutzbach A. Spectrum of gonococcal arthritis: evidence for sequential stages and clinical subgroups. J Rheumatol 1975;2:83–90.

[10] Holmes KK, Counts GW, Beaty HN. Disseminated gonococcal infection. Ann Intern Med 1971;74:979–93.

[11] Barr J, Danielsson D. Septic gonococcal dermatitis. BMJ 1971;1:482–5.

[12] Tronca E, Handsfield HH, Wiesner PJ, et al. Demonstration of *Neisseria gonorrhoeae* with fluorescent antibody in patients with disseminated gonococcal infection. J Infect Dis 1974; 129:583–6.

[13] Rothschild BM, Schrank GD. Histologic documentation of gonococcal infection in the absence of a culturable organism. Clin Rheumatol 1984;3:389–94.

[14] Gantz NM, McCormack WM, Laughlin LW, et al. Gonococcal osteomyelitis: an unusual complication of gonococcal arthritis. JAMA 1976;236:2431–2.

[15] Garcia-Kutzbach A, Dismuke SE, Masi AT. Gonococcal arthritis: clinical features and results of penicillin therapy. J Rheumatol 1974;1:210–21.

[16] Handsfield HH, Wiesner PJ, Holmes KK. Treatment of the gonococcal arthritis-dermatitis syndrome. Ann Intern Med 1976;84:661–7.

[17] Cooke CL, Owen DS Jr, Irby R, et al. Gonococcal arthritis: a survey of 54 cases. JAMA 1971;217:204–5.

[18] Walker LC, Ahlin TD, Tung KS, et al. Circulating immune complexes in disseminated gonorrheal infection. Ann Intern Med 1978;89:28–33.

[19] Ludivicio CL, Myers AR. Survey for immune complexes in disseminated gonococcal arthritis-dermatitis syndrome. Arthritis Rheum 1979;22:19–24.

[20] Manicourt DH, Orloff S. Gonococcal arthritis-dermatitis syndrome: study of serum and synovial fluid immune complex levels. Arthritis Rheum 1982;25:574–8.

[21] Fleming TJ, Wallsmith DE, Rosenthal RS. Arthropathic properties of gonococcal peptidoglycan fragments: implications for the pathogenesis of disseminated gonococcal disease. Infect Immun 1986;52:600–8.

[22] Knapp JS, Holmes KK. Disseminated gonococcal infections caused by *Neisseria gonorrhoeae* with unique nutritional requirements. J Infect Dis 1975;28:204–8.

[23] Knapp JS, Tam MR, Nowinsky RC, et al. Serological classification of *Neisseria gonorrhoeae* with use of monoclonal antibodies to gonococcal outer membrane protein I. J Infect Dis 1984;150:44–8.

[24] Schoolnik GK, Buchanan TM, Holmes KK. Gonococci causing disseminated gonococcal infection are resistant to the bactericidal action of normal human serum. J Clin Invest 1976; 58:1163–73.

[25] Ram S, McQuillen DP, Gulati S, et al. Binding of complement factor H to loop 5 of porin protein 1A: a molecular mechanism of serum resistance of non-sialylated *Neisseria gonorrhoeae*. J Exp Med 1998;188:671–80.

[26] Ram S, Cullinane M, Blom AM, et al. Binding of C4bp-binding protein to porin: a molecular mechanism of serum resistance of *Neisseria gonorrhoeae*. J Exp Med 2001; 193:281–95.

[27] Simpson SD, Ho Y, Rice PA, et al. T lymphocyte response to *Neisseria gonorrhoeae* Por in individuals with mucosal gonococcal infection. J Infect Dis 1999;180:762–73.

[28] Rice PA, Gulati S, McQuillen DP, et al. Is there protective immunity to gonococcal disease? In: Proceedings of the 10th International Pathogenic Neisseria Conference. Baltimore: National Institutes of Health; 1996. p. 3–8.

[29] Petersen BH, Graham JA, Brooks GF. Human deficiency of the eighth component of complement: the requirement of C8 for serum *Neisseria gonorrhoeae* bactericidal activity. J Clin Invest 1976;57:283–90.

[30] Petersen BH, Lee TJ, Snyderman R, et al. *Neisseria meningitidis* and *Neisseria gonorrhoeae* bacteremia associated with C6, C7, or C8 deficiency. Ann Intern Med 1979;90:917–20.

[31] Snyderman R, Durack DT, McCarty GA, et al. Deficiency of the fifth component of complement in human subjects: clinical, genetic and immunologic studies in a large kindred. Am J Med 1979;67:638–45.

[32] Holmes KK, Weisner PJ, Pedersen AH. The gonococcal arthritis-dermatitis syndrome. Ann Intern Med 1971;75:470–1.

[33] Keefer CS, Spink WW. Gonococcic arthritis: pathogenesis, mechanisms of recovery and treatment. JAMA 1937;109:1448–53.

[34] Brogadir SP, Schimmer BM, Myers AR. Spectrum of the gonococcal arthritis-dermatitis syndrome. Semin Arthritis Rheum 1979;8:177–83.

[35] Handsfield HH, Knapp JS, Diehr PK, et al. Correlation of auxotype and penicillin susceptibility of Neisseria gonorrhoeae with sexual preference and clinical manifestations of gonorrhoeae. Sex Transm Dis 1980;7:1–5.

[36] Kousa M, Saikku P, Richmond S, et al. Frequent association of chlamydial infection with Reiter's syndrome. Sex Transm Dis 1978;5:57–61.

[37] Rice PA, Handsfield HH. Arthritis associated with sexually transmitted diseases. In: Holmes KK, Sparling PF, Mardh P-A, et al. Sexually transmitted diseases. 3rd edition. New York: McGraw-Hill; 1999. p. 921–35.

[38] Goldenberg DL, Cohen AS. Acute infectious arthritis. Am J Med 1976;60:369–77.

[39] Cooke DB, Arensberg D, Felner JM, et al. Gonococcal endocarditis in the antibiotic era. Arch Intern Med 1979;139:1247–50.

[40] Ebright JR, Komorowski R. Gonococcal endocarditis associated with immune complex glomerulonephritis. Am J Med 1980;68:793–6.

[41] Johnston JI, Johnston JM. Gonococcal and pneumococcal vegetative endocarditis of the pulmonary valve. Am J Med Sci 1929;177:843–9.

[42] Thayer WS. Cardiac complications of gonorrhea. Bull Johns Hopkins Hosp 1922;33:361–72.

[43] Taubin HL, Landsberg L. Gonococcal meningitis. N Engl J Med 1971;285:504–5.

[44] van Hal SJ, Post JJ. An unusual case of an epidural abscess. Med J Aust 2004;6:40–1.

[45] Mendelson J, Portnoy J, Abel T, et al. Disseminated gonorrhea: diagnosis through contact tracing. Can Med Assoc J 1975;112:864–5.

[46] Centers for Disease Control and Prevention. Sexually transmitted diseases treatment guidelines. MMWR Morb Mortal Wkly Rep 2002;51:38–9.

[47] Centers for Disease Control and Prevention. Increases in fluoroquinolone-resistant Neisseria gonorrhoeae among men who have sex with men–United States, 2003, and revised recommendations for gonorrhea treatment, 2004. MMWR Morb Mortal Wkly Rep 2004; 53:335–8.

ELSEVIER
SAUNDERS

INFECTIOUS
DISEASE CLINICS
OF NORTH AMERICA

Infect Dis Clin N Am 19 (2005) 863–883

Reactive Arthritis

Danielle Lauren Petersel, MD[a],
Leonard H. Sigal, MD[a,b],*

[a]*Division of Rheumatology, Department of Medicine, University of Medicine and Dentistry of New Jersey, Robert Wood Johnson Medical School, MEB484, PO Box 19, New Brunswick, NJ 08903–0019, USA*
[b]*Pharmaceutical Research Institute, Bristol-Myers Squibb, J.3100, Route 206 and Province Line Road, PO Box 4000, Princeton, NJ 08543–4000, USA*

Reactive Arthritis (ReA) is a syndrome of asymmetric sterile oligoarthritis, predominantly affecting the lower limbs, primarily occurring in young adults, and following mucosal infections with certain enteric or genitourinary pathogens, particularly *Chlamydia*, *Shigella*, *Salmonella*, *Yersinia*, and *Campylobacter*. ReA is also commonly associated with spondylitis; sacroiliitis; and enthesitis (inflammation of tendinous and ligamentous insertions). Unlike most forms of arthritis, ReA has a known trigger, a defined genetic association, and a recognized cellular and immune response. Most ReA patients carry one of the HLA-B27 alleles, but not all HLA-B27 alleles are associated with ReA. Extra-articular symptoms associated with ReA include urethritis, uveitis, and skin manifestations, which may not be present in all patients. ReA is a sterile arthritis, not a septic arthritis; it represents an immunologic reaction to prior infection. Patients with ReA are predominantly male, although evidence suggests that many cases of ReA in women are missed, being either subclinical or misdiagnosed. Nonsteroidal anti-inflammatory drugs are the mainstay of therapy. Trials of long-term antibiotic therapy in ReA have shown little efficacy. There are limited data regarding the use of disease-modifying antirheumatic drugs and molecular biologic therapy.

Diagnostic criteria for reactive arthritis

ReA is classified with the spondyloarthropathies, a family of primarily articular inflammatory conditions. There is a common predilection for

---

* Corresponding author.
E-mail address: leonard.sigal@bms.com (L.H. Sigal).

0891-5520/05/$ - see front matter © 2005 Elsevier Inc. All rights reserved.
doi:10.1016/j.idc.2005.07.001

id.theclinics.com

spondylitis (vertebral inflammation), sacroiliitis, peripheral arthritis, extra-articular manifestations, and genetic associations with certain HLA-B27 alleles. The spondyloarthropathies include ankylosing spondylitis, psoriatic arthritis, and inflammatory bowel disease–related arthritis [1]. Most patients lack circulating serum rheumatoid factor. The fact that they are seronegative leads to another common term for these syndromes, the "seronegative spondyloarthropathies."

ReA is an immune-mediated aseptic inflammatory synovitis following specific bacterial exposures, associated with extra-articular manifestations, and affecting patients with a specific genetic predisposition. The clinical features of ReA may be diverse. The American College of Rheumatology (ACR) and the Third International Workshop on Reactive Arthritis in 1995 [2] established criteria for the diagnosis of ReA (Boxes 1 and 2). The Third International Workshop proposed that the diagnostic criteria should include specific clinical features, such as oligoarthritis or asymmetric arthritis of the lower limb, with or without inflammation of the sacroiliac joint or tendons, and evidence of gastrointestinal or genitourinary infection within the past 4 weeks with known ReA-inducing organisms. The ACR criteria require the presence of peripheral arthritis occurring in association with urethritis or cervicitis. Laboratory tests are not necessary for diagnosis.

Differential diagnosis

ReA should be part of the differential diagnosis of undifferentiated oligoarthritis or monoarthritis, particularly because the preceding enteric or genitourinary infection may be mild, or even asymptomatic, and likely has resolved by the onset of arthritis. The paramount consideration in such patients is that joint inflammation may represent active infection. Appropriate antibiotics should be given until septic arthritis is excluded

---

Box 1. American College of Rheumatology criteria for reactive arthritis

1. Arthritis for greater than 1 month with uveitis or cervicitis
2. Arthritis for greater than 1 month and other urethritis or cervicitis or bilateral conjunctivitis
3. Episode of arthritis and conjunctivitis
4. Episode of arthritis of more than 1 month, urethritis, and conjunctivitis

---

Adapted from ACR slide collection on the rheumatic diseases. 3rd edition. Atlanta: American College of Rheumatology; 2004.

Box 2. Third International Workshop diagnostic criteria

Peripheral arthritis
  Predominantly lower limb, asymmetric oligoarthritis
Plus
Evidence of preceding infection
  Diarrhea or urethritis in the prior 4 weeks
  No evidence of infection
Exclusion
  Other causes of monoarthritis or oligoarthritis excluded

Adapted from Kingsley G, Sieper J. Third International Workshop on Reactive Arthritis. 23–26 September 1995, Berlin, Germany. Ann Rheum Dis 1996;55: 564–84.

---

based on the results of synovial fluid aspiration, with Gram stain and culture.

The differential diagnosis of oligoarthritis or monoarthritis should also include crystalline arthropathy (gout and pseudogout); trauma (acute meniscal or ligamentous tear); other spondyloarthropathies (psoriatic arthritis, ankylosing spondylitis, inflammatory bowel disease–related arthritis); HIV arthropathy; Whipple's disease; Lyme arthritis; and immune polyarticular disease. Diagnostic tests must be performed to rule out these diseases before a diagnosis of ReA can be ensured (Table 1).

Reactive arthritis: history

The association of genital infection with arthritis, specifically of the lower extremities, has been known for centuries, a correlation until recently known as Reiter's syndrome. In 1916, Hans Reiter described a soldier who suffered from bloody diarrhea before developing the triad of urethritis, conjunctivitis, and arthritis, which he called "spirochaetosis arthritic" [3]. ReA is a general term that encompasses Reiter's syndrome, applied only when the preceding infection can be identified. Most patients with ReA lack the full triad of Reiter's syndrome [4]. The very term "Reiter's syndrome," however has fallen out of favor for two reasons.

The less serious reason is that Reiter was not the first to describe this syndrome. Van Forest in 1507 described knee swelling, arthritis, and urethral infection [5]. Brodie [6] in 1818 reported five patients with urethritis and associated polyarthritis. In 1916 Piessinger and Leroy described a similar postdysentery "oculo-urethro-synovial" syndrome. Arthritis as a complication of dysentery was also well described in the literature throughout the nineteenth century, especially during wartime.

Table 1
Differential diagnosis of reactive arthritis

Syndrome	Specific diagnosis	Suggested evaluation
Infectious arthritis	Gonorrhea	Gram stain and culture of synovial fluid, urethral swab
	Viral	
	Rheumatic fever	Anti-streptolysin titer
	anti-*Borrelia burgdorferi* arthritis	anti-*Borrelia burgdorferi* ELISA, anti-*Borrelia burgdorferi* Western blot
Spondyloarthropathies	Psoriatic arthritis	
	Ankylosing spondylitis	Associated clinical findings (rash, symmetric sacroiliitis, bamboo spine, colitis)
Enteritis and colitis-associated arthritis	Crohn's disease	
	Ulcerative colitis	
	Whipple's disease	Diarrhea, weight loss, colitis
Crystal disease	Gout, pseudogout	Crystals in synovial fluid
HIV	HIV arthritis	HIV and serostatus
Inflammatory	Rheumatoid arthritis	Rheumatoid factor and x-ray findings
Mechanical or degenerative	Trauma, osteoarthritis	X-ray and MRI

The more compelling reason to deny him eponymous immortalization was that Hans Reiter was an early and enthusiastic convert to Nazism and later a high-ranking Nazi official, who committed crimes against humanity, violated the precepts of the Hippocratic Oath, and planned and perpetrated abominable medical experiments in the concentration camps [7]. The evidence is sufficiently damning that international medical editors, and the Spondylitic Association of America, no longer accept the eponym in manuscripts, and recommend exclusive use of the term "reactive arthritis."

Epidemiology and genetics

The worldwide prevalence of ReA is 1 per 1000, with higher risk tied to specific genetic backgrounds and bacterial exposure. The prevalence of spondyloarthropathy among whites was found to be 1.9 per 1000, making it the most common inflammatory rheumatic disease to affect the white population in Europe [8]. The average age of onset is between 20 and 40 years. There is often an increased incidence during wartime, because conditions favor the spread of predisposing infections [9]. A Swedish study found that ReA had an annual incidence of 28 per 100,000, and with rheumatoid arthritis made up 45% of the national incidence of arthritides [10].

The incidence of ReA in the general population is 4.6 to 13 per 100,000 for genitourinary ReA, and 5 to 14 per 100,000 for gastrointestinal infection–related ReA [11]. The frequency of cases of ReA induced by a particular organism parallels the rate of primary infection with that organism within the population [12]. A recent study showed that ReA following *Campylobacter* had an annual incidence of 4.3 per 100,000 [13].

ReA has a male predilection when related to genitourinary infection, with a male to female ratio of 9:1 [14]. Enteric-related ReA has a male/female ratio of 1:1. This difference may be caused by overlooked urethral symptoms in women; misdiagnosis; or a possible deficient humoral response to bacterial antigens by males, specifically related to *C trachomatis* [15].

HLA–B27 has a frequency in the white Western European population of 9.3% [16]; 8% of American whites carry an HLA-B27 allele. The frequency of HLA-B27 varies with ethnicity, and corresponding differences are observed in the rates of ReA. There are at least 11 subtypes of HLA-B27 defined by genetic studies. A total of 65% to 95% of white patients with ReA carry the HLA-B27 allele (30%–50% of African Americans), but only 20% of HLA-B27 carriers ultimately develop signs of spondyloarthropathy. HLA-B27 subtypes associated with spondylarthropathy include the following:

B*2705: white, African, African-American, Native American (most common subtype)
B*2702: whites
B*2704: Eastern Asians; no association with spondyloarthropathy:
B*2703: West Africa
B*2706: Southeast Asians

There have been claims of an association between ReA and HIV infection. It seems that HIV does not cause ReA; the same pathogens that cause ReA are common in patients with HIV. It is clear, however, that ReA in HIV-positive individuals is often severe and explosive, with florid polyarthritis; enthesitis (especially plantar fasciitis); and extensive psoriasiform skin lesions. B27 positivity rates of 75% in this population have been reported.

Musculoskeletal manifestations

The classic features of ReA are an acute, asymmetric oligoarthritis associated with enthesitis (inflammation of tendinous or ligamentous insertions), and extra-articular signs, such as urethritis and conjunctivitis. The joints most commonly affected are the knees, ankles, and feet. The Third International Workshop on ReA proposed that the diagnosis of ReA did not require the triad of clinical features, but could be made in the presence of asymmetric oligoarthritis with or without enthesopathy and sacroiliitis, with evidence of infection within the past 4 weeks (Table 2).

Musculoskeletal symptoms usually begin 2 to 4 weeks following a gastrointestinal or genitourinary infection. Arthritis is usually the last of the clinical signs to present, usually preceded by uveitis. By the time articular symptoms appear, the gastrointestinal infection is usually cleared or resolved, so that the organism cannot be cultured from the stool.

Table 2
Extra-articular manifestations of reactive arthritis

Eye	
Conjunctivitis	30%–60% of affected reactive arthritis
Uveitis	Usually unilateral, iritis
Urogenital tract	
Urethritis	Part of clinical triad, associated with *Chlamydia*
Cervicitis	
Skin	
Circinate balanitis	
Oral ulcers	
Kertaoderma blenorrhagicum	Hyperkeratotic lesion with an erythematous base; usually on the palms and soles
Gastrointestinal	
Diarrhea	Usually presenting manifestation
Cardiac	Conduction abnormalities, aortic regurgitation
Peripheral joints	
Arthritis	Asymmetric sacroiliitis
	Enthesitis, dactylitis
	Peripheral arthritis, low back pain

The arthritis of ReA typically affects the large joints of the lower extremities, knees, foot joints, and ankles being the most common. Simultaneous involvement of many joints is often found. Some patients suffer from dactylitis, diffuse swelling of an entire digit, sometimes referred to as a "sausage digit" or "cigar digit." Dactylitis usually affects the toes, although the fingers may also be involved. It results from inflammation of the joint capsule and surrounding periarticular structures [17]. When hand arthritis occurs, it commonly affects the distal interphalangeal joints. As many as 50% of patients have lower back or buttock pain from asymmetric sacroiliitis, which may be mistaken for sciatica [18]. This is in marked contrast to the bilateral sacroiliitis of ankylosing spondylitis.

Heel pain is common, caused by enthesitis at the insertion of the Achilles tendon and plantar aponeurosis. Other locations for enthesitis are the ischial tuberosities, iliac crests, tibial tuberosities, and even the ribs [19].

Extra-articular manifestations

Ophthalmic

Extra-articular manifestations are generally more common with chlamydial ReA than postdysentery ReA. Conjunctivitis, which occurs in 30% to 60% of patients, is usually bilateral, and occurs early in the course of disease, but typically after urethritis. Conjunctivitis is more common with sexually acquired and after *Shigella* infection than with other postdysentery ReA syndromes [20]. There is a male/female ratio of 1.3:1. Chronic inflammation of the eye can lead to progressive intraocular damage and visual loss [17]. The uveitis is typically characterized by acute unilateral attacks of inflammation of the anterior chamber. Acute anterior uveitis is seen in approximately 5% of patients, presenting as ocular pain, erythema, and photophobia. The prognosis is favorable, but if untreated up to 11% of those affected may become legally blind [20].

Cardiac

Inflammation of the heart and coronary vessels can result in aortic regurgitation. ReA inflammatory aortic disease may be difficult to distinguish pathologically from syphilis, and may require surgical correction [21]. Screening echocardiography is warranted, however, only if ReA is chronic [22]. Severe conduction system abnormalities, and less commonly mitral regurgitation, may be associated with aortic involvement [23].

Weinberger and coworkers [3] described myocarditis in ReA causing asymptomatic atrioventricular (AV) node conduction abnormalities. This can be seen in 5% to 14% of patients. First-degree AV block is more common, but progression to second-degree AV block and even complete heart block can occur [12]. Carditis can occur in carriers of the HLA-B27 allele without being associated with ReA or ankylosing spondylitis.

Mucocutaneous

Cutaneous manifestations of ReA occur in up to 50% of patients. Keratoderma blennorrhagicum is a hyperkeratotic lesion seen in about 25% of affected men, usually on the soles of the feet or palms of the hands. It begins as a clear vesicle on an erythematous base, developing into nodules. It eventually crusts over, and adjacent lesions coalesce [18]. The cutaneous lesions are difficult to distinguish from pustular psoriasis, both clinically and histologically, and it is important to note that psoriatic and ReA skin and joint lesions may be hard to differentiate. Nail changes similar to those of psoriasis are seen in up to 15% of patients with ReA.

Circinate balanitis is a painless shallow erythematous ulcer of the glans penis, seen in up to 25% of men. In circumcised men it is dry, plaque-like, and hyperkeratotic, resembling psoriasis or keratoderma. In uncircumcised men it is typically a moist, shallow ulcer surrounding the meatus. Superficial, usually painless oral ulcers occur in approximately 5% to 15% of patients. They are typically located on the hard palate or tongue, but they may also be found on the soft palate, gingiva, and cheeks [24].

Pathogenesis

The development of ReA involves infectious and genetic factors. Approximately 4 weeks after the onset of the antecedent gastrointestinal or genitourinary infection, the bacteria have been cleared, but the systemic immune response causes an acute peripheral aseptic synovitis and associated characteristic features. Arthrocentesis and synovial fluid do not reveal live bacteria; a positive culture indicates septic arthritis requiring parenteral antibiotics. In such a circumstance, ReA is not the correct diagnosis.

Bacteria associated with reactive arthritis

Unlike most forms of arthritis, the role of exogenous antigen in triggering symptoms of ReA is quite clear. The four most common pathogens implicated in enteric-infection–related ReA are (1) *Yersinia*, (2) *Salmonella*, (3) *Campylobacter*, and (4) *Shigella*. Only specific species of these bacteria cause the ReA reaction (Box 3). These bacteria are believed to express arthritogenic antigens, which may find a reservoir in the synovium and synoviocytes, leading to an ongoing immune response to antigenic material lodged in the synovium.

Common features of arthritogenic bacteria

Yersinia, *Shigella*, *Campylobacter*, and *Salmonella* share some common features, perhaps accounting for their association with ReA. These bacteria

---

Box 3. Bacteria associated with reactive arthritis

Genitourinary
  Chlamydia trachomatis
  Chlamydia psittaci
  Possible: *Ureaplasma urealyticum*

Gastrointestinal
  Shigella flexneri
  Campylobacter jejuni
  Campylobacter fetus
  Salmonella typhimurium
  Salmonella enteritidis (less common: *S heidelberg, S choleraesuis, S paratyphi B*)
  Shigella sonnei
  Shigella dysenteriae
  Yersinia pseudotuberculosis
  Yersinia enterocolitica O:3 or O:9 (less common: *Y enterocolitica* O:8)
  Clostridium difficile

Adapted from Moreland LW, Koopman WJ. Infection as a cause of reactive arthritis, ankylosing spondylitis and rheumatic fever. Curr Opin Rheumatol 1992;4:534–42; Khan MA. Update on spondyloarthropathies. Ann Intern Med 2002;136:896–907.

are all either obligate or facultative intracellular bacteria. They are aerobic (*Campylobacter* is microaerophilic) and gram-negative, with a lipopolysaccharide-containing outer membrane. They are invasive and infect the gastrointestinal tract, with local colonic inflammation. Perhaps the most critical common feature is that they are all conveyed from the colonic mucosa to the joint by monocytes. Why ReA most commonly affects specific joints, usually of the lower extremity, is as yet unclear, but may relate to the fact that circulating mononuclear cells may preferentially exit the circulation at sites of inflammation. There is probably low-level inflammation in the repeatedly microtraumatized joints of the weight-bearing lower extremity.

There are many other bacteria with similar features that do not result in ReA. Fendler and coworkers [25] investigated 52 patients, all diagnosed with ReA, to find their causative pathogen. Through diagnostic testing, stool cultures, and antibody assays, 56% of the pathogens were identified, being *Yersinia*, *Shigella*, *Campylobacter*, and *C trachomatis*.

Salmonella

The incidence of *Salmonella*-induced ReA generally ranges from 1.2% to 8% of persons exposed to *Salmonella*, with approximately 22 of the 2000 known serotypes reported to trigger ReA [26,27]. Higher frequencies of ReA have been reported, however, in certain outbreaks. In a 1994 outbreak of *Salmonella enteritidis* in Washington State, of 217 cases of gastroenteritis identified, 29% had symptoms of ReA, with 3% having the full triad. Those patients who developed a more severe illness, with a longer duration of diarrhea resulting in hospital visits, were more likely to develop ReA [28]. In an outbreak in Copenhagen, Denmark, 17 (19%) of 91 persons exposed to *S enteritidis* developed ReA, with ankle and knee pain being the most frequent complaints [29]. Post-*Salmonella* exposure ReA is associated with the HLA-B27 allele.

Yersinia

The enteropathogenic *Yersinia* species, *Y enterocolitica* and *Y pseudotuberculosis*, cause a clinical syndrome of enterocolitis, sometimes with mesenteric adenitis and terminal ileitis, which may mimic appendicitis. *Y enterocolitica* is a sporadic cause of human disease, whereas *Y pseudotuberculosis* is a relatively rare human pathogen. Both are more common in northern Europe than North America. *Yersinia* occasionally cause ReA. In Scandinavia, 10% to 30% of *Y enterocolitica* cases are associated with ReA [30]. Hannu and coworkers [31] described an outbreak in Finland of *Y pseudotuberculosis* serotype O:3. There was a 15% incidence of musculoskeletal symptoms, with 12% fulfilling criteria for ReA. ReA associated with *Y pseudotuberculosis* seemed to be more severe than that associated with other pathogens.

An investigation of the immune response of HLA-B27–positive individuals to *Yersinia* found increased neutrophil chemotaxis in response to *Yersinia* antigen, compared with HLA-B27–negative controls [32]. Patients with HLA-B27 positivity usually have a more prolonged course of ReA and are more susceptible to recurrences [2].

Campylobacter

Campylobacter jejuni is now recognized as a leading cause of enteritis in humans worldwide [33]. The annual incidence of *Campylobacter* infection is approximately 4.3 per 100,000. ReA from *Campylobacter* follows a milder course, and has only a weak association with the HLA-B27 allele [34]. In one study of patients with stool cultures revealing *Campylobacter*, 7% had ReA, and 1% had tendonitis symptoms but not a full ReA picture [35].

Shigella

Most cases of ReA triggered by *Shigella* species are caused by *S flexneri*, with a few cases caused by *S sonnei* and *S dysenteriae* [36]. A cruise-ship outbreak exposed 205 passengers to *Shigella flexneri* 2a, with five developing ReA symptoms. Of the five affected, four were HLA-B27 positive [37]. In one Finnish study, 7% of patients with positive *Shigella* stool cultures had ReA symptoms. Of those patients, 36% were HLA-B27 positive. The major symptoms were low back pain and peripheral arthritis, the most commonly affected joint being the wrist [36].

Chlamydia

A common urogenital pathogen, *C trachomatis*, has been known for some time to cause ReA. In a 1978 study of 384 patients with *Chlamydia* urethritis, 16 had arthritic symptoms. Of those who developed arthritis, 40% were carriers of the HLA-B27 allele [38]. Inman and Chiu [39] created synovial cell lines infected with *Chlamydia*. The cells were placed into the joints of rats, which later developed inflammatory markers and arthritis, without evidence of active bacterial infection. This was interpreted as evidence that *Chlamydia* causes an inflammatory reaction persisting after the infection resolves.

Other bacteria

There is a smattering of case reports of other bacterial causes of ReA. *Clostridium difficile* has been associated with ReA. Enteric infection with *C difficile* in two adult patients resulted in ReA arthritis. One patient had HLA-B27 antigen. Outcomes were good in short-term follow-up [40]. Cases of ReA caused by leptospirosis and Q fever have been reported [41]. A single report of seven European cases suggested that *Borrelia burgdorferi* (the causative agent of Lyme disease) could cause true ReA [42]; this association has not been substantiated subsequently.

Persistence of antigen within the synovial space

In ReA, techniques to identify viable bacteria within the synovium have failed until recently. Studies using polymerase chain reaction have found DNA sequences of *Chlamydia* in the synovium of some ReA patients [43]. In another study, the synovium of eight patients with *Chlamydia*-associated inflammatory arthritis were inoculated with fluorescein-labeled monoclonal antibody to *C trachomatis*. Elementary bodies were found in the inflamed synovium [44]. These strands of evidence have led to the hypothesis that although viable organisms are no longer present, bacterial antigens persist within the synovium of affected joints, and that the immune response to the antigens is arthritogenic.

Similar evidence has been reported in ReA caused by other bacteria. In *Yersinia* ReA, polymorphonuclear leukocytes and macrophages from synovium contained *Yersinia* antigens in immunofluorescence studies. Investigation with Western blot analysis found some *Yersinia*-associated ReA patients had *Yersinia* antigens present in the affected synovial fluid [45]. Western blot analysis using monoclonal antibodies identified *Salmonella* lipopolysaccharide in the synovium of affected joints. Immunofluorescence studies were also positive for *Salmonella* antigens [46].

Immune responses

It is generally believed that ReA is not caused by active infection. Rather, infection with certain gastrointestinal and genitourinary pathogens is thought to precipitate either an autoimmune response to cross-reactive host antigens, or an immune response to slowly or incompletely cleared microbial antigens lodged in host tissues [2,47].

Given the HLA-B27 linkage in ReA, it is tempting to suspect that the immunopathogenesis of ReA is related to a $CD8^+$ T-cell response. HLA-B27, and other major histocompatibility complex class I molecules on antigen-presenting cells, typically interact with $CD8^+$ T cells. An attractive theory is that the HLA-B27 molecule is uniquely suited to present pathogen-derived peptides. Local immunodysregulation and inflammation can be sustained as long as the supply of such peptides is maintained. Alternatively, a poorly degradable pathogen-derived antigen might bind firmly to a molecule found uniquely within the tissues affected in ReA. In such a setting, the persisting foreign antigen could perpetuate long-lasting local inflammation. The absence of a defined antigen, however, has hampered the search for pathogenic T-cell clones. Another theory is that a pathogen-derived antigen resembles a host antigen. Such a host antigen might be found in the tissues affected in ReA, leading to a local autoimmune reaction.

Peculiarities of the heavy chain of HLA-B27 have also been implicated in the pathogenesis of ReA [48]. This heavy chain is prone to misfolding, perhaps allowing cryptic self-peptides to become available for expression as autoantigens. Further research is required to clarify the precise immune mechanisms of ReA.

HLA-B27

Although ReA occurs in the absence of HLA-B27, this allele is strongly associated with ReA. HLA-B27 may play a role in the antigen presentation of the unidentified arthritogenic antigen [12].

It is believed that the arthritogenic microbial peptide is presented to the T-cell receptor, and has cross-reactivity to autoantigens. One study demonstrated HLA-B27– positive cells infected with ReA-inducing bacteria show an increased presentation of certain self-peptides [49]. Intra-articular synthesis of IgG by B cells may contribute to the inflammatory response [50]. A study examining the activity of HLA-B27–positive polymorphonuclear leukocytes involved in *Yersinia* ReA showed an amplified reaction to chemotactic stimulus, possibly contributing to the more severe inflammatory symptoms in carriers of this allele [51].

HLA-B27 is not the only allele predisposing to spondyloarthropathies and ReA. In Mexican populations, one study found an association of HLA-DR1 and HLA-B15, independent of HLA-B27. HLA-B27 was associated with younger age of onset and increased severity of disease, and HLA-DR1 with older age of onset [52].

The HLA-B27 allele does not predispose the patient to infection or ReA, but it increases the risk of severe and prolonged ReA. Patients with this allele have a diminished ability to eliminate the infected bacterium, and may have increased intracellular survival of pathogens [53].

Laboratory studies

Although many nonspecific tests can corroborate the presence of inflammation, no single test or panel of tests allow a clinician to diagnose ReA. This caveat is especially directed at the indiscriminate use of the HLA-B27 test. The high frequency of this allele in the white population guarantees a high rate of false-positivity. Because only 20% of HLA-B27 positive individuals will ever develop a seronegative spondyloarthropathy, HLA-B27 has little diagnostic value, although it may have prognostic value.

Although the ACR and International Workshop criteria may be used as a guide, there are currently no uniformly accepted diagnostic or classification criteria for ReA. These criteria are based on physical findings and negative laboratory studies for other conditions. No laboratory studies assist the specific diagnosis of ReA. Mild normocytic anemia and leukocytosis are common. Nonspecific serum markers of inflammation, such as the erythrocyte sedimentation rate (ESR) and C-reactive protein, are elevated in association with the acute-phase response.

Stool cultures and urethral swabs should be performed to identify causative organisms, although they are rarely positive. It is not necessary to order HLA-B27, because it has no diagnostic or therapeutic value. HLA-B27, however, may predict a more prolonged course. The diagnostic work-up of a patient thought to have ReA should include the following:

Blood
    Complete blood count
    Erythrocyte sedimentation rate and C-reactive protein (inflammatory markers)
    Uric acid (crystal disease)
    Rheumatoid factor (if suspect rheumatoid arthritis)
Culture
    Urethral swab for chlamydia
    Stool culture
Synovial fluid
    Gram stain and culture (rule out infectious etiology)
    Crystal analysis

In patients with ReA severe enough to result in hospital admission, there is usually laboratory evidence of an acute-phase response, with an ESR >100, an elevated C-reactive protein, and neutrophilia. Other investigations are generally not helpful. Antinuclear antibodies and rheumatoid factor are generally absent. Antineutrophil cytoplasmic antibodies have been positive in some studies, but have no established diagnostic value [54].

Microscopic evaluation of the synovial fluid, and culture and gram stain, should be obtained to exclude infection and crystal-induced arthritis to avoid severe joint damage and possible systemic sepsis. In ReA, synovial fluid cultures are negative.

Eberl and coworkers [55] developed a composite score for measuring ReA activity. They found that swollen and tender joints, C-reactive protein, pain assessment by the patient, and global assessment by the physician were useful in grading the severity of disease and response to treatment.

Radiographic investigations

Early in ReA, plain radiographs are normal or may show soft tissue swelling and joint effusions. Evaluation with more sensitive techniques, such as MRI or CT, may show bony erosions and sclerosis, which progresses with time [56]. Late radiographic changes include new asymmetric bone proliferation at sites of inflammation. Linear periostitis may be observed along the metacarpophalangeal (MCP), metatarsophalangeal (MTP), and phalangeal shafts. The regions of insertion of tendons may show areas of calcification caused by enthesopathy. MRI or ultrasound can be used for the evaluation of enthesitis. Ultrasound can also assess for plantar fasciitis. The spine, particularly in the lower thoracic and upper lumbar regions, may show comma-shaped ossification on radiograph. The hallmark of ReA patients is asymmetric sacroiliitis, found in 70%.

Outcomes

Approximately 75% of patients with ReA have musculoskeletal symptoms persisting for more than 1 year, and up to 30% of those patients had symptoms after 6 years. The duration of joint symptoms is shorter, usually 3 to 5 months, with 15% of patients developing chronic symptoms. In some studies, 20% to 40% of patients have chronic indolent arthritis after 1 year, and 5% of those patients continue to have symptoms at 2 years.

Recurrent attacks are more common in patients with *Chlamydia* ReA and patients with the HLA-B27 allele. Patients with the full triad of symptoms usually have a longer duration of symptoms and more recurrences [12]. Enthesopathy and skin lesions may persist after joint symptoms resolve. Disease activity and arthritis are linked to increased type I collagen degradation [57], a possible future marker for disease activity of ReA.

Prognostic factors

Specific symptoms, genetics, and bacterial exposures predict poor outcome in ReA [24]. Hip arthritis and high ESR are associated with a more chronic course [58]. The prognosis of ReA is also affected by the inciting bacterium, the presence of HLA-B27, the gender of the patient, and the presence of recurrent symptoms [2]. Chronic intestinal inflammation and ReA induced by *Shigella, Salmonella*, and *Chlamydia* are associated with greater chronicity. In Finland, patients hospitalized with post-*Salmonella* arthritis had a high incidence of chronic disease, with HLA-B27 positivity predicting severity and chronicity [59]. Chronic symptoms persisted in most patients in a large cohort of patients with post-*Salmonella* ReA. Joint damage and radiographic evidence of enthesitis and sacroiliitis correlate with functional disability [60].

In one cohort study, 122 ReA patients were followed for a mean of 5.6 years. Eighty-three percent had some disease activity, 34% had chronic symptoms, and 11% were disabled from employment. Of all patients, 83% were HLA-B27; sacroiliitis and chronic uveitis were more common in the HLA-B27–positive group. Heel disease at baseline was the only poor prognostic predictor in this study [61]. In one study, male gender also influenced the disease course. Men were more likely to have a higher ESR,

HLA-B27 positivity, complete triad of symptoms, and longer duration of illness, compared with women [62].

Treatment

Treatment of ReA can be subdivided into treatment of acute joint inflammation, treatment of the triggering infection, and treatment of chronic arthritis. Therapeutic management of ReA includes the following:

Education
Physical therapy
Occupational therapy
Acute medication
 NSAIDs to relieve pain and inflammation
 Antibiotics (controversial), use if infection present
 Intra-articular steroid injection
Chronic medication
 Disease-modifying antirheumatic drugs
 Molecular biologic agent (eg, tumor necrosis factor–blocker)

Initial treatment focuses on pain management, primarily the use of anti-inflammatory medication. NSAIDs are usually used in high doses for short periods of time, and tapered to low daily doses for chronic pain. Medication should be given to treat pain adequately and adjusted for individual cases. For monoarticular or oligoarticular disease, intra-articular steroids can be used. Neither treatment with NSAIDs nor corticosteroids shortens the course or lessens the extent of disease. Physical therapy is also recommended.

Antibiotics

Because ReA is associated with prior bacterial exposure, many studies have examined the use of antibiotics either early or late in the disease course (Table 3). The overall evidence for antibiotic efficacy is conflicting, and not terribly encouraging. To create further confusion, it should be noted tetracycline antibiotics inhibit matrix metalloproteinases. They have anti-inflammatory effects independent of their antibiotic activity. Long-term tetracycline was associated with decreased duration and severity of symptoms in one study [2]. A double-blind study of chronic ReA patients given 3 months of ciprofloxacin showed that at 6-month follow-up, there was a decrease in clinical symptoms of arthralgia and morning stiffness [63]. In a double-blinded, placebo-controlled trial of ciprofloxacin given for 3 months to acute ReA patients, decreased symptoms were noted 4 to 7 years later in comparison with the placebo group, suggesting acute treatment may improve long-term prognosis [64]. In patients with *Yersinia*-triggered ReA, ciprofloxacin for 3 months was compared with placebo. Treated patients achieved faster remission and pain relief [65].

Table 3
Summary of clinical trials in reactive arthritis

Antibiotic	Bacteria	Duration	Result	Reference
Doxycylcline versus placebo	Chlamydia-induced ReA	3 mo	No improvement of pain or functional status	71
Doxycycline versus Doxy/Rifampin		9 mo	Combination showed decrease in morning stiffness	66
Ciprofloxacin versus placebo		3 mo	Acute treatment may be beneficial 4–7 y later	62
Ciprofloxacin		6 mo	Decrease in arthralgia and morning stiffness	61
Ciprofloxacin versus placebo	Yersinia ReA	3 mo	Faster remission and relief of pain with antibiotic	63
Sulfasalazine versus placebo		36 wk	Improvement in ESR and pain	69
Sulfasalazine versus placebo		6 mo	Improve only short-term outcome	72
Lymecylcline	Chlamydia-induced arthritis	3 mo	No change in the natural course of disease	67
Azithromycin		3 mo	Prolonged treatment is ineffective	65
Infliximab	Yersinia ReA		Inconclusive	70

Abbreviations: ESR, erythrocyte sedimentation rate; ReA, reactive arthritis.

A small double-blind randomized placebo-controlled trial of ciprofloxacin in the treatment of ReA and anterior uveitis found no difference between groups in terms of relapse time, joint inflammation, or enthesitis, and symptoms of anterior uveitis [66]. There are no large trials of ciprofloxacin that show any significant differences compared with placebo for the treatment of ReA symptoms.

A recent trial with azithromycin in ReA failed to produce any effect on duration and severity of symptoms. Weekly azithromycin given for 24 weeks failed to show changes in the outcome of the disease [67]. A study of doxycycline, compared with doxycycline and rifampin, for 9 months in a randomized controlled trial showed that combination therapy was effective in decreasing morning stiffness and Visual Analog Scale patient assessment of joint pain and stiffness [68]. A small double-blind controlled study of a 3-month course of lymecycline on long-term prognosis of ReA showed a decreased duration of arthritis in the subset of patients with C trachomatis–triggered ReA, but not ReA from other causes. Overall, lymecycline treatment did not alter the natural history of ReA [69,70]. This putative short-term benefit of antibiotics for the treatment of chlamydia-triggered ReA was not observed in another randomized, controlled trial [71]. Early antibiotic treatment of chlamydial urethritis may prevent the later development of ReA [72].

Present evidence does not support the use of long-term antibiotics to treat ReA caused by enteric organisms [73]. Definitive evidence of benefit of short- or long-term antibiotic therapy in chlamydial ReA is also lacking [67,71]. Patients with ReA and their sexual partners, however, should receive antibiotic therapy adequate to cure genital *Chlamydia* infection.

Disease-modifying antirheumatic drugs

For more severe and prolonged disease course (symptoms lasting longer than 3 months), disease-modifying antirheumatic drug therapy has been used. Sulfasalazine has been shown to be effective in some cases, specifically for peripheral joint involvement. In controlled trials, it produced improvement in the intensity and duration of symptoms compared with placebo, but only in the short term, and with a significant risk of adverse events, primarily gastrointestinal [74]. Clegg and coworkers [75] compared the effects on spondyloarthropathy of sulfasalazine, 2 g/d, versus placebo over a 36-week period. Although the axial disease did not respond, peripheral articular disease showed a statistically significant improvement. Methotrexate and azathioprine have also been used, and in placebo trials show a shortened duration of symptoms. Disease-modifying antirheumatic drug therapy, because of side effects and variable efficacy, should only be considered in those patients with chronic inflammation that is not responsive to anti-inflammatory medication.

Molecular biologic therapies

The effect of molecular biologic therapy, such as tumor necrosis factor-blockers, on ReA has only been examined in small studies. Two patients with ReA caused by *Yersinia* were given infliximab, one of the patients having acute ReA. The acute inflammation of ReA responded well to the initial infusion, but during the study the patient required alternate disease-modifying antirheumatic treatment for his symptoms [76]. The influence of biologics in treatment of ReA still remains to be evaluated. NSAIDs and physiotherapy are the mainstay of treatment, and only in severe cases are disease-modifying antirheumatics and molecular biologic therapy initiated.

Summary

ReA consists of sterile axial or peripheral articular inflammation, enthesitis, and extra-articular manifestations. Most patients are HLA-B27 positive, although determining the B27 status of an individual patient is irrelevant. Exposure to specific bacterial antigens is usually the inciting factor. Diagnosis usually can be made by clinical examination and history. The current standard therapy is NSAIDs and physiotherapy, but molecular biologic treatment may ultimately become the mainstay in recalcitrant and severe ReA.

References

[1] Miceli-Richard C, van der Heijde D, Dougados M. Spondyloarthropathy for practicing rheumatologists: diagnosis, indication for disease controlling antirheumatic therapy, and evaluation of the response. Rheum Dis Clin North Am 2003;29:449–62.

[2] Kingsley G, Sieper J. Third International Workshop on Reactive Arthritis. 23–26 September 1995, Berlin, Germany. Ann Rheum Dis 1996;55:564–84.

[3] Weinberger HW, Ropes MW, Kulka JP, et al. Reiter's syndrome, clinical and pathologic observations: a long term study of 16 cases. Medicine (Baltimore) 1962;41:35–91.

[4] Taurog JD. The role of bacteria in HLA-B27-associated reactive arthritis. Cliniguide Rheum 1995;5:1–8.

[5] Keat A. Reiter's syndrome and reactive arthritis in perspective. N Engl J Med 1983;309: 1606–15.

[6] Brodie BC. Pathologic and surgical observations of disease of joints. London: Longman; 1818.

[7] Panush RS, Paraschiv D, Dorff RE. The tainted legacy of Hans Reiter. Semin Arthritis Rheum 2003;32:231–6.

[8] Braun J, Bollow M, Remlinger G, et al. Prevalence of spondylarthropathies in HLA-B27 positive and negative blood donors. Arthritis Rheum 2004;41:58–61.

[9] Paronen J. Reiter's disease: a study of 344 cases observed in Finland [doctoral thesis]. Acta Med Scand 1948;S212:1–112.

[10] Soderlin MK, Borjesson O, Kautiainen H, et al. Annual incidence of inflammatory joint diseases in a population based study in southern Sweden. Ann Rheum Dis 2002; 61:911–5.

[11] Kvien TK, Glennas A, Melby K, et al. Reactive arthritis: incidence, triggering agents and clinical presentation. J Rheumatol 1994;21:115–22.

[12] Colmegna I, Cuchacovich R, Espinoza LR. HLA-B27-associated reactive arthritis: pathogenetic and clinical considerations. Clin Microbiol Rev 2004;17:348–69.

[13] Hannu T, Mattila L, Rautelin H, et al. *Campylobacter*-triggered reactive arthritis: a population-based study. Rheumatology (Oxford) 2002;41:312–8.

[14] Khan MA. Update on spondyloarthropathies. Ann Intern Med 2002;136:896–907.

[15] Bas S, Scieux C, Vischer TL. Male sexual predominance in *Chlamydia trachomatis* sexually acquired reactive arthritis: are women more protected by anti-chlamydia antibodies? Ann Rheum Dis 2001;60:605–11.

[16] Yu DTY, Fan PT. Spondyloarthropathy and reactive arthritis. In: Harris ED Jr, Budd RC, Firestein GS, et al, editors. Kelley's textbook of rheumatology. 7th edition. Philadelphia: Elsevier; 2005. p. 1142–54.

[17] Khan MA, Sieper J. Reactive arthritis. In: Koopman WJ, Moreland LW, editors. Arthritis and allied conditions: a textbook of rheumatology. 15th edition. Philadelphia: Lippincott Williams & Wilkins; 2005. p. 1336–55.

[18] Hill Gaston JS, Lillicrap MS. Arthritis and enteric infection. Best Pract Res Clin Rheumatol 2003;17:219–39.

[19] Sholkofff SD, Glickman MG, Steinbach HL. The radiographic pattern of polyarthritis in Reiter's syndrome. Arthritis Rheum 1971;14:551–5.

[20] Monnet D, Breban M, Hudry C, et al. Ophthalmic findings and frequency of extraocular manifestations in patients with HLA-B27 uveitis: a study of 175 cases. Ophthalmology 2004; 111:802–9.

[21] Hoogland YT, Alexander EP, Patterson RH, et al. Coronary artery stenosis in Reiter's syndrome: a complication of aortitis. J Rheumatol 1994;21:757–9.

[22] Hannu T, Nieminen MS, Swan H, et al. Cardiac findings of reactive arthritis: an observational echocardiographic study. Rheumatol Int 2002;21:169–72.

[23] Bergfeldt L. HLA-B27-associated cardiac disease. Ann Intern Med 1997;127(8 Pt 1):621–9.

[24] Arnett FC. Seronegative spondylarthropathies. Bull Rheum Dis 1987;37:1–12.

[25] Fendler C, Laitko S, Sorensen H, et al. Frequency of triggering bacteria in patients with reactive arthritis and undifferentiated oligoarthritis and the relative importance of the tests used for diagnosis. Ann Rheum Dis 2001;60:337–43.

[26] Maki-Ikola O, Granfors K. *Salmonella*-triggered reactive arthritis. Lancet 1992;339:1096–7.

[27] Hannu T, Mattila L, Siitonen A, et al. Reactive arthritis following an outbreak of *Salmonella typhimurium* phage type 193 infection. Ann Rheum Dis 2002;61:264–6.

[28] Dworkin MS, Shoemaker PC, Goldoft MJ, et al. Reactive arthritis and Reiter's syndrome following an outbreak of gastroenteritis caused by *Salmonella enteritidis*. Clin Infect Dis 2001;33:1010–4.

[29] Locht H, Molbak K, Krogfelt KA. High frequency of reactive joint symptoms after an outbreak of *Salmonella enteritidis*. J Rheumatol 2002;29:767–71.

[30] van der Heijden IM, Res PC, Wilbrink B, et al. *Yersinia enterocolitica*: a cause of chronic polyarthritis. Clin Infect Dis 1997;25:831–7.

[31] Hannu T, Mattila L, Nuorti JP, et al. Reactive arthritis after an outbreak of *Yersinia pseudotuberculosis* serotype O:3 infection. Ann Rheum Dis 2003;62:866–9.

[32] Leirisalo M, Repo H, Tiilikainen A, et al. Chemotaxis in yersinia arthritis: HLA-B27 positive neutrophils show high stimulated motility in vitro. Arthritis Rheum 1980;23: 1036–44.

[33] Blaser MJ, Reller LB. *Campylobacter* enteritis. N Engl J Med 1981;305:1444–52.

[34] Hannu T, Kauppi M, Tuomala M, et al. Reactive arthritis following an outbreak of *Campylobacter jejuni* infection. J Rheumatol 2004;31:528–30.

[35] Hannu T, Mattila L, Rautelin H, et al. *Campylobacter*-triggered reactive arthritis: a population based study. Rheumatology (Oxford) 2004;41:312–8.

[36] Hannu T, Mattila L, Siitonen A, et al. Reactive arthritis attributable to *Shigella* infection: a clinical and epidemiological nationwide study. Ann Rheum Dis 2005;64:594–8.

[37] Finch M, Rodey G, Lawrence D, et al. Epidemic Reiter's syndrome following an outbreak of shigellosis. Eur J Epidemiol 1986;2:26–30.

[38] Keat AC, Maini RN, Nkwazi GC, et al. Role of *Chlamydia trachomatis* and HLA-B27 in sexually acquired reactive arthritis. BMJ 1978;1:605–7.

[39] Inman RD, Chiu B. Synoviocyte-packaged *Chlamydia trachomatis* induces a chronic aseptic arthritis. J Clin Invest 1998;102:1776–82.

[40] Atkinson MH, McLeod BD. Reactive arthritis associated with *Clostridium difficile* enteritis. J Rheumatol 1988;15:520–2.

[41] Pappas G, Akritidis N, Christou L, et al. Unusual causes of reactive arthritis: *Leptospira* and *Coxiella burnetii*. Clin Rheumatol 2003;22:343–6.

[42] Weyand CM, Goronzy JJ. Immune responses to *Borrelia burgdorferi* in patients with reactive arthritis. Arthritis Rheum 1989;32:1057–64.

[43] Cuchacovich R, Japa S, Huang WQ, et al. Detection of bacterial DNA in Latin American patients with reactive arthritis by polymerase chain reaction and sequencing analysis. J Rheumatol 2002;29:1426–9.

[44] Keat A, Thomas B, Dixey J, et al. *Chlamydia trachomatis* and reactive arthritis: the missing link. Lancet 1987;1:72–4.

[45] Granfors K, Jalkanen S, von Essen R, et al. *Yersinia* antigens in synovial-fluid cells from patients with reactive arthritis. N Engl J Med 1989;320:216–21.

[46] Granfors K, Jalkanen S, Lindberg AA, et al. *Salmonella* lipopolysaccharide in synovial cells from patients with reactive arthritis. Lancet 1990;335:685–8.

[47] Yu D, Kuipers J. Role of bacteria and HLA-B27 in the pathogenesis of reactive arthritis. Rheum Dis Clin North Am 2003;29:21–36.

[48] Mear JP, Schreiber KL, Munz C, et al. Misfolding of HLA-B27 as a result of its B pocket suggests a novel mechanism for its role in susceptibility to spondyloarthropathies. J Immunol 1999;163:6665–70.

[49] Ringrose JH, Muijsers AO, Pannekoek Y, et al. Influence of infection of cells with bacteria associated with reactive arthritis on the peptide repertoire presented by HLA-B27. J Med Microbiol 2001;50:385–9.

[50] Bas S, Muzzin P, Fulpius T, et al. Indirect evidence of intra-articular immunoglobulin G synthesis in patients with *Chlamydia trachomatis* reactive arthritis. Rheumatology (Oxford) 2001;40:801–5.

[51] Leirisalo M, Repo H, Tiilikainen A, et al. Chemotaxis in *Yersinia* arthritis: HLA-B27 positive neutrophils show high stimulated motility in vitro. Arthritis Rheum 1980;23:1036–44.

[52] Vargas-Alarcon G, Londono JD, Hernandez-Pacheco G, et al. Effect of HLA-B and HLA-DR genes on susceptibility to and severity of spondyloarthropathies in Mexican patients. Ann Rheum Dis 2002;61:714–7.

[53] Sigal LH. Update on reactive arthritis. Bull Rheum Dis 2001;50:1–4.

[54] Locht H, Skogh T, Kihlstrom E. Anti-lactoferrin antibodies and other types of anti-neutrophil cytoplasmic antibodies (ANCA) in reactive arthritis and ankylosing spondylitis. Clin Exp Immunol 1999;117:568–73.

[55] Eberl G, Studnicka-Benke A, Hitzelhammer H, et al. Development of a disease activity index for the assessment of reactive arthritis (DAREA). Rheumatology (Oxford) 2000;39:148–55.

[56] Ford DK. Reactive arthritis: a viewpoint rather than a review. Clin Rheum Dis 1986;12:389–401.

[57] Kotaniemi A, Risteli J, Aho K, et al. Increased type I collagen degradation correlates with disease activity in reactive arthritis. Clin Exp Rheumatol 2003;21:95–8.

[58] Amor B, Santos RS, Nahal R. Predictive factors for the long-term outcome of spondyloarthropathies. J Rheumatol 1994;21:1883–7.

[59] Leirisalo-Repo M, Helenius P, Hannu T, et al. Long term prognosis of reactive salmonella arthritis. Ann Rheum Dis 1997;56:516–20.

[60] Thomson GT, DeRubeis DA, Hodge MA, et al. Post-*Salmonella* reactive arthritis: late clinical sequelae in a point source cohort. Am J Med 1995;98:13–21.

[61] Fox R, Calin A, Gerber RC, et al. The chronicity of symptoms and disability in Reiter's syndrome: an analysis of 131 consecutive patients. Ann Intern Med 1979;91:190–3.

[62] Yli-Kerttula UI. Clinical characteristics in male and female uro-arthritis or Reiter's syndrome. Clin Rheumatol 1984;3:351–60.

[63] Toivanen A, Yli-Kerttula T, Luukkainen R, et al. Effect of antimicrobial treatment on chronic reactive arthritis. Clin Exp Rheumatol 1993;11:301–7.

[64] Yli-Kerttula T, Luukkainen R, Yli-Kerttula U, et al. Effect of a three month course of ciprofloxacin on the late prognosis of reactive arthritis. Ann Rheum Dis 2003;62:880–4.

[65] Hoogkamp-Korstanje JA, Moesker H, Bruyn GA. Ciprofloxacin v placebo for treatment of *Yersinia enterocolitica* triggered reactive arthritis. Ann Rheum Dis 2000;59:914–7.

[66] Wakefield D, McCluskey P, Verma M, et al. Ciprofloxacin treatment does not influence course or relapse rate of ReA arthritis and anterior uveitis. Arthritis Rheum 1999;42:1894–7.

[67] Kvien TK, Gaston JS, Bardin T, et al. Three month treatment of reactive arthritis with azithromycin: a EULAR double blind, placebo controlled study. Ann Rheum Dis 2004;63:1113–9.

[68] Carter JD, Valeriano J, Vasey FB. Doxycycline versus doxycycline and rifampin in undifferentiated spondyloarthropathy, with special reference to chlamydia-induced arthritis: a prospective, randomized 9-month comparison. J Rheumatol 2004;31:1973–80.

[69] Lauhio A, Leirisalo-Repo M, Lähdevirta J, et al. Double-blind, placebo-controlled study of three-month treatment with lymecycline in reactive arthritis, with special reference to chlamydia arthritis. Arthritis Rheum 1991;34:6–14.

[70] Laasila K, Laasonen L, Leirisalo-Repo M. Antibiotic treatment and long term prognosis of reactive arthritis. Ann Rheum Dis 2003;62:655–8.

[71] Smieja M, MacPherson DW, Kean W, et al. Randomised, blinded, placebo controlled trial of doxycycline for chronic seronegative arthritis. Ann Rheum Dis 2001;60:1088–94.

[72] Bardin T, Enel C, Cornelis F, et al. Antibiotic treatment of venereal disease and Reiter's syndrome in a Greenland population. Arthritis Rheum 1992;35:190–4.

[73] Leirisalo-Repo M. Are antibiotics of any use in reactive arthritis? APMIS 1993;101:575–81.

[74] Egsmose C, Hansen TM, Andersen LS, et al. Limited effect of sulphasalazine treatment in reactive arthritis: a randomized double blind placebo controlled trial. Ann Rheum Dis 1997; 56:32–6.

[75] Clegg DO, Reda DJ, Abdellatif M. Comparison of sulfasalazine and placebo for the treatment of axial and peripheral articular manifestations of the seronegative spondylarthropathies: a Department of Veterans Affairs cooperative study. Arthritis Rheum 1999;42: 2325–9.

[76] Oili KS, Niinisalo H, Korpilahde T, et al. Treatment of reactive arthritis with infliximab. Scand J Rheumatol 2003;32:122–4.

ELSEVIER
SAUNDERS

INFECTIOUS
DISEASE CLINICS
OF NORTH AMERICA

Infect Dis Clin N Am 19 (2005) 885–914

Prosthetic Joint Infections

Irene G. Sia, MD[a,*], Elie F. Berbari, MD[a],
Adolf W. Karchmer, MD[b]

[a]*Division of Infectious Diseases, Mayo Clinic College of Medicine,
200 First Street, SW, Rochester, MN 55905, USA*
[b]*Department of Medicine, Division of Infectious Diseases, Beth Israel Deaconess
Medical Center, 330 Brookline Avenue, Boston, MA 02215, USA*

Infections associated with prosthetic joint implantations occur in only a small proportion of joint recipients. Prosthetic joint infection is a dreaded complication, however, resulting in pain, reoperation, potential loss of the prosthesis, and in some instances loss of limb or life. Additionally, prosthetic joint infection is an economic burden; the estimated cost of treating an infected prosthetic joint is $50,000 to $60,000 [1]. In general, the risk for infection is higher for knee arthroplasty (1%–2%) than hip (0.3%–1.3%) or shoulder (less than 1%) arthroplasty [2–4]. The infection rate is even higher after revision procedures (3% for hips and 6% for knees). The risk of prosthesis infection after joint replacement is also higher in patients with rheumatoid arthritis (2.2%) compared with those with osteoarthritis (1.2%) [5].

Clinical presentation

The clinical presentation of patients with infection involving a prosthetic joint is highly variable. Prosthesis infection may occur early as a complication of an overt wound infection. Here the challenge is to determine if the wound infection extends to the prosthesis. Alternatively, infection can be indolent and present months after surgery with pain as the primary symptom. Differentiating a painful prosthesis secondary to mechanical loosening from that resulting from occult infection remains difficult, and the consequences of misdiagnosis may be considerable. Finally, stable functioning prosthetic joints are occasionally infected hematogenously from infection at a remote site. These infections frequently present as acute septic arthritis.

---

* Corresponding author.
E-mail address: sia.irene@mayo.edu (I.G. Sia).

The history and physical examination of patients with a suspected prosthesis infection may be unrevealing. Nonetheless, careful attention to the history of perioperative events may establish conditions and events that are associated with an increased risk for infection. Well-established risk factors include postoperative surgical site infection or hematoma formation, wound healing complications, a high National Nosocomial Infections Surveillance System surgical risk score, presence of malignant disease, a prior joint arthroplasty with a large prosthesis, prior surgery or infection of the joint or adjacent bone, perioperative nonarticular infection, and rheumatoid arthritis [6,7]. Less well documented risk factors are diabetes mellitus, steroid use, obesity, extreme age, poor nutrition, psoriasis, hemophilia, sickle cell hemoglobinopathy, and prolonged preoperative hospitalization.

A consistent symptom of prosthetic joint infection is pain at the implant site, occurring in over 90% of cases. During the initial postoperative month, infection typically manifests with acute onset of joint pain and effusion or wound complications. The wound may be swollen, erythematous, warm and tender, with purulent drainage; associated systemic symptoms may vary. A sinus tract that extends to the joint is a definitive sign of prosthesis infection, but such is not always present. Early, more aggressive infection, although not common, is frequently caused by virulent microorganisms, such as *Staphylococcus aureus*, β-hemolytic streptococci, and aerobic gram-negative bacteria.

Chronic low-grade infection usually occurring several months to 2 years after prosthesis implantation is encountered more commonly. This presents with subtle signs and symptoms, if any, of infection, but rather with chronic pain and implant loosening. This type of infection is often caused by less virulent microorganisms, such as coagulase-negative staphylococci and *Propionibacterium acnes*. It is difficult to differentiate delayed indolent infection involving the implanted device from mechanical aseptic loosening of the total joint replacement. Typically, pain associated with chronic infection worsens with time and is accompanied by deterioration in function.

Patients with sudden onset of pain late after implantation may have hematogenous seeding of the prosthesis. The most frequent sources are skin, dental, respiratory tract, and urinary tract infections [8–10]. The first 2 years after joint replacement is the most critical period for hematogenous seeding [11]. Patients with rheumatoid arthritis seem to be at risk for late hematogenous *S aureus* implant infection [12]. *S aureus* bacteremia in patients with stable prostheses is associated with a 34% rate of implant infection [13].

Diagnosis

The diagnosis of prosthetic joint infection is obvious when it occurs in conjunction with a wound infection and sinus track extending to the joint, and is similar to septic arthritis when it results from hematogenous seeding. Diagnosis can be challenging when the onset of infection is delayed. The importance of accurate preoperative differentiation of aseptic mechanical loosening from infection of a joint arthroplasty cannot be overemphasized. Treatment of these two entities is radically different. Clinical examination, laboratory studies, plain radiographs, nuclear scans, and the cytologic features of aspirated synovial fluid cannot be relied on to demonstrate accurately the presence of infection. Making the correct diagnosis requires the synthesis of information from multiple investigations. Ultimately, only the identification of the causative microorganism from aspirated synovial fluid or periprosthetic tissue, or a biopsy confirming the presence of acute inflammatory cells, establishes the diagnosis of prosthetic joint infection.

Laboratory studies -

White blood cell count, erythrocyte sedimentation rate, and C-reactive protein are the most commonly used screening tools for the diagnosis of prosthetic joint infections. These tests, however, do not reliably predict the presence or absence of infection [14–17]. The white blood cell count rarely aids in the diagnosis of indolent-presenting joint prosthesis infection; the lack of a systemic inflammatory response accounts for a normal white blood cell count in most patients. Both erythrocyte sedimentation rate and C-reactive protein are nonspecific markers of acute inflammation. Both may be elevated in association with inflammatory conditions, some of which, such as rheumatoid arthritis, may have been the disease process that resulted in joint replacement. These tests are often used to exclude infection; the combination of a normal erythrocyte sedimentation rate and C-reactive protein has been shown to be a reliable indicator for the absence of infection [16]. Patients with chronic low-grade infection on suppressive antibiotics, however, may have false-negative results. Compared with erythrocyte sedimentation rate, C-reactive protein is more sensitive and specific for prosthetic joint infection [18].

Preoperative joint aspiration for the diagnosis of joint prosthesis infection is usually done as a corollary to other preoperative investigations [19,20]. Aspirations of the hip joint should be done under fluoroscopic or ultrasonographic guidance to confirm the position of the needle. Joint fluid should be sent for cell count, Gram's stain, and culture. Interpretive criteria of cell count and differential in synovial fluid for the diagnosis of implant infection are not well defined. The results of a prospective study in patients undergoing revision surgery for aseptic failure of total knee arthroplasty (TKA) showed that synovial fluid white blood cell count and percentage polymorphonuclear leukocytes are similar to those reported for unimplanted joints with similar primary diagnoses [21]. That is, in patients with orthopedic implants for osteoarthritis, synovial fluid white blood cell count less than 2×10^9 per liter and a differential with less 50% neutrophils have a 98% predictive value for the absence of infection. A larger prospective study of patients undergoing revision hip arthroplasty demonstrated that the presence of more than 50×10^9 white blood cell per liter and more than 80% neutrophils had positive predictive values of 91% and 52%, respectively, for infection [16].

A more recent study describing the preoperative synovial fluid analysis of patients with failed TKAs showed that synovial fluid leukocyte count and neutrophil percentage were significantly higher in those with infected arthroplasties than those with aseptic failure [22]. In patients without underlying inflammatory joint diseases, synovial fluid white blood cell count of more than 1.7×10^9 per liter and greater than 65% neutrophils had sensitivities of 94% and 97%, and specificities of 88% and 98%, respectively, for infection. Using these cutoff values for diagnosing an infected prosthetic joint, the synovial fluid white blood cell count is, in sensitivity and specificity, comparable with culture and histopathology of intraoperative tissue.

Synovial fluid analysis must be accompanied by synovial fluid culture to identify the causative microorganism and to guide appropriate drug selection for patients with systemic infection requiring antimicrobial therapy before surgery, for antimicrobial impregnation into cement, and in the choice of suppressive treatment if the patient is not a candidate for surgical revision.

Radiologic studies

Various imaging studies have been used for the detection of prosthetic implant infections. Plain radiographs may show prosthetic loosening or dislocation, lucency at the bone-cement interface, bony erosion, or subperiosteal bone growth [23], although these findings are neither sensitive nor specific (Fig. 1). Serial studies performed over time may be of greater use [24]. Demonstrating sinus tracts extending to the bone or device by arthrography is specific for infection [25].

Radionuclide imaging is the current imaging modality of choice for evaluation of suspected joint prosthesis infection; it is not hindered by the presence of metallic hardware [26]. Nuclear scintigraphy detects inflammation in the periprosthetic tissue; it is widely available and easily performed (Fig. 2). Bone scintigraphy with technetium-99m–labeled methylene diphosphonate (^{99m}Tc-MDP) is highly sensitive but lacks specificity for infection [27]. Tracer uptake is dependent on blood flow and rate of new bone formation; consequently, any process causing accelerated new bone formation may result in positive bone images. In addition to infection, fracture, previous surgery, arthritis, and heterotopic bone formation may be abnormal on scintigram. Because of increased periprosthetic bone remodeling, technetium bone scan can remain positive for more than a year after implantation or after infection, especially around knee prosthesis [28,29]. Nonetheless, bone imaging is useful because a normal result is strong

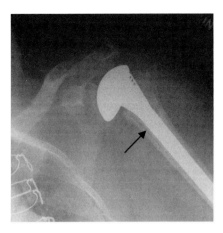

Fig. 1. Bone-cement interface lucency 2 years after humeral endoprosthesis, suggestive of infection.

evidence for the absence of prosthetic joint infection [30]. The overall accuracy of radionuclide bone imaging in the evaluation of infection in prosthetic joints is around 50% to 70% [31].

Sequential bone and gallium scanning is performed to increase the specificity of bone scintigraphy. The uptake of ^{67}gallium-citrate (^{67}Ga) is contingent on inflammation and not specific for infection. Infection is present when the distributions of the two tracers in sequential bone-gallium images are spatially incongruent, or when their distributions are spatially congruent and the intensity of gallium uptake exceeds that of the bone agent [31]. This approach has an overall accuracy of 70% to 80% in determining an infected prosthesis [30].

Labeled leukocyte imaging is most useful in detecting neutrophil-mediated inflammatory processes [31]. Leukocytes are labeled with ^{111}indium-oxyquinoline (^{111}In) or ^{99m}Tc-hexamethylpropyleneamine oxime (^{99m}Tc-HMPAO). Labeled leukocytes accumulate in areas where neutrophils congregate, which differentiates an infected prosthesis from an aseptically loosened prosthesis. Increased periprosthetic activity compared with adjacent bone activity is generally interpreted as indicating infection. Labeled leukocytes also accumulate in bone marrow, however, making it difficult to distinguish leukocyte-uptake in infection from uptake in aberrantly located normal marrow [31]. The addition of complementary bone marrow imaging with ^{99m}Tc sulfur colloid provides greater than 95% accuracy in determining prosthetic joint infections [32,33]. Both labeled leukocytes and sulfur colloid accumulate in the bone marrow, but only labeled leukocytes accumulate in infection; infection results in activity on labeled leukocyte images without corresponding activity on sulfur colloid [31]. There are, however, significant limitations with the combined leukocyte-marrow scintigraphy. The process is labor-intensive, time-consuming, costly, not always available, and

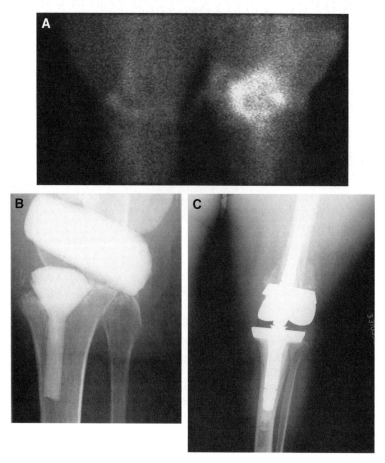

Fig. 2. (*A*) Nuclear bone scan showing intense uptake around the left knee. (*B*) The knee is now resected and an antimicrobial spacer is in place. (*C*) Knee is reimplanted with long tibia and femoral components.

requires contact with blood products. Several methods of labeling leukocytes in vivo using peptides and antigranulocyte antibodies or antibody fragments are currently being investigated [26].

The utility of F-18 fluorodeoxyglucose positron emission tomography for detecting infections associated with hip and knee prostheses might become feasible in the near future [34]. Fluorodeoxyglucose uptake is dependent on glucose metabolism, which is increased in infection. This method is exceptionally sensitive, but it does not differentiate infection from inflammation associated with an aseptically loosened prosthesis and is less accurate than labeled leukocyte-marrow imaging [35]. A novel approach that is being investigated is the use of radiolabeled antibiotics [36,37]. ^{99m}Tc-ciprofloxacin is the prototype tracer being studied; increased tracer uptake is presumed to reflect the presence of microorganisms.

CT and MRI are not routinely useful for diagnosing infection in prosthetic joints because of hardware-induced imaging artifacts. Additionally, MRI can be performed only in patients with titanium or tantalum implants.

Radionuclide bone imaging is best used as a screening procedure for suspected infection in a joint prosthesis. Combined leukocyte-marrow imaging is currently the procedure of choice for the diagnosis of infected prosthesis [38]. A negative bone imaging study effectively rules out a prosthetic complication, whereas a positive test requires further investigation.

Microbiologic studies

Making a microbiologic diagnosis is crucial for optimal antimicrobial therapy of prosthetic joint infection. Identifying the specific etiologic microorganism and its antimicrobial susceptibility relies on adequate specimen collection and handling before initiation of therapy.

Positive cultures for the same microorganism from multiple specimens, which are obtained separately, either from preoperative joint aspiration or tissues obtained intraoperatively, provide the most useful diagnostic information. Preoperative joint aspiration is a reliable method for diagnosing infection [39]. In the absence of prior antimicrobial therapy, a positive culture from a preoperative joint aspiration has 55% to 86% sensitivity and 94% to 96% specificity for infection in hip and knee arthroplasties [16,19]. Although a positive Gram's stain of synovial fluid has high specificity, the test has extremely low sensitivity (12%–19%) [16,40].

Multiple intraoperative specimens should be obtained for culture immediately after the pseudocapsule is opened; these should include tissues from the joint capsule, synovial lining, curetted intramedullary material, bone-cement interface, bone fragments, and samples from purulent material or sequestrum that may be present. Here too, recovery of the same microorganism from multiple specimens is diagnostic for prosthetic joint infection. To increase detection of microorganisms, the implant or its components can be cultured in its entirety in enrichment broth; however, the risk of contamination during specimen processing is high [41]. A minimum of three intraoperative tissue specimens should be sent for culture [40]. Routine cultures for aerobic and anaerobic bacteria are recommended when infection in the joint prosthesis is suspected [42]. Intraoperative Gram's stains have not been found to be useful for prosthetic joint infection diagnosis [17,40,43]. False-negative results of culture may occur because of prior antimicrobial exposure including antimicrobial-impregnated bone cement, a low number of microorganisms, an inappropriate culture medium, infection with adherent or fastidious organisms, or prolonged transport time to the microbiology laboratory [44]. Preoperative antimicrobial therapy may cause false-negative culture results in more than 50% of cases [16]. To avoid false-negative results, antimicrobial therapy should be withheld for at least

1 month before any attempt at establishing a microbiologic diagnosis [45]. At the time of revision arthroplasty, if the index of suspicion for joint prosthesis infection is high, perioperative antimicrobial prophylaxis should be delayed until after culture specimens have been collected. When the suspected cause of infection includes unusual microorganisms, which are difficult to culture, such as small-colony variants of staphylococci, *Abiotrophia defectiva* or *Granulicatella adiacens* (formerly classified as nutritionally variant streptococci), fungi, and mycobacteria, special culture techniques may be necessary. False-positive results are frequently caused by contaminants, such as coagulase-negative staphylococci or *Corynebacterium* spp [40].

Definitive diagnosis of joint prosthesis infection is made by recovering the same microorganism from either repeated joint aspirations [19], or in three of five periprosthetic specimens obtained at surgery [40,46]. It is reported that when three or more specimens are submitted for culture, the finding of no positive culture denotes a 3.4% probability of infection; one positive culture has a probability of 13.3%, two positive cultures a probability of 20.4%, and three or more positive cultures a 94.8% probability [40].

The most common pathogens causing prosthetic joint infections are listed in Table 1. Gram-positive cocci account for most cases; *S aureus* and coagulase-negative staphylococci are the most commonly reported microorganisms in both early (within 2 years following surgery) and late (beyond 2 years) infections, in both total hip arthroplasty (THA) and TKA. Polymicrobial infection is reported in 12% to 19% of cases. Aerobic gram-negative bacilli and anaerobic bacteria are less frequently encountered. Microbiologic cause remains unknown in up to 11% of cases. Unusual pathogens, such as *Candida* spp, *Brucella* spp, and various mycobacteria, have been reported. Establishing a microbiologic diagnosis is imperative because the type of infecting organism often affects the approach to therapy [42].

Except when *S aureus* is isolated, cultures of superficial wounds or sinus tracts do not provide a reliable bacteriologic diagnosis of chronic

Table 1
Common pathogens in infected joint arthroplasty

Pathogens	% Frequency
Staphylococcus aureus	20–25
Coagulase-negative staphylococci	20–30
Polymicrobial	12–19
Gram-negative bacilli	6–11
Streptococci	8–10
Anaerobes	4–10
Enterococcus species	3
Other or unknown	2–11

Data from Steckelberg J, Osmon D. Prosthetic joint infections. In: Waldvogel F, Bisno A, editors. Infections associated with indwelling medical devices. 3rd edition. Washington: American Society for Microbiology Press; 2000. p. 173–209; and Widmer AF. New developments in diagnosis and treatment of infection in orthopedic implants. Clin Infect Dis 2001;33:1.

osteomyelitis, because of bacterial colonization of the surrounding skin [47]. Results of sinus or wound cultures in prosthetic joint infection may not reflect the bacteriology in the deep tissues layers.

Histopathology

Histopathologic evaluation of periprosthetic tissue at the time of surgery is often necessary to confirm the presence of infection in prosthetic joints. Because there is considerable variation in the degree of inflammation within the tissues, samples from multiple areas should be obtained. Tissue samples from bone-cement or prosthesis-bone interface and from abnormal-appearing areas should be examined. Intraoperative frozen sections are examined for evidence of acute inflammation. Neutrophils are usually absent in aseptic loosening but invariably present in large numbers in infection [14,48]. The finding of at least five polymorphonuclear leukocytes per high-power field on frozen section has a sensitivity of 82% to 84% and a specificity of 93% to 96% for infection [49,50]. Using a higher cutoff value of 10 polymorphonuclear leukocytes per high-power field significantly increases the positive predictive value of the frozen sections from 70% to 89% [50]. The 98% negative predictive value when using either criterion is very good. There is, however, a high degree of interobserver variability in the interpretation of intraoperative frozen sections. As is the case with synovial fluid, in addition to histopathologic studies, tissue specimens must be cultured to identify the microbial pathogen, which is essential in the selection of appropriate antimicrobial therapy.

Novel diagnostic techniques

Advances in molecular technology have made possible the detection of bacterial genetic material from specimens when conventional cultures are negative [51,52]. Polymerase chain reaction is the most widely used nucleic acid amplification technique; it has a rapid turnaround time and is extremely sensitive [41]. Amplification of the 16S rRNA gene allows detection of bacteria that may be present in very low inoculum, or that do not grow [53]. Polymerase chain reaction techniques have not been standardized for joint assessment. Diagnostic tests to improve bacterial recovery by using methods to disrupt biofilm are being explored. Ultrasonication of the implant may increase culture yield by dislodging adherent bacteria; this technique is routinely done in some centers [54]. More research is necessary, however, to evaluate the use of these tests in the diagnosis of infected joint prosthesis.

Treatment

The management of an infected joint prosthesis is uniquely challenging. The objectives in the care of patients with infected joint prosthesis are to cure the infection, prevent its recurrence, preserve body function, and reduce the risk of death. To accomplish these goals usually involves multiple surgeries and an extended course of antimicrobial therapy [55]. Essential for the successful management of these complex infections is the close co-operation between surgeons and infectious diseases physicians. The ultimate goal of therapy is to achieve adequate mobility through a functional and pain-free joint.

A number of host, biomaterial, and microbial factors are unique to the initiation, persistence, and treatment of prosthetic joint infections. Biofilm formation is characteristic of infections associated with orthopedic pros-theses and is a major contributor to the difficulty in eradicating the infection with antimicrobial therapy alone [56,57]. Infecting bacteria are enmeshed in the biofilm wherein they persist in the stationary phase of the growth cycle. In this state, they are resistant to killing by many antimicrobials [58]. Additionally, bacterial shedding from the biofilm to planktonic state in the synovial fluid is reduced, and isolation of organisms from synovial fluid also is reduced.

Microbial colonization of the prosthesis can occur at the time of implantation, as a result of direct spread from a contiguous focus or from hematogenous seeding. The therapeutic approach to these infections takes into account several factors including symptom duration, stability and age of the prosthesis, host's immune and medical conditions, condition of bone and soft tissues, and the infecting pathogen and its antimicrobial susceptibility. The duration of infection is an important factor in deter-mining optimal treatment. Early postoperative and acute hematogenous infections encountered after brief periods of symptoms are less likely to be associated with the development of biofilm or prosthesis loosening; the chance of cure without prosthesis removal is higher in these cases compared with those with indolent disease or those presenting after longer symptomatic periods. Also, the overall treatment strategy must be guided by the patient's ability to tolerate surgical procedures and their projected longevity.

Surgical treatment

Surgical procedures for treating infections involving total joint arthro-plasty include resection arthroplasty with reimplantation either at the time of resection (one-stage replacement) or in a second surgery (two-stage replacement); debridement with retention of prosthesis; definitive resection arthroplasty with or without arthrodesis; and amputation [59]. In choosing the optimal surgical procedure, consideration must be given to the type of infection, condition of the bone stock and soft tissues, virulence and antimicrobial susceptibility of the infecting microorganism, the patient's overall health, and the experience of the surgeon. For selected patients, long-term suppressive oral antimicrobial therapy alone may be an acceptable option. The one-stage procedure is most often used in the management of prosthetic joint infection in Europe [44], whereas two-stage procedure is preferred in the United States [60]. When feasible, two-stage exchange is the most desirable method because this is associated with the greatest likelihood of long-term improved functional outcome and greater patient satisfaction [61].

Two-stage replacement arthroplasty

The two-stage replacement procedure entails removal of the prosthesis with debridement of all infected tissue followed by administration of antimicrobial therapy, and subsequent delayed reimplantation of a second prosthesis. Having adequate bone stock and medical fitness to undergo multiple surgical procedures are prerequisites for a two-stage procedure. Antimicrobials are administered for 4 to 6 weeks following resection, depending on the infecting microorganism. The time interval between the two surgical procedures is highly variable. Confirmation of successful eradication of infection is usually required before implantation of a new prosthesis. Several days to weeks before anticipated reimplantation, antimicrobials are stopped and biopsies are obtained for culture and histopathology, either at the time of reimplantation or as a separate surgery (ie, as a three-stage procedure).

Two-stage exchange is the standard in the treatment of TKA infections and chronic THA infections. It is the procedure of choice in patients with sinus tracts, deep abscess formation, or infections with virulent micro-organisms. A review of selected studies totaling 1077 infected joint prosthesis managed by this strategy showed an overall success rate of 87% (Table 2) [14,62–90]. The two-stage replacement strategy has been successful in 98% of patients with prosthetic joint infections caused by *S aureus* [62]. Studies on uncemented revision arthroplasty for THA infection have a reported success rate of 92% [63,64]. For TKA infection, outcome is guarded even with two-stage exchange and is worsened by premature reimplantation. Early reimplantation (ie, within 2 weeks of removal of the infected prosthesis) was successful in only 35% of patients with infected TKA [65]. Delaying reimplantation with more extensive antimicrobial therapy resulted in treatment success in 69% to 92% [66–68]. The best outcomes have been in those presenting with infection following a primary arthroplasty (92%) [67], and when antimicrobial-impregnated cement was used for prosthesis fixation at revision surgery (95%) [68]. Identifying patients with persistent infection and excluding them from reimplantation improves the outcome in patients with infection of a TKA [69]. Whereas the two-stage approach provides a high success rate for the eradication of infection, it entails the morbidity associated with multiple surgeries and prolonged immobilization, and may be unacceptable for frail older patients [91].

Although not evaluated in randomized controlled trials, antimicrobial-impregnated cement fixation and spacers are often used in the management

Table 2

Outcome of infection in patients managed by two-stage exchange arthroplasty

Study	Type and number of joint	Number free of infection	% free of infection
Brandt et al 1999 [62]	22 THA and 16 TKA	37	98
Fehring et al 1999 [64]	25 THA	23	92
Fitzgerald and Jones 1985 [71]	131 THA	115	88
Haddad et al 2000 [63]	50 THA	46	92
Hanssen et al 1994 [68]	89 TKA	79	89
Hirakawa et al 1998 [67]	54 TKA	41	92[a] and 41[b]
Insall et al 2002 [72]	11 TKA	10	91
Ivarsson et al 1994 [73]	5 THA	4	80
Jhoa and Jiang 2003 [74]	7 TKA	7	100
Kramhoft et al 1994 [75]	15 TKA	11	73
Lieberman et al 1994 [76]	32 THA	29	91
McDonald et al 1989 [77]	82 THA	71	87
McPherson 1997 [78]	21 TKA	20	95
Mont et al 2000 [69]	69 TKA	61	88
Nelson et al 1993 [79]	25 THA	23	92
Nestor et al 1994 [80]	34 THA	28	82
Pagnano et al 1997 [81]	11 THA	8	73[c]
Rand and Bryan 1983 [65]	14 TKA	8	57
Rand et al 1986 [70]	61 TKA	38	63
Rosenberg et al 1988 [82]	26 TKA	26	100
Salvati et al 1982 [83]	28 THA	28	100
Segawa et al 1999 [66]	45 TKA	31	69
Teeny et al 1990 [84]	9 TKA	9	100
Tsukayama et al 1996 [14]	41 THA	39	95
Wang 1997 [85]	9 TKA	9	100
Wang and Chen 1997 [86]	22 THA	20	91
Wilde and Ruth 1988 [87]	15 TKA	12	80
Wilson and Doss 1989 [88]	22 THA	20	91
Windsor et al 1990 [89]	38 TKA	37	97
Younger et al 1997 [90]	48 THA	45	94
Total	1077	935	87

Abbreviations: THA, total hip arthroplasty; TKA, total knee arthroplasty.
[a] Infection occurred after primary arthroplasty.
[b] After multiple previous knee operations.
[c] All with previous infection.

of joint prosthesis infection with two-stage replacement surgery. Cementless fixation offers the advantages of preserving bone stock and avoidance of the use of foreign material that may have a deleterious effect on the immune system. Long-term effects of both cemented and uncemented devices are yet to be determined.

One-stage replacement arthroplasty

This procedure, often referred to as "direct exchange," involves excision of all prosthetic components and infected bone and soft tissues, and implantation of a new prosthesis during the same surgery. Intravenous antimicrobial therapy is usually administered for a variable period of time following surgery. In practice, one-stage exchange is applied mainly for managing infected hip prostheses.

Success rates of one-stage exchange arthroplasty seem comparable for infected hip (75%–100%) and knee (75%–100%) arthroplasties (Table 3) [7,92–107]. Caution should be exercised when interpreting these results because almost all the studies, particularly those reporting the treatment of infected knee prostheses, included small numbers of selected patients with follow-up durations that were highly variable. Whereas the one-stage procedure provides the advantages of a single procedure, lower cost and earlier mobility, it carries the risk for reinfection of the newly implanted prosthesis by residual microorganism. Successful outcome of one-stage exchange arthroplasty is more likely when infection is caused by low virulence microorganism that is highly susceptible to antimicrobial agents, there is no sinus formation, all infected tissues are fully débrided, prolonged postsurgery antimicrobial therapy is provided, and when a bone graft is not necessary [60]. Bone cement loaded with a targeted antimicrobial agent is often used for fixation of the new prosthesis.

Debridement with retention of prosthesis

Debridement with retention of the prosthesis involves debridement of infected tissues, exchange of polyethylene insert, and large-volume irrigation followed by prolonged antimicrobial therapy. This procedure has the

Table 3
Outcome of infection in patients managed with one-stage exchange arthroplasty

Study	Type and number of joint	Number free of infection	% free of infection
Bengtson and Knutson 1991 [7]	69 TKA	52	75
Buchholz et al 1981 [92]	135 THA	104	77
Buechel et al 2004 [94]	22 TKA	20	91
Callaghan et al 1999 [95]	24 THA	22	92
Carlsson et al 1978 [96]	77 THA	69	90
Freeman et al 1985 [97]	8 TKA	8	100
Goksan and Freeman 1992 [98]	18 TKA	16	89
Hope et al 1989 [93]	72 THA	63	87
Hughes et al 1979 [99]	26 THA	22	85
Miley et al 1982 [100]	101 THA	14	86
Raut et al 1994 [101]	57 THA	49	86
Raut et al 1995 [102]	183 THA	154	84
Raut et al 1996 [103]	15 THA	14	93
Sanzen et al 1988 [104]	102 THA	77	75
Silva et al 2002 [105]	37 TKA	33	89
Ure et al 1998 [106]	20 THA	20	100
Wroblewski 1986 [107]	102 THA	93	91
Total	1068	830	78

Abbreviations: THA, total hip arthroplasty; TKA, total knee arthroplasty.

advantage of more limited surgery that preserves both prosthesis and bone stock [91], but carries the risk of leaving an infected foreign body in place. Even with prolonged intravenous and oral antimicrobial therapy, this approach has failure rates of 14% to 86% (Table 4) [14,66,84,108–121]. Over 60% of prosthetic joint infections caused by *S aureus* treated with debridement and retention failed; delayed debridement 2 days after symptom onset is associated with a higher probability of failure [108]. Similarly, an association between duration of symptoms and successful treatment with debridement and prosthesis retention was demonstrated in another study; the mean duration of symptoms in those successfully treated was 4.85 days [109]. Patients with infected joint prostheses caused by penicillin-susceptible streptococci, having well-fixed prostheses and short duration of symptoms, seemed to do well following debridement and retention. The reported failure rate was only 11% in a 19-patient study [110]. Failure of the debridement with retention strategy has been associated with the presence of a sinus tract, duration of symptoms greater than 7 days before debridement, infections caused by *S aureus*, insertion of prosthesis without antimicrobial-impregnated cement, and compromised immune status [14,66,108,109,111]. For patients with early postoperative infection (less than 4 weeks after the index procedure), or late acute hematogenous infection wherein the prosthesis is well-fixed and symptoms are of short duration (less than 2 weeks), debridement with retention of prosthesis may

Table 4

Outcome of infection in patients managed by debridement with retention of prosthesis

Study	Type and number of joint	Number free of infection	% free of infection
Brandt et al 1997 [108]	7 THA and 26 TKA	12	21
Burger et al 1991 [117]	39 TKA	7	18
Crockarell et al 1998 [112]	42 THA	6	14
Drancourt et al 1993 [114]	22 THA and 15 TKA	17 and 9	70
Marculescu et al 2003 [111]	52 TKA and 47 THA	46	60
Meehan et al 2003 [110]	13 TKA and 6 THA	17	89
Rasul et al 1991 [118]	11 TKA	7	64
Schoifet and Morrey 1990 [119]	31 TKA	7	23
Segawa et al 1999 [66]	17 TKA	10	59
Segreti et al 1998 [115]	6 THA and 12 TKA	15	83
Soriano et al 2003 [120]	30 THA	20	67
Tattevin et al 1999 [109]	34 TKA and THA[a]	13	38
Teeny et al 1990 [84]	21 TKA	6	29
Tsukayama et al 1991 [116]	8 TKA and 5 THA	3	23
Tsukayama et al 1996 [14]	41 THA	32	78
Waldman et al 2000 [121]	16 TKA	6	38
Zimmerli et al 1998 [113]	24 implants[b]	19	79
Total	525	252	48

Abbreviations: THA, total hip arthroplasty; TKA, total knee arthroplasty.
[a] Not specified.
[b] Including THA and TKA and other fixation devices.

be a potentially successful option [44,122]. In a study of 42 patients managed with this strategy, 6 (26%) of 23 with early onset or hematogenous THA infection had satisfactory outcome, particularly if debrided within 14 days of noting symptoms; two remained on chronic suppressive antibiotics [112]. The remaining 19 patients who had late chronic infection were deemed to have failed debridement and prosthesis retention. In other reports, successful outcomes using this strategy for TKA and THA infections were achieved in 50% and 71% of cases, respectively [14,66,111]. There is one report of a randomized placebo-controlled trial of patients with staphylococcal orthopedic device–related infections with abbreviated symptoms and stable devices managed by debridement with retention and either a prolonged fluoroquinolone-rifampin regimen or a fluoroquinolone alone [113]. Among patients with infected TKA, THA, and fracture fixation devices, 12 (67%) of 18 treated with fluoroquinolone-rifampin and 7 (47%) of 15 treated with fluoroquinolone alone were cured. Because of the relatively small number of patients studied, results with the debridement-retention strategy should be interpreted with caution. Nevertheless, using a mathematical model to simulate the projected lifetime clinical course of patients with THA infection caused by staphylococcal or streptococcal pathogens, debridement with retention of fixed prosthesis was shown to be cost-effective and provided greater quality-adjusted life expectancy gains in older persons with shorter life expectancy [91].

Resection arthroplasty

Resection arthroplasty involves the definitive removal of all infected components and tissue (prosthesis, cement, bone, and soft tissues) with no subsequent implantation. Resection is usually followed by treatment with an antimicrobial regimen for 4 to 6 weeks. With this procedure, successful eradication of infection can be achieved in 60% to 100% of THA infections [123–127] and 89% of TKA infections [128]. Patients treated with resection arthroplasty have shortened limbs and poor functional level, however, and are less satisfied with the clinical outcome.

The functional results following excision arthroplasty and creation of a pseudarthrosis as a salvage procedure for infection of a hip prosthesis are generally poor [124,126]. Once considered the standard therapeutic modality, resection arthroplasty currently has limited indications. Established indications include poor quality of bone and soft tissue, recurrent infections, infection with multidrug-resistant microorganisms, medical conditions precluding major surgery, and failure of exchange arthroplasty [129]. This may also be an acceptable alternative for elderly nonambulatory patients.

Arthrodesis

Arthrodesis is designed to provide bony ankylosis of a joint. This procedure is used when subsequent joint reimplantation is not feasible because of poor bone stock, active or recurrent infection, or in patients who have undergone multiple surgical procedures for treatment of infection with virulent microorganisms [130]. Currently, salvage of a failed TKA infection is the most frequent indication for arthrodesis. Eradication of infection and bony fusion is achieved in 71% to 95% of cases [7,70,131,132]. Adequate bone apposition and rigid fixation are essential to achieve successful bony fusion. The extent of bone loss seems to be an important determinant of the likelihood of achieving bony fusion of a primary arthrodesis [132].

External fixation has been used in active TKA infection, with variable success rate. Successful fusion with an external fixator using the Ilizarov technique ranged from 93% to 100% in some studies [130,133,134]. Unfortunately, external fixators are usually cumbersome and may result in a number of complications, such as pin tract infection, bone fracture at a pin site, pin loosening, and nonunion [135]. The use of intramedullary nails for stabilization achieves a stable fusion in a high percentage (80%–100%) of patients [136–138]. Complications from intramedullary nail fusion include nail migration, delayed union or nonunion, nail breakage, and distal tibial fracture [139–141]. Arthrodesis for failed TKA caused by gram-negative bacillus or mixed infections is associated with a lower fusion rate [142]. In these cases, arthrodesis using a two-stage procedure is advocated by some experts because it may lead to a higher probability for bony fusion [131,143]. An initial stage of thorough debridement and antimicrobial therapy is followed by a second stage that provides rigid stability until fusion is obtained. When successful, arthrodesis of the knee provides excellent pain relief and a stable leg [144]. Significant functional drawbacks may result, however, from limb shortening or deformity.

Amputation

Amputation above a TKA may be required in selected cases when other treatment options have failed to control the infection. In some instances, amputation may be indicated for intractable pain, in the presence of severe bone loss or vascular compromise, or when other limb salvage procedures have failed [145,146]. Some experts advocate earlier consideration for arthrodesis rather than multiple attempts at revision to avert amputation [145].

Antimicrobial therapy

Antimicrobial therapy for infected prosthetic joints may be curative when the infected joint is removed and periprosthetic tissue debrided. The importance of obtaining satisfactory specimens for culture and establishing a microbiologic diagnosis before administering empiric antimicrobial therapy cannot be overemphasized. Unless patients present with overwhelming sepsis, antimicrobials should be withheld until aspiration or intraoperative cultures are obtained. Initial empiric therapy should cover the most common pathogens (ie, staphylococcal species). A first-generation cephalosporin (eg, cefazolin) is adequate initial empirical treatment in most cases. In patients with a history of immediate hypersensitivity reaction to penicillin, vancomycin can be used as an alternative. Vancomycin is also preferred in institutions and locales with a high incidence of infection with methicillin-resistant *S aureus*. Following identification of the causative pathogen and in vitro antimicrobial susceptibility testing, the antimicrobial regimen should be modified.

Suggested regimens for common pathogens, few of which have been subjected to comparative trials, are summarized in Table 5. Antimicrobials are given systemically by parenteral or, if fully bioavailable, by oral administration and locally by temporary implantation of antimicrobial-impregnated cement beads. The optimal duration of antimicrobial therapy varies with the surgical procedure and the infecting pathogen; most authorities favor a minimum of 4 weeks of treatment. Vancomycin use should be restricted to methicillin-resistant staphylococcal infections and to patients who cannot tolerate β-lactam antibiotics. Some fluoroquinolones can be administered orally because of their excellent bioavailability. In vitro studies and animal models of device-related infections demonstrated rifampin to be effective against adherent and stationary-phase staphylococci [146–148]. Rifampin should never be used as monotherapy, however, because this often leads to the emergence of resistance. The ability of both rifampin and fluoroquinolones to achieve high concentrations in bone and soft tissues makes this combination an attractive regimen for treatment of prosthetic joint infections caused by susceptible bacteria [113,114]. Clinical studies showed that combination of rifampin with ciprofloxacin or a β-lactam antibiotic in selected cases of staphylococcal implant-related infections was successful in 60% to 82% of stable implants following initial debridement [113,114,149]. One study showed comparable treatment success using oral rifampin-fusidic acid or rifampin-fluoroquinolone for staphylococcal orthopedic implant infections [150]. The results of these studies should be interpreted with caution because of the small number of patients in each study, variations in inclusion criteria, inclusion of various types of orthopedic device infections, and differences in duration of follow-up.

Linezolid, a new oxazolidinone synthetic antibacterial agent, is active against aerobic gram-positive bacteria and has an excellent oral bioavailability. Successful outcome in 90% of patients with orthopedic infections treated with linezolid has been reported [151]. Reversible myelosuppression, however, occurred in 40% of patients. Moreover, long-term linezolid use has been associated with irreversible peripheral and optic neuropathy that may be severely debilitating [152]. The role of daptomycin, the first in the class of lipopeptide antibiotics, for the treatment of orthopedic infections is yet to be defined. It is a promising alternative for patients with infections caused by resistant gram-positive cocci, or when allergy or side effects preclude the use of vancomycin and linezolid.

Table 5
Suggested antimicrobial treatment of common pathogens causing prosthetic joint infections

Microorganism	First choice[a]	Alternative[a]
Staphylococcus spp, oxacillin-susceptible	Nafcillin sodium, 1.5–2 g IV q 4 h or Cefazolin, 1–2 g IV q 8 h	Vancomycin, 15 mg/kg IV q 12 h or Levofloxacin, 500–750 mg PO or IV q 24 h + rifampin, 300–450 mg PO q 12 h[b]
Staphylococcus spp, oxacillin-resistant	Vancomycin, 15 mg/kg IV q 12 h	Linezolid, 600 mg PO or IV q 12 h or Levofloxacin, 500–750 mg PO or IV q 24 h + rifampin, 300–450 mg PO q 12 h[b]
Enterococcus spp, penicillin-susceptible[c]	Aqueous crystalline penicillin G, 24–30 million units IV q 24 h continuously or in six divided doses or Ampicillin sodium, 12 g IV q 24 h continuously or in six divided doses	Vancomycin, 15 mg/kg IV q 12 h
Enterococcus spp, penicillin-resistant[c]	Vancomycin, 15 mg/kg IV q 12 h	Linezolid, 600 mg PO or IV q 12 h
Pseudomonas aeruginosa[d]	Cefepime, 1–2 g IV q 12 h or Meropenem, 1 g IV q 8 h or Imipenem, 500 mg IV q 6–8 h	Ciprofloxacin, 750 mg PO or 400 mg IV q 12 h or Ceftazidime, 2 g IV q 8 h
Enterobacter spp	Meropenem, 1 g IV q 8 h or Imipenem, 500 mg IV q 6–8 h	Cefepime, 1–2 g IV q 12 h or Ciprofloxacin, 750 mg PO or 400 mg IV q 12 h
β-hemolytic streptococci	Aqueous crystalline penicillin G, 20–24 million units IV q 24 h by continuous infusion or in six divided doses or Ceftriaxone, 1–2 g IV q 24 h	Vancomycin, 15 mg/kg IV q 12 h

Table 5 (continued)

Microorganism	First choice[a]	Alternative[a]
Propionibacterium acnes and Corynebacterium spp	Aqueous crystalline penicillin G, 20–24 million units IV q 24 h by continuous infusion or in six divided doses or Ceftriaxone 1–2 g IV q 24 h or Vancomycin, 15 mg/kg IV q 12 h	Clindamycin, 600–900 mg IV q 8 h

[a] Dose adjustment necessary for renal impairment.
[b] Levofloxacin-rifampin combination therapy for patients managed by debridement with retention. See reference regarding prolong duration of therapy.
[c] Addition of aminoglycoside for bactericidal synergy is optional. Considerations in choice of an agent are similar to those noted for treatment of enterococcal endocarditis.
[d] Addition of an aminoglycoside is option.

Suppressive antimicrobial therapy

Long-term, potentially indefinite, suppressive antimicrobial therapy may play a role in the treatment of selected patients with prosthetic joint infection. Among patients undergoing two-stage replacement who are noted at reimplantation to have residual acute inflammation in tissue, long-term oral suppressive therapy is associated with better implant survival [153]. Similarly, in many patients treated successfully by debridement and prosthesis retention, therapy included long-term suppressive antimicrobials [111,115,154,155]. Occasionally, surgery may not be feasible and long-term suppressive antimicrobial therapy without surgery may be the only available alternative. Indications for this treatment approach include contraindications to surgery because of poor health, terminal illness, unacceptable functional results from removal of the prosthesis, well-fixed prosthesis that is difficult to remove, or patient's refusal for further surgical procedures.

The goal of long-term suppressive antimicrobial therapy as primary treatment is to provide symptomatic relief, maintain a functioning joint, and prevent the systemic spread of infection rather than eradicate infection. The clinical efficacy of this strategy has been limited with reported success rates of only 10% to 25% [116,123,156]. Prerequisites for a successful outcome include a well-fixed and functional prosthesis, infection with a highly sensitive microorganism, absence of systemic infection, and patient's tolerance to long-term oral antimicrobial treatment [154]. Complications related to suppressive antimicrobial therapy occur in 8% to 22% of patients [115,155]. The ideal regimen and optimal duration of oral suppressive treatment has not been well-established, and the potential toxicities of antimicrobials considered for long-term suppressive therapy are significant (Table 6). Suppressive antimicrobial therapy as primary therapy should be considered only in patients who are old and frail, and those who refuse surgery.

Table 6
Selected side effects and considerations regarding antimicrobials of potential use

Antimicrobial	Long-term side effects and cautions
Minocycline	Photosensitivity, discoloration of skin; permanent discoloration of teeth when used in early childhood; drug-induced lupus; dizziness, light-headedness, vertigo; rarely, pseudotumor cerebri; should not be taken with antacids or iron-containing preparations; caution with concurrent anticoagulant therapy; may decrease contraceptive efficacy.
Trimethoprim-sulfamethoxazole	Myelosuppression; elevated creatinine; nephrotoxicity, crystalluria; possible disulfiram-like reactions; may enhance hypoglycemic effects of sulfonylureas.
β-Lactam	Antibiotic-associated diarrhea, pseudomembranous colitis; genital moniliasis; hepatic dysfunction.
Rifampin	Orange discoloration of body secretions; hepatotoxicity; should not be used as monotherapy; significant drug-drug interactions; increased requirement for anticoagulant drugs; may decrease contraceptive efficacy.
Linezolid	Myelosuppression; peripheral and optic neuropathy; potential interaction with adrenergic and serotonergic agents; avoid tyramine-containing food.
Fluoroquinolones	Phototoxicity; tendon rupture; very rarely, arrhythmia; may cause disturbances in blood glucose levels and lower seizure threshold; should not be taken with antacids.
Metronidazole	Peripheral neuropathy; ataxia; disulfiram-like reaction; caution with concurrent anticoagulant therapy.
Fluconazole	Hepatotoxicity; prolongation of QT interval; drug-drug interactions.

Antimicrobial-impregnated devices

The use of antimicrobial-impregnated cement in the treatment of prosthetic joint and other orthopedic device-related infections is widespread. There is significant practice variations, however, in the type of cement and antimicrobial used [157]. Bone cement implants may take the form of solid spacers [68], beads [14], or temporary arthroplasties that allow some function [158]. These devices offer the advantage of achieving high concentrations of antibiotic directly at the site of infection [159]. Success rates of 77% to 87% have been reported with the use of antimicrobial-loaded bone cement for one-stage hip exchange arthroplasty [92,93]. Cement spacers also reduce dead space, provide joint stability, and may improve patient mobility while awaiting reimplantation [158,160]. The PROSTALAC (Prosthesis of Antibiotic-Loaded Acrylic Cement; DePuy Orthopaedics Inc., Warsaw, NJ) is a temporary prosthesis initially developed for the hip [161,162] and subsequently for the knees [163]. The system consists of articulating components made primarily of antibiotic-loaded bone cement. It allows continuous rehabilitation, and can provide early mobilization and shorter hospitalization. With this system, reinfection occurred in 9% of two-stage revision for infected TKA [164]. Using antibiotic-loaded beads in the femur and an antibiotic-loaded cement spacer in the acetabulum, 8% of infected THA experienced reinfection [63].

Aminoglycosides, mainly tobramycin and gentamicin, with or without vancomycin, are most commonly used in impregnated devices. Penicillin and cephalosporins are generally avoided because of their potential allergenicity. Ciprofloxacin use is currently experimental but may be limited because of potential interference with bone and soft tissue healing [165,166], and widespread resistance among staphylococci. In vitro studies show that fluconazole and amphotericin B retain their antimicrobial activity when mixed with bone cement [167]. The antimicrobial effect of daptomycin eluted from polymethylmethacrylate beads is comparable with vancomycin [168]. Ideally, the antimicrobial loaded into cement should be selected based on culture results.

Despite the promising reports on the value of antimicrobial-loaded cement, other factors may influence its use in clinical practice. Addition of high doses of antimicrobial agents may result in lower mechanical properties of bone cement [169,170]. There are also concerns regarding allergic reactions to impregnated antibiotics and the potential for emergence of antibiotic-resistant bacteria [170]. Further research is needed to establish the value of antimicrobial-loaded bone cements in the treatment of prosthetic joint infections.

Special situations

Culture-negative prosthetic joint infection

Prior antimicrobial exposure is perhaps the most frequent cause of culture-negative prosthetic joint infection. Accordingly, in the absence of systemic sepsis, antimicrobial therapy should be withheld until appropriate cultures are taken. Biofilm-embedded microorganisms may not grow in routine cultures. Slow growing, small-colony S aureus variants could easily be missed on routine solid media cultures [171]. Although their role in causing prosthesis infection is not well described, they have been associated with persistent and relapsing infections in patients with chronic osteomyelitis [172,173]. When routine aerobic and anaerobic bacterial cultures are sterile, specimens should be cultured in specific media for fungi, mycobacteria, and fastidious bacteria, and periprosthetic tissues should be examined using acid-fast bacillus, fungal, and Giemsa stains. Finally, noninfectious etiologies of joint inflammation could mimic culture-negative prosthetic joint infection; examples include inflammatory arthritides secondary to rheumatoid arthritis and systemic lupus erythematosus.

Recurrent prosthetic joint infection

The therapeutic approach to recurrent infection differs in some aspects from treatment of infections after a primary arthroplasty. Risks of losing further bone stock and soft tissues may outweigh the benefits of another revision arthroplasty. Treatment of recurrent prosthetic joint infections often yields poor outcomes. Among 24 patients with recurrent TKA infection, there were 10 successful knee arthrodesis and 1 uninfected total knee prosthesis after an average of 3.7 surgical procedures [174]. Repeated attempts at reimplantation in the face of recurrent infection should be viewed with caution. Instead, early resection arthroplasty or arthrodesis should be considered.

Infection with unusual microorganisms

A wide variety of unusual microorganisms have been reported to cause infection in prosthetic joints. Pneumococcal prosthetic joint infection can be cured with a combination of long-term antibiotic therapy and drainage [175]. Infection of prosthetic joints caused by anaerobes is uncommon; metronidazole may be effective following debridement or prosthesis removal. Fungal infections of joint prostheses are difficult to cure with medical therapy alone. Patients with candidal infections susceptible to oral azole therapy may be successfully treated by debridement with delayed reimplantation arthroplasty after appropriate antifungal therapy [176]. Although uncommon, successful outcome with standard antituberculosis treatment of *Mycobacterium tuberculosis* prosthetic joint infection without implant removal has been reported [177]. Often, treatment requires both medical and surgical approach [178]. Other causes of prosthetic joint infection include *Brucella* spp [179], *Mycobacterium fortuitum* [180], *Listeria monocytogenes* [181], *Haemophilus parainfluenzae* [182], *Yersinia enterocolitica* [183], *Campylobacter fetus* [184], *Tropheryma whippelii* [185], *Pasteurella multocida* [186], and *Clostridium difficile* [187]. This diversity of pathogens highlights the importance of an accurate microbiologic diagnosis to design the optimal antimicrobial treatment.

Summary

Success in the treatment of infected orthopedic prosthesis requires the best surgical approach in combination with prolonged optimum targeted antimicrobial therapy. In choosing the surgical option, one must consider the type of infection, condition of the bone stock and soft tissue, the virulence and antimicrobial susceptibility of the pathogen, the general health and projected longevity of the patient, and the experience of the surgeon. If surgery is not possible, an alternative is long-term oral antimicrobial suppression to maintain a functioning prosthesis. Treatment must be individualized for a specific infection in a specific patient.

References

[1] Sculco TP. The economic impact of infected joint arthroplasty. Orthopedics 1995;18:871–3.

[2] Lidgren L, Knutson K, Stefansdottir A. Infection and arthritis: infection of prosthetic joints. Best Pract Res Clin Rheumatol 2003;17:209–18.

[3] Hanssen AD, Rand JA. Evaluation and treatment of infection at the site of a total hip or knee arthroplasty. Instr Course Lect 1999;48:111–22.

[4] Sperling JW, Kozak TK, Hanssen AD, et al. Infection after shoulder arthroplasty. Clin Orthop 2001;382:206–16.

[5] Robertsson O, Knutson K, Lewold S, et al. The Swedish Knee Arthroplasty Register 1975–1997: an update with special emphasis on 41,223 knees operated on in 1988–1997. Acta Orthop Scand 2001;72:503–13.

[6] Berbari EF, Hanssen AD, Duffy MC, et al. Risk factors for prosthetic joint infection: case-control study. Clin Infect Dis 1998;27:1247–54.

[7] Bengston S, Knutson K. The infected knee arthroplasty: a 6-year follow-up of 357 cases. Acta Orthop Scand 1991;62:301–11.

[8] Maderazo EG, Judson S, Pasternak H. Late infections of total joint prostheses: a review and recommendations for prevention. Clin Orthop 1988;229:131–42.

[9] Deacon JM, Pagliaro AJ, Zelicof SB, et al. Prophylactic use of antibiotics for procedures after total joint replacement. J Bone Joint Surg Am 1996;78:1755–70.

[10] Rubin R, Salvati EA, Lewis R. Infected total hip replacement after dental procedures. Oral Surg Oral Med Oral Pathol 1976;41:18–23.

[11] Hanssen AD, Osmon DR, Nelson CL. Prevention of deep periprosthetic joint infection. Instr Course Lect 1997;46:555–67.

[12] Bengtson S, Blomgren G, Knutson K, et al. Hematogenous infection after knee arthroplasty. Acta Orthop Scand 1987;58:529–34.

[13] Murdoch DR, Roberts SA, Fowler VG Jr, et al. Infection of orthopedic prostheses after *Staphylococcus aureus* bacteremia. Clin Infect Dis 2001;32:647–9.

[14] Tsukayama DT, Estrada R, Gustilo RB. Infection after total hip arthroplasty: a study of the treatment of one hundred and six infections. J Bone Joint Surg Am 1996;78:512–23.

[15] Sanzen L, Sundberg M. Periprosthetic low-grade hip infections: erythrocyte sedimentation rate and C-reactive protein in 23 cases. Acta Orthop Scand 1997;68:461–5.

[16] Spangehl MJ, Masri BA, O'Connell JX, et al. Prospective analysis of preoperative and intraoperative investigations for the diagnosis of infection at the sites of two hundred and two revision total hip arthroplasties. J Bone Joint Surg Am 1999;81:672–83.

[17] Spangehl MJ, Younger AS, Masri BA, et al. Diagnosis of infection following total hip arthroplasty. Instr Course Lect 1998;47:285–95.

[18] Bernard L, Lubbeke A, Stern R, et al. Value of preoperative investigations in diagnosing prosthetic joint infection: retrospective cohort study and literature review. Scand J Infect Dis 2004;36:410–6.

[19] Barrack RL, Jennings RW, Wolfe MW, et al. The value of preoperative aspiration before total knee revision. Clin Orthop 1997;345:8–16.

[20] Mulcahy DM, Fenelon GC, McInerney DP. Aspiration arthrography of the hip joint: its uses and limitations in revision hip surgery. J Arthroplasty 1996;11:64–8.

[21] Kersey R, Benjamin J, Marson B. White blood cell counts and differential in synovial fluid of aseptically failed total knee arthroplasty. J Arthroplasty 2000;15:301–4.

[22] Trampuz A, Hanssen AD, Osmon DR, et al. Synovial fluid leukocyte count and differential for the diagnosis of prosthetic knee infection. Am J Med 2004;117:556–62.

[23] Cuckler JM, Star AM, Alavi A, et al. Diagnosis and management of the infected total joint arthroplasty. Orthop Clin North Am 1991;22:523–30.

[24] Stumpe KD, Notzli HP, Zanetti M, et al. FDG PET for differentiation of infection and aseptic loosening in total hip replacements: comparison with conventional radiography and three-phase bone scintigraphy. Radiology 2004;231:333–41.

[25] Lyons CW, Berquist TH, Lyons JC, et al. Evaluation of radiographic findings in painful hip arthroplasties. Clin Orthop 1985;195:239–51.

[26] Love C, Palestro CJ. Radionuclide imaging of infection. J Nucl Med Technol 2004;32: 47–57.
[27] Smith SL, Wastie ML, Forster I. Radionuclide bone scintigraphy in the detection of significant complications after total knee joint replacement. Clin Radiol 2001;56:221–4.
[28] Kantor SG, Schneider R, Insall JN, et al. Radionuclide imaging of asymptomatic versus symptomatic total knee arthroplasties. Clin Orthop 1990;260:118–23.
[29] Hofmann AA, Wyatt RW, Daniels AU, et al. Bone scans after total knee arthroplasty in asymptomatic patients: cemented versus cementless. Clin Orthop 1990;251:183–8.
[30] Palestro CJ, Torres MA. Radionuclide imaging in orthopedic infections. Semin Nucl Med 1997;27:334–45.
[31] Love C, Tomas MB, Marwin SE, et al. Role of nuclear medicine in diagnosis of the infected joint replacement. Radiographics 2001;21:1229–38.
[32] Palestro CJ, Swyer AJ, Kim CK, et al. Infected knee prosthesis: diagnosis with In-111 leukocyte, Tc-99m sulfur colloid, and Tc-99m MDP imaging. Radiology 1991;179:645–8.
[33] Palestro CJ, Kim CK, Swyer AJ, et al. Total-hip arthroplasty: periprosthetic indium-111-labeled leukocyte activity and complementary technetium-99m-sulfur colloid imaging in suspected infection. J Nucl Med 1990;31:1950–5.
[34] Zhuang H, Duarte PS, Pourdehnad M, et al. The promising role of 18F-FDG PET in detecting infected lower limb prosthesis implants. J Nucl Med 2001;42:44–8.
[35] Love C, Marwin SE, Tomas MB, et al. Diagnosing infection in the failed joint replacement: a comparison of coincidence detection 18F-FDG and 111In-labeled leukocyte/99mTc-sulfur colloid marrow imaging. J Nucl Med 2004;45:1864–71.
[36] Larikka MJ, Ahonen AK, Niemela O, et al. Comparison of 99mTc ciprofloxacin, 99mTc white blood cell and three-phase bone imaging in the diagnosis of hip prosthesis infections: improved diagnostic accuracy with extended imaging time. Nucl Med Commun 2002;23: 655–61.
[37] Larikka MJ, Ahonen AK, Niemela O, et al. 99m Tc-ciprofloxacin (Infecton) imaging in the diagnosis of knee prosthesis infections. Nucl Med Commun 2002;23:167–70.
[38] Palestro CJ. Nuclear medicine, the painful prosthetic joint, and orthopedic infection. J Nucl Med 2003;44:927–9.
[39] Wilde AH. Management of infected knee and hip prostheses. Curr Opin Rheumatol 1993;5: 317–21.
[40] Atkins BL, Athanasou N, Deeks JJ, et al. Prospective evaluation of criteria for microbiological diagnosis of prosthetic-joint infection at revision arthroplasty. The OSIRIS Collaborative Study Group. J Clin Microbiol 1998;36:2932–9.
[41] Trampuz A, Steckelberg JM, Osmon DR, et al. Advances in the laboratory diagnosis if prosthetic joint infection. Rev Clin Microbiol 2003;14:1–14.
[42] Steckelberg J, Osmon D. Prosthetic joint infections. In: Waldvogel F, Bisno A, editors. Infections associated with indwelling medical devices. 3rd edition. Washington: American Society for Microbiology Press; 2000. p. 173–209.
[43] Chimento GF, Finger S, Barrack RL. Gram stain detection of infection during revision arthroplasty. J Bone Joint Surg Br 1996;78:838–9.
[44] Zimmerli W, Trampuz A, Ochsner PE. Prosthetic-joint infections. N Engl J Med 2004;351: 1645–54.
[45] Berbari EF, Steckelberg JM, Osmon DR. Osteomyelitis. In: Mandell GL, Bennett JE, Dolin R, editors. Mandell, Douglas and Bennett's principles and practice of infectious diseases, vol. 1. Sixth edition. Philadelphia: Elsevier Churchill Livingstone; 2005. p. 1322–32.
[46] Kamme C, Lindberg L. Aerobic and anaerobic bacteria in deep infections after total hip arthroplasty: differential diagnosis between infectious and non-infectious loosening. Clin Orthop 1981;154:201–7.
[47] Mackowiak PA, Jones SR, Smith JW. Diagnostic value of sinus-tract cultures in chronic osteomyelitis. JAMA 1978;239:2772–5.

[48] Della Valle CJ, Bogner E, Desai P, et al. Analysis of frozen sections of intraoperative specimens obtained at the time of reoperation after hip or knee resection arthroplasty for the treatment of infection. J Bone Joint Surg Am 1999;81:684–9.

[49] Pace TB, Jeray KJ, Latham JT Jr. Synovial tissue examination by frozen section as an indicator of infection in hip and knee arthroplasty in community hospitals. J Arthroplasty 1997;12:64–9.

[50] Lonner JH, Desai P, Dicesare PE, et al. The reliability of analysis of intraoperative frozen sections for identifying active infection during revision hip or knee arthroplasty. J Bone Joint Surg Am 1996;78:1553–8.

[51] Mariani BD, Martin DS, Levine MJ, et al. Polymerase chain reaction detection of bacterial infection in total knee arthroplasty. Clin Orthop 1996;331:11–22.

[52] Mariani BD, Tuan RS. Advances in the diagnosis of infection in prosthetic joint implants. Mol Med Today 1998;4:207–13.

[53] Tunney MM, Patrick S, Curran MD, et al. Detection of prosthetic hip infection at revision arthroplasty by immunofluorescence microscopy and PCR amplification of the bacterial 16S rRNA gene. J Clin Microbiol 1999;37:3281–90.

[54] Tunney MM, Patrick S, Gorman SP, et al. Improved detection of infection in hip replacements: a currently underestimated problem. J Bone Joint Surg Br 1998;80: 568–72.

[55] Lentino JR. Prosthetic joint infections: bane of orthopedists, challenge for infectious disease specialists. Clin Infect Dis 2003;36:1157–61.

[56] Costerton JW, Stewart PS, Greenberg EP. Bacterial biofilms: a common cause of persistent infections. Science 1999;284:1318–22.

[57] Khardori N, Yassien M. Biofilms in device-related infections. J Ind Microbiol 1995;15: 141–7.

[58] Widmer AF. New developments in diagnosis and treatment of infection in orthopedic implants. Clin Infect Dis 2001;33:1.

[59] Garvin KL, Hanssen AD. Infection after total hip arthroplasty: past, present, and future. J Bone Joint Surg Am 1995;77:1576–88.

[60] Wilde AH. Management of infected knee and hip prostheses. Curr Opin Rheumatol 1994;6: 172–6.

[61] Hanssen AD, Rand JA. Evaluation and treatment of infection at the site of a total hip or knee arthroplasty. J Bone Joint Surg Am 1998;80:910–22.

[62] Brandt CM, Duffy MC, Berbari EF, et al. *Staphylococcus aureus* prosthetic joint infection treated with prosthesis removal and delayed reimplantation arthroplasty. Mayo Clin Proc 1999;74:553–8.

[63] Haddad FS, Muirhead-Allwood SK, Manktelow AR, et al. Two-stage uncemented revision hip arthroplasty for infection. J Bone Joint Surg Br 2000;82:689–94.

[64] Fehring TK, Calton TF, Griffin WL. Cementless fixation in 2-stage reimplantation for periprosthetic sepsis. J Arthroplasty 1999;14:175–81.

[65] Rand JA, Bryan RS. Reimplantation for the salvage of an infected total knee arthroplasty. J Bone Joint Surg Am 1983;65:1081–6.

[66] Segawa H, Tsukayama DT, Kyle RF, et al. Infection after total knee arthroplasty: a retrospective study of the treatment of eighty-one infections. J Bone Joint Surg Am 1999; 81:1434–45.

[67] Hirakawa K, Stulberg BN, Wilde AH, et al. Results of 2-stage reimplantation for infected total knee arthroplasty. J Arthroplasty 1998;13:22–8.

[68] Hanssen AD, Rand JA, Osmon DR. Treatment of the infected total knee arthroplasty with insertion of another prosthesis: the effect of antibiotic-impregnated bone cement. Clin Orthop 1994;309:44–55.

[69] Mont MA, Waldman BJ, Hungerford DS. Evaluation of preoperative cultures before second-stage reimplantation of a total knee prosthesis complicated by infection: a comparison-group study. J Bone Joint Surg Am 2000;82-A:1552–7.

[70] Rand JA, Bryan RS, Morrey BF, et al. Management of infected total knee arthroplasty. Clin Orthop 1986;205:75–85.

[71] Fitzgerald RH, Jones DR. Hip implant infection: treatment with resection arthroplasty and late total hip arthroplasty. Am J Med 1985;78:225–8.

[72] Insall JN, Thompson FM, Brause BD. Two-stage reimplantation for the salvage of infected total knee arthroplasty. J Bone Joint Surg Am 2002;84-A:490.

[73] Ivarsson I, Wahlstrom O, Djerf K, et al. Revision of infected hip replacement: two-stage procedure with a temporary gentamicin spacer. Acta Orthop Scand 1994;65:7–8.

[74] Jhao C, Jiang CC. Two-stage reimplantation without cement spacer for septic total knee replacement. J Formos Med Assoc 2003;102:37–41.

[75] Kramhoft M, Bodtker S, Carlsen A. Outcome of infected total knee arthroplasty. J Arthroplasty 1994;9:617–21.

[76] Lieberman JR, Callaway GH, Salvati EA, et al. Treatment of the infected total hip replacement with a two-stage reimplantation protocol. Clin Orthop 1994;301:205–12.

[77] McDonald DJ, Fitzgerald RH Jr, Ilstrup DM. Two-stage reconstruction of a total hip arthroplasty because of infection. J Bone Joint Surg Am 1989;71:828–34.

[78] McPherson EJ, Patzakis MJ, Gross JE, et al. Infected total knee arthroplasty. Two-stage reimplantation with a gastrocnemius rotational flap. Clin Orthop 1997;341:73–81.

[79] Nelson CL, Evans RP, Blaha JD, et al. A comparison of gentamicin-impregnated polymethylmethacrylate bead implantation to conventional parenteral antibiotic therapy in infected total hip and knee arthroplasty. Clin Orthop 1993;295:96–101.

[80] Nestor BJ, Hanssen AD, Ferrer-Gonzalez R, et al. The use of porous prostheses in delayed reconstruction of total hip replacements that have failed because of infection. J Bone Joint Surg Am 1994;76:349–59.

[81] Pagnano MW, Trousdale RT, Hanssen AD. Outcome after reinfection following reimplantation hip arthroplasty. Clin Orthop 1997;338:192–204.

[82] Rosenberg AG, Haas B, Barden R, et al. Salvage of infected total knee arthroplasty. Clin Orthop 1988;226:29–33.

[83] Salvati EA, Chekofsky KM, Brause BD, et al. Reimplantation in infection: a 12-year experience. Clin Orthop 1982;170:62–75.

[84] Teeny SM, Dorr L, Murata G, et al. Treatment of infected total knee arthroplasty: irrigation and debridement versus two-stage reimplantation. J Arthroplasty 1990;5:35–9.

[85] Wang CJ. Management of infected total knee arthroplasty. Changgeng Yi Xue Za Zhi 1997;20:1–10.

[86] Wang JW, Chen CE. Reimplantation of infected hip arthroplasties using bone allografts. Clin Orthop 1997;335:202–10.

[87] Wilde AH, Ruth JT. Two-stage reimplantation in infected total knee arthroplasty. Clin Orthop 1988;236:23–35.

[88] Wilson MG, Dorr LD. Reimplantation of infected total hip arthroplasties in the absence of antibiotic cement. J Arthroplasty 1989;4:263.

[89] Windsor RE, Insall JN, Urs WK, et al. Two-stage reimplantation for the salvage of total knee arthroplasty complicated by infection: further follow-up and refinement of indications. J Bone Joint Surg Am 1990;72:272–8.

[90] Younger AS, Duncan CP, Masri BA, et al. The outcome of two-stage arthroplasty using a custom-made interval space to treat the infected hip. J Arthroplasty 1997;12:615–23.

[91] Fisman DN, Reilly DT, Karchmer AW, et al. Clinical effectiveness and cost-effectiveness of 2 management strategies for infected total hip arthroplasty in the elderly. Clin Infect Dis 2001;32:419–30.

[92] Buchholz HW, Elson RA, Engelbrecht E, et al. Management of deep infection of total hip replacement. J Bone Joint Surg Br 1981;63-B:342–53.

[93] Hope PG, Kristinsson KG, Norman P, et al. Deep infection of cemented total hip arthroplasties caused by coagulase-negative staphylococci. J Bone Joint Surg Br 1989;71: 851–5.

[94] Buechel FF, Femino FP, D'Alessio J. Primary exchange revision arthroplasty for infected total knee replacement: a long-term study. Am J Orthop 2004;33:190–8 [discussion: 198].

[95] Callaghan JJ, Katz RP, Johnston RC. One-stage revision surgery of the infected hip: a minimum 10-year followup study. Clin Orthop 1999;369:139–43.

[96] Carlsson AS, Josefsson G, Lindberg L. Revision with gentamicin-impregnated cement for deep infections in total hip arthroplasties. J Bone Joint Surg Am 1978;60:1059–64.

[97] Freeman MA, Sudlow RA, Casewell MW, et al. The management of infected total knee replacements. J Bone Joint Surg Br 1985;67:764–8.

[98] Goksan SB, Freeman MA. One-stage reimplantation for infected total knee arthroplasty. J Bone Joint Surg Br 1992;74:78–82.

[99] Hughes PW, Salvati EA, Wilson PD, et al. Treatment of subacute sepsis of the hip by antibiotics and joint replacement criteria for diagnosis with evaluation of twenty-six cases. Clin Orthop 1979;141:143–57.

[100] Miley GB, Scheller AD, Turner RH. Medical and surgical treatment of the septic hip with one-stage revision arthroplasty. Clin Orthop 1982;170:76–82.

[101] Raut VV, Siney PD, Wroblewski BM. One-stage revision of infected total hip replacements with discharging sinuses. J Bone Joint Surg Br 1994;76:721–4.

[102] Raut VV, Siney PD, Wroblewski BM. One-stage revision of total hip arthroplasty for deep infection: long-term followup. Clin Orthop 1995;321:202–7.

[103] Raut VV, Orth MS, Orth MC, et al. One stage revision arthroplasty of the hip for deep gram negative infection. Int Orthop 1996;20:12–4.

[104] Sanzen L, Carlsson AS, Josefsson G, et al. Revision operations on infected total hip arthroplasties: two- to nine-year follow-up study. Clin Orthop 1988;229:165–72.

[105] Silva M, Tharani R, Schmalzried TP. Results of direct exchange or debridement of the infected total knee arthroplasty. Clin Orthop 2002;404:125–31.

[106] Ure KJ, Amstutz HC, Nasser S, et al. Direct-exchange arthroplasty for the treatment of infection after total hip replacement: an average ten-year follow-up. J Bone Joint Surg Am 1998;80:961–8.

[107] Wroblewski BM. One-stage revision of infected cemented total hip arthroplasty. Clin Orthop 1986;211:103–7.

[108] Brandt CM, Sistrunk WW, Duffy MC, et al. *Staphylococcus aureus* prosthetic joint infection treated with debridement and prosthesis retention. Clin Infect Dis 1997;24:914–9.

[109] Tattevin P, Cremieux AC, Pottier P, et al. Prosthetic joint infection: when can prosthesis salvage be considered? Clin Infect Dis 1999;29:292–5.

[110] Meehan AM, Osmon DR, Duffy MC, et al. Outcome of penicillin-susceptible streptococcal prosthetic joint infection treated with debridement and retention of the prosthesis. Clin Infect Dis 2003;36:845–9.

[111] Marculescu C, Berbari E, Hanssen A, et al. Outcome of PJI treated with debridement and retention of components [abstract 493]. Presented at the 41st Annual Meeting of Infectious Diseases Society of America. San Diego, CA, October 9–12, 2003.

[112] Crockarell JR, Hanssen AD, Osmon DR, et al. Treatment of infection with debridement and retention of the components following hip arthroplasty. J Bone Joint Surg Am 1998;80:1306–13.

[113] Zimmerli W, Widmer AF, Blatter M, et al. Role of rifampin for treatment of orthopedic implant-related staphylococcal infections: a randomized controlled trial. Foreign-Body Infection (FBI) Study Group. JAMA 1998;279:1537–41.

[114] Drancourt M, Stein A, Argenson JN, et al. Oral rifampin plus ofloxacin for treatment of staphylococcus-infected orthopedic implants. Antimicrob Agents Chemother 1993;37:1214–8.

[115] Segreti J, Nelson JA, Trenholme GM. Prolonged suppressive antibiotic therapy for infected orthopedic prostheses. Clin Infect Dis 1998;27:711–3.

[116] Tsukayama DT, Wicklund B, Gustilo RB. Suppressive antibiotic therapy in chronic prosthetic joint infections. Orthopedics 1991;14:841–4.

[117] Burger RR, Basch T, Hopson CN. Implant salvage in infected total knee arthroplasty. Clin Orthop 1991;273:105–12.

[118] Rasul AT, Tsukayama DT, Gustilo RB. Effect of time of onset and depth of infection on the outcome of total knee arthroplasty infections. Clin Orthop 1991;273:98–104.

[119] Schoifet SD, Morrey BF. Treatment of infection after total knee arthroplasty by debridement with retention of the components. J Bone Joint Surg Am 1990;72:1383–90.

[120] Soriano A, Garcia S, Ortega M, et al. Treatment of acute infection of total or partial hip arthroplasty with debridement and oral chemotherapy. Med Clin (Barc) 2003;121: 81–5.

[121] Waldman BJ, Hostin E, Mont MA, et al. Infected total knee arthroplasty treated by arthroscopic irrigation and debridement. J Arthroplasty 2000;15:430–6.

[122] Bernard L, Hoffmeyer P, Assal M, et al. Trends in the treatment of orthopaedic prosthetic infections. J Antimicrob Chemother 2004;53:127–9.

[123] Canner GC, Steinberg ME, Heppenstall RB, et al. The infected hip after total hip arthroplasty. J Bone Joint Surg Am 1984;66:1393–9.

[124] Kantor GS, Osterkamp JA, Dorr LD, et al. Resection arthroplasty following infected total hip replacement arthroplasty. J Arthroplasty 1986;1:83–9.

[125] Grauer JD, Amstutz HC, O'Carroll PF, et al. Resection arthroplasty of the hip. J Bone Joint Surg Am 1989;71:669–78.

[126] McElwaine JP, Colville J. Excision arthroplasty for infected total hip replacements. J Bone Joint Surg Br 1984;66:168–71.

[127] Bittar ES, Petty W. Girdlestone arthroplasty for infected total hip arthroplasty. Clin Orthop 1982;170:83–7.

[128] Falahee MH, Matthews LS, Kaufer H. Resection arthroplasty as a salvage procedure for a knee with infection after a total arthroplasty. J Bone Joint Surg Am 1987;69:1013–21.

[129] Gillespie WJ. Prevention and management of infection after total joint replacement. Clin Infect Dis 1997;25:1310–7.

[130] Manzotti A, Pullen C, Deromedis B, et al. Knee arthrodesis after infected total knee arthroplasty using the Ilizarov method. Clin Orthop 2001;389:143–9.

[131] Bengston S, Knutson K, Lidgren L. Treatment of infected knee arthroplasty. Clin Orthop 1989;245:173–8.

[132] Rand JA, Bryan RS, Chao EY. Failed total knee arthroplasty treated by arthrodesis of the knee using the Ace-Fischer apparatus. J Bone Joint Surg Am 1987;69:39–45.

[133] David R, Shtarker H, Horesh Z, et al. Arthrodesis with the Ilizarov device after failed knee arthroplasty. Orthopedics 2001;24:33–6.

[134] Oostenbroek HJ, van Roermund PM. Arthrodesis of the knee after an infected arthroplasty using the Ilizarov method. J Bone Joint Surg Br 2001;83:50–4.

[135] Wiedel JD. Salvage of infected total knee fusion: the last option. Clin Orthop 2002;404: 139–42.

[136] Donley BG, Matthews LS, Kaufer H. Arthrodesis of the knee with an intramedullary nail. J Bone Joint Surg Am 1991;73:907–13.

[137] Incavo SJ, Lilly JW, Bartlett CS, et al. Arthrodesis of the knee: experience with intramedullary nailing. J Arthroplasty 2000;15:871–6.

[138] Waldman BJ, Mont MA, Payman KR, et al. Infected total knee arthroplasty treated with arthrodesis using a modular nail. Clin Orthop 1999;367:230–7.

[139] Wilde AH, Stearns KL. Intramedullary fixation for arthrodesis of the knee after infected total knee arthroplasty. Clin Orthop 1989;248:87–92.

[140] Ellingsen DE, Rand JA. Intramedullary arthrodesis of the knee after failed total knee arthroplasty. J Bone Joint Surg Am 1994;76:870–7.

[141] Rand JA. Alternatives to reimplantation for salvage of the total knee arthroplasty complicated by infection. J Bone Joint Surg Am 1993;75:282–9.

[142] Damron TA, McBeath AA. Arthrodesis following failed total knee arthroplasty: comprehensive review and meta-analysis of recent literature. Orthopedics 1995;18:361–8.

[143] Kaufer H, Matthews LS. Resection arthroplasty: an alternative to arthrodesis for salvage of the infected total knee arthroplasty. Instr Course Lect 1986;35:283–9.

[144] Benson ER, Resine ST, Lewis CG. Functional outcome of arthrodesis for failed total knee arthroplasty. Orthopedics 1998;21:875–9.

[145] Isiklar ZU, Landon GC, Tullos HS. Amputation after failed total knee arthroplasty. Clin Orthop 1994;299:173–8.

[146] Sierra RJ, Trousdale RT, Pagnano MW. Above-the-knee amputation after a total knee replacement: prevalence, etiology, and functional outcome. J Bone Joint Surg Am 2003; 85-A:1000–4.

[147] Widmer AF, Frei R, Rajacic Z, et al. Correlation between in vivo and in vitro efficacy of antimicrobial agents against foreign body infections. J Infect Dis 1990;162:96–102.

[148] Blaser J, Vergeres P, Widmer AF, et al. In vivo verification of in vitro model of antibiotic treatment of device-related infection. Antimicrob Agents Chemother 1995;39:1134–9.

[149] Widmer AF, Gaechter A, Ochsner PE, et al. Antimicrobial treatment of orthopedic implant-related infections with rifampin combinations. Clin Infect Dis 1992;14:1251–3.

[150] Drancourt M, Stein A, Argenson JN, et al. Oral treatment of *Staphylococcus* spp. infected orthopaedic implants with fusidic acid or ofloxacin in combination with rifampicin. J Antimicrob Chemother 1997;39:235–40.

[151] Razonable RR, Osmon DR, Steckelberg JM. Linezolid therapy for orthopedic infections. Mayo Clin Proc 2004;79:1137–44.

[152] Rho JP, Sia IG, Crum BA, et al. Linezolid-associated peripheral neuropathy. Mayo Clin Proc 2004;79:927–30.

[153] Marculescu C, Berbari E, Hanssen A, et al. Significance of acute inflammation in joint tissue at reimplantation arthroplasty in patients with prosthetic joint infection treated with two-stage exchange [abstract 283]. Presented at the 41st Annual Meeting of Infectious Diseases Society of America. San Diego, CA, October 9–12, 2003.

[154] Goulet JA, Pellicci PM, Brause BD, et al. Prolonged suppression of infection in total hip arthroplasty. J Arthroplasty 1988;3:109–16.

[155] Rao N, Crossett LS, Sinha RK, et al. Long-term suppression of infection in total joint arthroplasty. Clin Orthop 2003;414:55–60.

[156] Johnson DP, Bannister GC. The outcome of infected arthroplasty of the knee. J Bone Joint Surg Br 1986;68:289–91.

[157] Heck D, Rosenberg A, Schink-Ascani M, et al. Use of antibiotic-impregnated cement during hip and knee arthroplasty in the United States. J Arthroplasty 1995;10:470–5.

[158] Hofmann AA, Kane KR, Tkach TK, et al. Treatment of infected total knee arthroplasty using an articulating spacer. Clin Orthop 1995;321:45–54.

[159] Hendriks JG, Neut D, van Horn JR, et al. The release of gentamicin from acrylic bone cements in a simulated prosthesis-related interfacial gap. J Biomed Mater Res 2003;64B:1–5.

[160] Magnan B, Regis D, Biscaglia R, et al. Preformed acrylic bone cement spacer loaded with antibiotics: use of two-stage procedure in 10 patients because of infected hips after total replacement. Acta Orthop Scand 2001;72:591–4.

[161] Duncan CP, Beauchamp C. A temporary antibiotic-loaded joint replacement system for management of complex infections involving the hip. Orthop Clin North Am 1993;24:751–9.

[162] Duncan CP, Masri B. Antibiotic depots. J Bone Joint Surg Br 1993;75:349–50.

[163] Masri BA, Kendall RW, Duncan CP, et al. Two-stage exchange arthroplasty using a functional antibiotic-loaded spacer in the treatment of the infected knee replacement: the Vancouver experience. Semin Arthroplasty 1994;5:122–36.

[164] Haddad FS, Masri BA, Campbell D, et al. The PROSTALAC functional spacer in two-stage revision for infected knee replacements: prosthesis of antibiotic-loaded acrylic cement. J Bone Joint Surg Br 2000;82:807–12.

[165] Perry AC, Prpa B, Rouse MS, et al. Levofloxacin and trovafloxacin inhibition of experimental fracture-healing. Clin Orthop 2003;414:95–100.

[166] Huddleston PM, Steckelberg JM, Hanssen AD, et al. Ciprofloxacin inhibition of experimental fracture healing. J Bone Joint Surg Am 2000;82:161–73.

[167] Silverberg D, Kodali P, Dipersio J, et al. In vitro analysis of antifungal impregnated polymethylmethacrylate bone cement. Clin Orthop 2002;403:228–31.

[168] Hall EW, Rouse MS, Jacofsky DJ, et al. Release of daptomycin from polymethylmethacrylate beads in a continuous flow chamber. Diagn Microbiol Infect Dis 2004;50: 261–5.

[169] Hendriks JG, van Horn JR, van der Mei HC, et al. Backgrounds of antibiotic-loaded bone cement and prosthesis-related infection. Biomaterials 2004;25:545–56.

[170] Joseph TN, Chen AL, Di Cesare PE. Use of antibiotic-impregnated cement in total joint arthroplasty. J Am Acad Orthop Surg 2003;11:38–47.

[171] von Eiff C, Proctor RA, Peters G. *Staphylococcus aureus* small colony variants: formation and clinical impact. Int J Clin Pract Suppl 2000;115:44–9.

[172] von Eiff C, Proctor RA, Peters G. Small colony variants of staphylococci: a link to persistent infections. Berl Munch Tierarztl Wochenschr 2000;113:321–5.

[173] Proctor RA, van Langevelde P, Kristjansson M, et al. Persistent and relapsing infections associated with small-colony variants of *Staphylococcus aureus*. Clin Infect Dis 1995;20: 95–102.

[174] Hanssen AD, Trousdale RT, Osmon DR. Patient outcome with reinfection following reimplantation for the infected total knee arthroplasty. Clin Orthop 1995;321:55–67.

[175] Ross JJ, Saltzman CL, Carling P, et al. Pneumococcal septic arthritis: review of 190 cases. Clin Infect Dis 2003;36:319–27.

[176] Phelan DM, Osmon DR, Keating MR, et al. Delayed reimplantation arthroplasty for candidal prosthetic joint infection: a report of 4 cases and review of the literature. Clin Infect Dis 2002;34:930–8.

[177] Spinner RJ, Sexton DJ, Goldner RD, et al. Periprosthetic infections due to *Mycobacterium tuberculosis* in patients with no prior history of tuberculosis. J Arthroplasty 1996;11: 217–22.

[178] Berbari EF, Hanssen AD, Duffy MC, et al. Prosthetic joint infection due to *Mycobacterium tuberculosis*: a case series and review of the literature. Am J Orthop 1998;27:219–27.

[179] Weil Y, Mattan Y, Liebergall M, et al. Brucella prosthetic joint infection: a report of 3 cases and a review of the literature. Clin Infect Dis 2003;36:e81–6.

[180] Herold RC, Lotke PA, MacGregor RR. Prosthetic joint infections secondary to rapidly growing *Mycobacterium fortuitum*. Clin Orthop 1987;216:183–6.

[181] Weiler PJ, Hastings DE. Listeria monocytogenes: an unusual cause of late infection in a prosthetic hip joint. J Rheumatol 1990;17:705–7.

[182] Jellicoe PA, Cohen A, Campbell P. *Haemophilus parainfluenzae* complicating total hip arthroplasty: a rapid failure. J Arthroplasty 2002;17:114–6.

[183] Iglesias L, Garcia-Arenzana JM, Valiente A, et al. *Yersinia enterocolitica* O:3 infection of a prosthetic knee joint related to recurrent hemarthrosis. Scand J Infect Dis 2002;34:132–3.

[184] Bates CJ, Clarke TC, Spencer RC. Prosthetic hip joint infection due to *Campylobacter fetus*. J Clin Microbiol 1994;32:2037.

[185] Fresard A, Guglielminotti C, Berthelot P, et al. Prosthetic joint infection caused by *Tropheryma whippelii* (Whipple's bacillus). Clin Infect Dis 1996;22:575–6.

[186] Maradona JA, Asensi V, Carton JA, et al. Prosthetic joint infection by *Pasteurella multocida*. Eur J Clin Microbiol Infect Dis 1997;16:623–5.

[187] McCarthy J, Stingemore N. *Clostridium difficile* infection of a prosthetic joint presenting 12 months after antibiotic-associated diarrhoea. J Infect 1999;39:94–6.

INFECTIOUS
DISEASE CLINICS
OF NORTH AMERICA

ELSEVIER
SAUNDERS

Infect Dis Clin N Am 19 (2005) 915–929

Management of Open Fractures

Charalampos G. Zalavras, MD[a],
Michael J. Patzakis, MD[a],*, Paul D. Holtom, MD[a],
Randy Sherman, MD[b]

[a]*Keck School of Medicine of University of Southern California, 2025 Zonal Avenue,
GNH 3900, Los Angeles, CA 90089-9312, USA*
[b]*Keck School of Medicine of University of Southern California, 2000 Doheny Eye Institute
Los Angeles, CA 90089-9224, USA*

An open fracture is characterized by soft tissue disruption that results in communication of the fracture site with the outside environment [1]. Open fractures are severe injuries with a potential for serious complications, such as infection and nonunion, and they constitute a challenging problem for the treating physician. During the past 3 decades, improved understanding of infection and fracture biology principles, new devices for fracture stabilization, and development of microsurgical procedures for reconstruction of the soft tissue envelope have considerably improved open fracture management, which aims to prevent infection at the fracture site, achieve fracture union, and restore function.

Principle-based intervention can play a critical role in reducing the morbidity and improving the prognosis. The main principles of open fracture management include careful evaluation of the injury, prevention of infection, wound management with soft tissue coverage, fracture stabilization, and promotion of healing by early bone grafting or other supplemental procedures. Antibiotic administration should start as soon as possible after the injury, and surgical management should begin as soon as the patient has been adequately evaluated and resuscitated. Delayed surgical management in children [2] and adults [3,4] has not been associated with an increased infection rate in patients who received early antibiotic therapy.

* Corresponding author.
E-mail address: edkwong@usc.edu (M.J. Patzakis).

0891-5520/05/$ - see front matter © 2005 Elsevier Inc. All rights reserved.
doi:10.1016/j.idc.2005.08.001
id.theclinics.com

Evaluation and classification

Open fractures usually result from high-energy trauma, with motorcycle, motor vehicle, and auto versus pedestrian injuries accounting for most cases [5,6]. Open fractures can be accompanied by potentially life-threatening trauma of other organ systems, or by musculoskeletal injuries elsewhere. Associated injuries involving intra-abdominal organs, chest, skull, pelvis, and major blood vessels are seen in 50% of open fracture patients [5]. Therefore, detailed evaluation and appropriate resuscitation of the patient presenting with an open fracture is necessary.

The neurovascular status of the injured extremity should be carefully assessed and documented. Open fractures are complicated by compartment syndrome in up to 9% of cases, especially in injuries with a severe crushing component [7].

The surrounding soft tissues are by definition disrupted to a variable degree in all open fractures. The associated soft tissue injury has several adverse consequences. Exposed bone, articular cartilage, tendons, and nerves will desiccate, and exposed hardware will facilitate infection. Soft tissue injury compromises vascularity at the fracture site, thus diminishing the healing potential and host immune response to infection. Finally, communication of the fracture site with the outside environment leads to contamination with infectious microorganisms [4,8,9] or even introduction of foreign bodies into the wound.

High-energy trauma can result in comminution and displacement of bone fragments, which may be stripped from their soft tissue attachments. Loss of bone fragments at the time of injury is also possible. Thus, the structural integrity and viability of the injured bone may be severely compromised depending on the severity of injury.

Classification systems

The severity of injury can vary considerably between cases. Therefore, a classification system of open fractures based on the earlier evaluation will help describe the injury, provide guidelines for treatment, determine prognosis, and compare various treatment methods for research purposes. The classification system of Gustilo and Anderson [8], subsequently modified by Gustilo and colleagues [10], has been widely used and comprises the following types:

Type I: Puncture wound of 1 cm or less, with minimal contamination or muscle crushing.
Type II: Laceration more than 1 cm long with moderate soft tissue damage and crushing. Bone coverage is adequate and comminution is minimal.
Type IIIA: Extensive soft tissue damage, often caused by a high-energy injury with a severe crushing component. Massively contaminated

wounds and severely comminuted or segmental fractures are included in this subtype. Bone coverage is adequate.

Type IIIB: Extensive soft tissue damage with periosteal stripping and bone exposure, usually with severe contamination and bone comminution. Flap coverage is required.

Type IIIC: Arterial injury requiring repair.

However, the reliability of this classification has been questioned. Evaluation of the responses of orthopaedic surgeons asked to classify open fractures of the tibia on the basis of videotaped case presentations showed that the average agreement among the observers to be 60% overall [11]. It is important to emphasize that the true extent and severity of the injury cannot be accurately assessed in the emergency department. Classification of the fracture should be conducted only in the operating room, after wound exploration and debridement. The degrees of contamination and soft tissue crushing are important factors for classifying an open fracture that may be mistakenly overlooked in a wound of small size.

Reconstruction or amputation?

Reconstruction and salvage of a severely traumatized extremity, although possible with advances in microsurgical techniques, are not always indicated. The treating surgeon may be confronted with the dilemma of salvage versus amputation of a nonviable extremity with a type IIIC open fracture or a mangled extremity with a IIIB fracture. Recovery of function in a salvaged but severely injured extremity may be limited or absent, despite multiple reconstructive procedures with associated morbidity and prolonged hospitalization. Moreover, leg prostheses offer satisfactory restoration of function, especially for below-knee amputations, thereby making the appropriate decision difficult. Georgiadis and colleagues [12] concluded that early below-knee amputation resulted in faster recovery and reduced long-term disability compared with successful limb-salvage. However, Bosse an colleagues [13] reported that reconstruction of extremities at high risk for amputation resulted in 2-year outcomes equivalent to those of amputation.

In deciding how to best treat the mangled extremity, patient and extremity factors should be considered. Patient factors include the general condition and age of the patient. Pre-existing medical problems and associated injuries resulting in cardiopulmonary or hemodynamic compromise militate against a lengthy salvage procedure, especially in a patient of advanced age. Conditions adversely affecting the blood vessels, such as diabetes mellitus, vasculitis, and smoking, will increase the risk for anastomosis failure. The occupation, functional requirements, and socioeconomic background of the patient are important because the salvage attempt is accompanied by prolonged disability time, increased psychologic distress, and financial demands [12].

Important extremity factors include the time elapsed since injury, the severity of the injury, and the previous functional status of the extremity. Warm ischemia time greater than 6 hours leads to irreversible changes in cellular structure of muscle. Revascularization of a limb with prolonged ischemia may lead to acidosis, hyperkalemia, and rhabdomyolysis. Severe crushing and avulsion compromise the functional result. Tibial nerve disruption deprives the sole of the foot from protective sensation. Finally, a history of major trauma, neurologic disease, or congenital deformity resulting in impaired function may not justify a salvage attempt.

Specialized scoring systems, such as the mangled extremity severity score (MESS), appear to offer guidelines for decision making in lower extremity injuries [14]. However, the final decision should be an individualized one, based on sound judgment and assessment of patient and extremity parameters [15]. The patient should be informed of the potential risks and benefits of surgery and the possibility of early or late amputation.

Prevention of infection

Prevention of infection is a main goal of open fracture management. Approximately 65% of patients who have open fractures have wound contamination with microorganisms [4,8,9].Therefore, antibiotics are not used for prophylaxis but rather for treatment of wound contamination. The risk for infection depends on the severity of injury and ranges from 0% to 2% for type I open fractures, 2% to 10% for type II, and 10% to 50% for type III fractures [4,8].

Prevention of infection is based on immediate antibiotic administration and wound debridement. Tetanus prophylaxis may be necessary based on the patient's immunization status.

Wound cultures

The usefulness of wound cultures obtained at patient presentation or intraoperatively has been controversial because the cultures often fail to identify the organism causing the infection [16,17]. A randomized controlled trial reported that only 3 (18%) of 17 infections that developed in a series of 171 open fractures were caused by an organism identified by the initial cultures [18]. Wound cultures obtained before wound debridement have a very low predictive value and are no longer recommended [16]. The results of postdebridement cultures and sensitivity testing may help in selecting the best agents for subsequent procedures or in the case of an early infection.

Systemic antibiotic therapy

Antibiotic therapy decreases the risk for infection in patients who have open fractures, and the early administration of antibiotics is an important factor in reducing the infection rate. Patzakis and colleagues [9] established the role of antibiotics in a prospective randomized study that showed a marked decrease of the infection rate when cephalothin was administered before debridement (2.3%, 2/84 fractures) compared with no antibiotics (13.9%, 11/79 fractures).

The selected antibiotic therapy should target the organisms likely to cause infection. In most cases, the organisms initially present in the wound are not the ones that cause infection later. Most infections are caused by staphylococci and aerobic gram-negative bacilli, therefore antibiotic therapy should target gram-positive and gram-negative pathogens.

An effective and commonly used regimen consists of a first-generation cephalosporin (eg, cefazolin) that is active against gram-positive organisms, combined with an aminoglycoside (eg, gentamicin or tobramycin) that is active against gram-negative organisms. Alternatives to aminoglycosides include quinolones, aztreonam, third-generation cephalosporins, or other antibiotics with gram-negative coverage. Systemic administration of aminoglycosides is not necessary if aminoglycoside-impregnated beads are used for local antibiotic delivery.

Anaerobic infections, such as clostridial myonecrosis (gas gangrene), are a particular concern in injuries occurring in farms that may result in contamination with clostridial organisms, and in vascular injuries that may create conditions of ischemia and low oxygen tension. Therefore, ampicillin or penicillin should be added to the antibiotic regimen in these cases to provide coverage against anaerobes.

Some investigators have proposed administration of cefazolin as a single agent in type I open fractures [19]. However, this regimen does not provide reliable coverage against contaminating gram-negative organisms. In addition, a type IIIA open fracture with a small wound size may be misclassified, and thus mistakenly treated only with a cephalosporin. Patzakis and Wilkins [4] reported that in open tibia fractures, combination therapy reduced the infection rate (4.5%, 5/109) compared with cephalosporin only (13%, 25/192). Type I and II fractures were not analyzed separately, but the distribution of fracture types was comparable between the two groups.

Fluoroquinolones may be useful in this setting based on their broad-spectrum antimicrobial coverage, bactericidal properties, high oral bioavailability, and good tolerability. Ciprofloxacin as a single agent was shown in a randomized prospective study to be effective in the management of type I and II open fractures, resulting in a similar infection rate (6%) compared with combination therapy with cefamandole and gentamicin [18]. However, in type III open fractures, ciprofloxacin was associated with a higher infection rate of 31% (8/26) compared with 7.7% (2/26) in the combination therapy group. Therefore, in type III open fractures, ciprofloxacin can be used instead of an aminoglycoside and combined with a cephalosporin, but should not be used as monotherapy. In open fracture wounds secondary to low-velocity gunshot injuries, oral ciprofloxacin was found to be as effective as intravenous administration of cephapirin sodium and gentamicin

[20]. However, quinolones have been associated with inhibition of osteoblasts and experimental bone healing [21,22]. Healing potential is compromised in open fractures, so further investigation is needed to clarify the clinical benefit of quinolone use.

Antibiotic administration should be started promptly, as delay of more than 3 hours increases the risk for infection [4]. The optimal duration of antibiotic therapy remains controversial. The length of antibiotic therapy is generally 3 days, although 1 day has been proposed by some investigators [23,24]. The duration of therapy should be limited to 3 days because prolonged therapy may select for resistant organisms. An additional 3-day administration of antibiotics is recommended for subsequent surgical procedures, such as wound coverage and bone grafting [4,19].

The growing problem of antimicrobial resistance in bacteria is complicating the management of open fractures. Methicillin-resistant *S aureus* has become a community-acquired pathogen and a nosocomial hazard. Multidrug-resistant gram-negative bacilli are increasing in frequency. Vancomycin-resistant *Enterococcus faecium* has become an important nosocomial pathogen in the United States, but thus far has been rarely seen in osteomyelitis. The greatest concern is the development of vancomycin-resistant *S aureus* (VRSA). Although infections with VRSA have been rarely reported, bone infections with this organism could be catastrophic as it is resistant to the standard antibiotics used in empiric therapy.

Local antibiotic therapy

Local therapy with antibiotic-impregnated delivery vehicles has been used as an adjunct to systemic antibiotic therapy in the treatment of open fractures. The most commonly used delivery vehicle is polymethylmethacrylate (PMMA) cement, which can be molded to bead-resembling spheres with a diameter ranging from 5 to 10 mm, or to spacer blocks of larger size. The spherical shape of the beads increases the surface area, thereby promoting the release of antibiotics and facilitating drainage of secretions. Bioabsorbable delivery vehicles, such as calcium sulfate, synthetic polymers, and fibrin clots, appear to be a promising alternative and are currently under investigation [25–27].

Many antimicrobial agents have been successfully incorporated into PMMA cement for local delivery, including aminoglycosides, vancomycin, and cephalosporins [28]. An antibiotic appropriate for local delivery must be available in powder form because antibiotics in aqueous solution inhibit the polymerization process. It must also be heat-stable to withstand the temperatures generated during the exothermic polymerization reaction, and should be active against the targeted microbial pathogens. In open fractures, aminoglycosides are common choices because of their broad spectrum of activity, heat stability, and low allergenicity.

The release of antibiotic from the delivery vehicle to the surrounding tissues is called *elution* and is determined by the difference in the concentration of antibiotics between the antibiotic delivery system and its environment. Elution is facilitated by an increased surface–area-to-volume ratio of the delivery vehicle [29] and by a high concentration of antibiotic in the beads or spacer [30]. The type of antibiotic is also important, and tobramycin has superior elution properties compared with vancomycin [31]. A fluid medium is necessary for elution of antibiotics, and the rate of fluid turnover influences the elution and local antibiotic concentration [32]. Elution of antibiotics from PMMA beads follows a biphasic pattern, with an initial rapid phase and a secondary slow phase [33].

Although gentamicin-impregnated PMMA beads are commercially available in Europe (Septopal, Biomet-Merck, Bridgend, UK), the Food and Drug Administration has not approved a similar antibiotic-impregnated product for use in the United States. The delivery system has to be prepared in the operating room by the surgeon immediately before use [28]. The PMMA powder is mixed with the antibiotic in powder form, polymerized, and formed into beads that are then incorporated on a 24-gauge wire. Usually 3.6 g of tobramycin are mixed with 40 g of PMMA cement. Vancomycin is not recommended as an initial agent because of concerns regarding resistant enterococci. Antibiotic-impregnated PMMA beads are inserted in the open fracture wound, which is subsequently sealed by OpSite (Smith and Nephew, Hull, UK) or a similar semipermeable barrier so that the eluted antibiotic remains at the involved area to achieve a high local concentration.

The bead-pouch technique has unique advantages. First, a high local concentration of antibiotics is achieved, which is often 10 to 20 times higher than with systemic administration and decreases the need for systemic use of aminoglycosides. Second, the systemic concentration remains low, thus minimizing the adverse effects of aminoglycosides. Finally, the sealing of the wound from the external environment by the semipermeable barrier prevents secondary contamination by nosocomial pathogens and may safely extend the period for soft tissue transfers. In addition, OpSite establishes an aerobic wound environment, which is important for avoiding catastrophic anaerobic infections; maintains the local antibiotic within the wound; and promotes patient comfort by avoiding painful dressing changes.

The antibiotic bead pouch technique has been shown to reduce the infection rate when used in addition to systemic antibiotics for management of open fractures [34–38]. In a series of 1085 open fractures, Ostermann and colleagues [37] compared systemic antibiotics alone with combined treatment with systemic antibiotics and the bead pouch technique. The infection rate was 3.7% (31/845 fractures) in the antibiotic bead pouch group, which was considerably lower than the 12% (29/240 fractures) infection rate in open fractures treated with local antibiotics. Analysis of the results based on the severity of the open fracture showed that the reduction of infection was statistically significant in type III fractures only (6.5% for the antibiotic bead pouch versus 20.6% for systemic antibiotics alone). However, in this study wound treatment was not identical between the two groups. In the systemic antibiotic group, only 37% of wounds were closed primarily and the remaining wounds were left open initially, thereby predisposing the wounds to secondary contamination. In the antibiotic bead pouch group, 95% of wounds were either closed primarily or sealed with OpSite. Therefore, the relative contribution of the local antibiotic versus the sealing of the wound cannot be determined.

In a randomized controlled trial, Moehring and colleagues [39] compared antibiotic beads as the only method of antibiotic therapy (after a single systemic dose in the emergency department) with systemic antibiotics in open fractures and observed an infection rate of 8.3% (2/24 fractures) versus 5.3% (2/38 fractures), respectively. However, an unanticipated third group of patients emerged, with 18% (12/67) of patients treated with beads and systemic antibiotics secondary to limb-threatening injuries or for nonorthopedic reasons.

Wound management

Wound management includes debridement, irrigation, and subsequent wound closure if adequate coverage can be achieved with the soft tissues available, or soft tissue reconstruction with local or free muscle flaps.

Debridement

Thorough surgical debridement plays a critical role in the management of open fractures because devitalized tissue and foreign material promote the growth of microorganisms and constitute a barrier for the host's defense mechanisms. Debridement should be performed in the operating room. When the injury wound is insufficient for thorough assessment of the injury, such as in type I and II open fractures, the existing wound should be extended. Surgical extension of the wound should respect the vascularity of soft tissue flaps and facilitate fracture fixation and anticipated reconstructive procedures. Skin and subcutaneous tissue are sharply debrided back to bleeding edges. Muscle is debrided until bleeding is visualized. Viable muscle can be identified by its bleeding, color, and contractility. Bone fragments without soft tissue attachments are avascular and should be discarded. Articular fragments, however, should be preserved even if they have no attached blood supply, provided they are large enough and the surgeon believes reconstruction of the involved joint is possible. A repeat debridement can be performed after 24 to 48 hours, based on the degree of contamination and soft tissue damage. The goal is a clean wound with viable tissues and no infection. In injuries requiring flap coverage, debridement should also be repeated at the time of the soft tissue procedure.

Irrigation

Irrigation mechanically removes foreign bodies and reduces the bacterial concentration. Although consensus exists on the need for irrigation, the irrigation solution and delivery pressure remain controversial. Antiseptic solutions may be toxic to host cells and are best avoided. Antibiotic solutions have been shown in animal and in vitro studies to be more effective than saline alone, but clinical data on open fracture wounds are lacking. Detergent solutions help remove bacteria and appear to be a promising alternative [40].

High-pressure pulsatile lavage was associated in experimental studies with a detrimental effect on early new bone formation [41] and damage to bone architecture with bacterial seeding into the intramedullary canal [42]. Low-pressure lavage, however, may not be as effective in removing adherent bacteria if more than 6 hours have elapsed since the injury [43]. No clinical studies have yet addressed the effects of different irrigation methods on infection and fracture healing. The authors advocate irrigating the wound with 10 L of saline by gravity tubing, and adding 50,000 units of bacitracin and 1 million units of polymyxin in the last liter of irrigation fluid.

Wound closure

The optimal time for wound closure is still debated [44]. Primary wound closure following a thorough debridement is not associated with an increased rate of infection, may prevent secondary contamination, and may reduce surgical morbidity, hospital stay, and cost [4,45]. However, the main disadvantage of primary closure is the potential for gas gangrene. Gas gangrene (clostridial myonecrosis) is a catastrophic complication that may lead to loss of the limb or even to death of the patient [46]. Primary wound closure, inadequate debridement, and inadequate antibiotic therapy increase the risk for this complication [47].

Delayed wound closure—within 3 to 7 days—prevents anaerobic conditions in the wound, permits drainage, allows for repeat debridements at 24- to 48-hour intervals, gives time to tissues of questionable viability to declare themselves, and facilitates use of the antibiotic bead-pouch technique. Sealing of the wound with OpSite prevents secondary contamination, makes delayed wound closure even more preferable, and possibly prolongs the time window to closure.

The additional surgical wound, created to assess the condition of the bone and soft tissues and facilitate debridement, can be safely closed primarily in type I and II open fractures, leaving the injury wound open. If the injury wound is directly over the bone, it can be closed and the wound away from the fracture site left open. Patzakis and colleagues coined the phrase *partial wound closure* to describe this technique [48]. In type III injuries, the wound should be left open in its entirety.

Soft tissue reconstruction

When extensive damage to the soft tissues is present, as in type IIIB open fractures, adequate coverage may not be possible and soft tissue reconstruction should be performed. The importance of a viable soft tissue envelope cannot be overemphasized. The soft tissue envelope is a source of vascularity at the fracture site, promoting fracture healing, antibiotic delivery, and host defense mechanisms. It provides durable coverage, preventing secondary contamination of the wound and desiccation of bone, articular cartilage, tendons, and nerves. The selection of coverage depends on the location and magnitude of the soft tissue defect [49–51]. Soft tissue reconstruction is usually achieved with local or free tissue transfers, and a microvascular surgeon should always evaluate an open fracture with extensive soft tissue damage and participate in its management.

Local pedicle muscle flaps include the gastrocnemius for proximal third tibia fractures and the soleus for middle third fractures. In distal third tibia fractures, free muscle flaps such as the latissimus dorsi, the rectus abdominis, and the gracilis muscle are necessary [52,53]. Free muscle flaps may be considered even in more proximally located fractures for two reasons. First, the local muscles usually participate in the zone of injury, thus their viability may be compromised. Pollak and colleagues [53] concluded that use of a free flap in limbs with a severe osseous injury was associated with fewer wound complications necessitating operative treatment compared with a rotational flap. Second, even if local muscles are not damaged, their transfer will deprive the already traumatized leg of function [54]. On the other hand, free muscle transfer is more demanding, technically for the surgeon and physiologically for the patient. In injuries with exposed tendons, fasciocutaneous flaps, such as the radial forearm flap, are preferred to facilitate tendon gliding.

Soft tissue reconstruction should be performed early, within the first 7 days. Delays beyond 7 to 10 days have been associated with increased flap and infectious complications [17,55]. Godina [56] even argued in favor of flap coverage within 72 hours. He observed flap failure in less than 1% (1/134) of early cases compared with 12% (20/167) in patients operated on within 4 to 90 days. The infection rate was only 1.5% (2/134) in the early group, whereas it increased to 17.5% (29/167) in the other one. Gopal and colleagues [52] also used an early aggressive protocol in type IIIB and IIIC open fractures and observed deep infection in 6% (4/63) of fractures that were covered within 72 hours, compared with 29% (6/21) in the ones covered beyond 72 hours. It should be stressed that in all these studies the antibiotic bead pouch had not been used, and therefore secondary contamination was a factor contributing to the infectious complications.

Fracture fixation

Stable fracture fixation is necessary in open fractures, preventing further injury to the soft tissues and enhancing the host response to infectious organisms despite the presence of implants [57]. In addition, stable fixation facilitates wound and patient care and allows early motion and functional rehabilitation of the extremity. Fracture stabilization can be accomplished with intramedullary nailing, external fixation, or plate and screw fixation. The choice of method depends on the fractured bone, location of the fracture (eg, intra-articular, metaphyseal, diaphyseal), soft tissue injury, and surgeon's expertise.

Intramedullary nailing is an effective method for stabilizing diaphyseal fractures of the lower extremity [58–60]. Statically interlocked intramedullary nailing maintains length and alignment of the fracture bone, is biomechanically superior to other methods, and does not interfere with soft tissue management. However, it is technically more demanding and disrupts the endosteal bone circulation to a variable degree, depending on the extent of reaming of the medullary canal.

External fixation is useful in wounds with severe soft tissue damage and contamination, as in type IIIB and IIIC open fractures, because no hardware is implanted and the vascularity of the fracture is not disturbed [61–63]. It is applied in a technically easy, safe, and expedient way with minimal blood loss at a site distant to the injury, and does not interfere with wound management. External fixation is particularly suitable for diaphyseal tibia fractures because of the subcutaneous location of the bone. Ring or transarticular fixators may be used for periarticular fractures. The disadvantages of the technique are the necessity for patient compliance and the associated complications of pin tract infections.

Plate and screw fixation is useful in intraarticular and metaphyseal fractures because it allows restoration of joint congruency and orientation, and in upper extremity diaphyseal fractures without massive contamination. Plate and screw fixation has the advantage of accurate restoration of the anatomy. Screw fixation can be used for fixation of intra-articular fragments, either alone or in conjunction with a ring or transarticular fixator.

Early secondary procedures to stimulate healing

In the presence of bone defects or delayed healing, the authors advocate early bone grafting. The preferred timing for bone grafting ranges in the literature from 2 to 6 weeks after soft tissue coverage [61,64]. The authors elect to wait for 6 weeks following a soft tissue transfer to ensure the absence of infection and the restoration of the soft tissue envelope. Then, the existing defect is bone grafted. Early bone grafting is also beneficial when healing is delayed and no callus is apparent on radiographs by 8 to 12 weeks. Grafts are applied either at the fracture site beneath a flap or posterolaterally away from the site of injury. Exchange nailing is another option to stimulate healing in cases of delayed union, provided no infection or bone defect is present. Infection necessitates additional debridement, whereas bone defects should be managed with bone grafting. In the presence of large bone defects, specialized reconstructive procedures are required, such as vascularized bone grafts [65] or distraction osteogenesis [66].

Summary

Open fractures are high-energy injuries that require a principle-based approach, starting with detailed evaluation of patient status and injury severity. Early, systemic, wide-spectrum antibiotic therapy should cover gram-positive and gram-negative organisms, and a common regimen is a 3-day administration of a first-generation cephalosporin and an aminoglycoside, supplemented with ampicillin or penicillin to cover anaerobes in farm or vascular injuries. Local antibiotic delivery with the bead pouch technique increases the local concentration of antibiotics, minimizes systemic toxicity, and prevents secondary wound contamination. Thorough irrigation and surgical debridement is critical for prevention of infection. Primary wound closure remains controversial because of concerns for gas gangrene. Partial wound closure is an alternative, with delayed wound closure within 3 to 7 days. In the presence of extensive soft tissue damage, local or free muscle flaps should be transferred to achieve coverage. Stable fracture fixation should be achieved with a method suitable for the bone and soft tissue characteristics. Early bone grafting is indicated for bone defects, unstable fractures treated with external fixation, and delayed union. A management plan guided by the above principles will achieve the goals of prevention of infection, fracture healing, and restoration of function in most of these challenging injuries.

References

[1] Zalavras CG, Patzakis MJ. Open fractures: evaluation and management. J Am Acad Orthop Surg 2003;11:212–9.
[2] Skaggs DL, Friend L, Alman B, et al. The effect of surgical delay on acute infection following 554 open fractures in children. J Bone Joint Surg Am 2005;87:8–12.
[3] Harley BJ, Beaupre LA, Jones CA, et al. The effect of time to definitive treatment on the rate of nonunion and infection in open fractures. J Orthop Trauma 2002;16:484–90.
[4] Patzakis MJ, Wilkins J. Factors influencing infection rate in open fracture wounds. Clin Orthop Relat Res 1989;243:36–40.
[5] Gustilo RB. Management of open fractures. An analysis of 673 cases. Minn Med 1971;54: 185–9.

[6] Court-Brown CM, Rimmer S, Prakash U, et al. The epidemiology of open long bone fractures. Injury 1998;29:529–34.

[7] Blick SS, Brumback RJ, Poka A, et al. Compartment syndrome in open tibial fractures. J Bone Joint Surg Am 1986;68:1348–53.

[8] Gustilo RB, Anderson JT. Prevention of infection in the treatment of one thousand and twenty-five open fractures of long bones: retrospective and prospective analyses. J Bone Joint Surg Am 1976;58:453–8.

[9] Patzakis MJ, Harvey JP Jr, Ivler D. The role of antibiotics in the management of open fractures. J Bone Joint Surg Am 1974;56:532–41.

[10] Gustilo RB, Mendoza RM, Williams DN. Problems in the management of type III (severe) open fractures: a new classification of type III open fractures. J Trauma 1984;24:742–6.

[11] Brumback RJ, Jones AL. Interobserver agreement in the classification of open fractures of the tibia. The results of a survey of two hundred and forty-five orthopaedic surgeons. J Bone Joint Surg Am 1994;76:1162–6.

[12] Georgiadis GM, Behrens FF, Joyce MJ, et al. Open tibial fractures with severe soft-tissue loss. Limb salvage compared with below-the-knee amputation. J Bone Joint Surg Am 1993;75:1431–41.

[13] Bosse MJ, MacKenzie EJ, Kellam JF, et al. An analysis of outcomes of reconstruction or amputation after leg-threatening injuries. N Engl J Med 2002;347:1924–31.

[14] Johansen K, Daines M, Howey T, et al. Objective criteria accurately predict amputation following lower extremity trauma. J Trauma 1990;30:568–72 [discussion: 572–63].

[15] Tornetta P III, Olson SA. Amputation versus limb salvage. Instr Course Lect 1997;46:511–8.

[16] Lee J. Efficacy of cultures in the management of open fractures. Clin Orthop Relat Res 1997; 339:71–5.

[17] Fischer MD, Gustilo RB, Varecka TF. The timing of flap coverage, bone-grafting, and intramedullary nailing in patients who have a fracture of the tibial shaft with extensive soft-tissue injury. J Bone Joint Surg Am 1991;73:1316–22.

[18] Patzakis MJ, Bains RS, Lee J, et al. Prospective, randomized, double-blind study comparing single-agent antibiotic therapy, ciprofloxacin, to combination antibiotic therapy in open fracture wounds. J Orthop Trauma 2000;14:529–33.

[19] Templeman DC, Gulli B, Tsukayama DT, et al. Update on the management of open fractures of the tibial shaft. Clin Orthop Relat Res 1998;350:18–25.

[20] Knapp TP, Patzakis MJ, Lee J, et al. Comparison of intravenous and oral antibiotic therapy in the treatment of fractures caused by low-velocity gunshots. A prospective, randomized study of infection rates. J Bone Joint Surg Am 1996;78:1167–71.

[21] Huddleston PM, Steckelberg JM, Hanssen AD, et al. Ciprofloxacin inhibition of experimental fracture healing. J Bone Joint Surg Am 2000;82:161–73.

[22] Holtom PD, Pavkovic SA, Bravos PD, et al. Inhibitory effects of the quinolone antibiotics trovafloxacin, ciprofloxacin, and levofloxacin on osteoblastic cells in vitro. J Orthop Res 2000;18:721–7.

[23] Dellinger EP, Caplan ES, Weaver LD, et al. Duration of preventive antibiotic administration for open extremity fractures. Arch Surg 1988;123:333–9.

[24] Dellinger EP, Miller SD, Wertz MJ, et al. Risk of infection after open fracture of the arm or leg. Arch Surg 1988;123:1320–7.

[25] Kanellakopoulou K, Giamarellos-Bourboulis EJ. Carrier systems for the local delivery of antibiotics in bone infections. Drugs 2000;59:1223–32.

[26] Mader JT, Stevens CM, Stevens JH, et al. Treatment of experimental osteomyelitis with a fibrin sealant antibiotic implant. Clin Orthop Relat Res 2002;403:58–72.

[27] McKee MD, Wild LM, Schemitsch EH, et al. The use of an antibiotic-impregnated, osteoconductive, bioabsorbable bone substitute in the treatment of infected long bone defects: early results of a prospective trial. J Orthop Trauma 2002;16:622–7.

[28] Zalavras CG, Patzakis MJ, Holtom P. Local antibiotic therapy in the treatment of open fractures and osteomyelitis. Clin Orthop Relat Res 2004;427:86–93.

[29] Holtom PD, Warren CA, Greene NW, et al. Relation of surface area to in vitro elution characteristics of vancomycin-impregnated polymethylmethacrylate spacers. Am J Orthop 1998; 27:207–10.

[30] Baker AS, Greenham LW. Release of gentamicin from acrylic bone cement. Elution and diffusion studies. J Bone Joint Surg Am 1988;70:1551–7.

[31] Greene N, Holtom PD, Warren CA, et al. In vitro elution of tobramycin and vancomycin polymethylmethacrylate beads and spacers from Simplex and Palacos. Am J Orthop 1998; 27:201–5.

[32] Holtom PD, Patzakis MJ. Newer methods of antimicrobial delivery for bone and joint infections. Instr Course Lect 2003;52:745–9.

[33] Torholm C, Lidgren L, Lindberg L, et al. Total hip joint arthroplasty with gentamicin-impregnated cement. A clinical study of gentamicin excretion kinetics. Clin Orthop Relat Res 1983;181:99–106.

[34] Henry SL, Ostermann PA, Seligson D. The prophylactic use of antibiotic impregnated beads in open fractures. J Trauma 1990;30:1231–8.

[35] Henry SL, Ostermann PA, Seligson D. The antibiotic bead pouch technique. The management of severe compound fractures. Clin Orthop Relat Res 1993;295:54–62.

[36] Ostermann PA, Henry SL, Seligson D. The role of local antibiotic therapy in the management of compound fractures. Clin Orthop Relat Res 1993;295:102–11.

[37] Ostermann PA, Seligson D, Henry SL. Local antibiotic therapy for severe open fractures. A review of 1085 consecutive cases. J Bone Joint Surg Br 1995;77:93–7.

[38] Keating JF, Blachut PA, O'Brien PJ, et al. Reamed nailing of open tibial fractures: does the antibiotic bead pouch reduce the deep infection rate? J Orthop Trauma 1996;10:298–303.

[39] Moehring HD, Gravel C, Chapman MW, et al. Comparison of antibiotic beads and intravenous antibiotics in open fractures. Clin Orthop Relat Res 2000;372:254–61.

[40] Burd T, Christensen GD, Anglen JO, et al. Sequential irrigation with common detergents: a promising new method for decontaminating orthopedic wounds. Am J Orthop 1999;28: 156–60.

[41] Dirschl DR, Duff GP, Dahners LE, et al. High pressure pulsatile lavage irrigation of intraarticular fractures: effects on fracture healing. J Orthop Trauma 1998;12:460–3.

[42] Bhandari M, Adili A, Lachowski RJ. High pressure pulsatile lavage of contaminated human tibiae: an in vitro study. J Orthop Trauma 1998;12:479–84.

[43] Bhandari M, Schemitsch EH, Adili A, et al. High and low pressure pulsatile lavage of contaminated tibial fractures: an in vitro study of bacterial adherence and bone damage. J Orthop Trauma 1999;13:526–33.

[44] Weitz-Marshall AD, Bosse MJ. Timing of closure of open fractures. J Am Acad Orthop Surg 2002;10:379–84.

[45] DeLong WG Jr, Born CT, Wei SY, et al. Aggressive treatment of 119 open fracture wounds. J Trauma 1999;46:1049–54.

[46] Patzakis MJ. Clostridial myonecrosis. Instr Course Lect 1990;39:491–3.

[47] Patzakis MJ, Dorr LD, Hammond W, et al. The effect of antibiotics, primary and secondary closure on clostridial contaminated open fracture wounds in rats. J Trauma 1978;18: 34–7.

[48] Patzakis MJ, Wilkins J, Moore TM. Considerations in reducing the infection rate in open tibial fractures. Clin Orthop Relat Res 1983;178:36–41.

[49] Sherman R. Soft tissue coverage. In: Browner BD, Jupiter JB, Levine AM, et al, editors. Skeletal trauma. 3rd edition. Philadelphia: WB Saunders; 2003. p. 320–49.

[50] Yaremchuk MJ. Acute management of severe soft-tissue damage accompanying open fractures of the lower extremity. Clin Plast Surg 1986;13:621–32.

[51] Shepherd LE, Costigan WM, Gardocki RJ, et al. Local or free muscle flaps and unreamed interlocked nails for open tibial fractures. Clin Orthop Relat Res 1998;350:90–6.

[52] Gopal S, Majumder S, Batchelor AG, et al. Fix and flap: the radical orthopaedic and plastic treatment of severe open fractures of the tibia. J Bone Joint Surg Br 2000;82:959–66.

[53] Pollak AN, McCarthy ML, Burgess AR. Short-term wound complications after application of flaps for coverage of traumatic soft-tissue defects about the tibia. The Lower Extremity Assessment Project (LEAP) Study Group. J Bone Joint Surg Am 2000;82-A:1681–91.

[54] Kramers-de Quervain IA, Lauffer JM, Kach K, et al. Functional donor-site morbidity during level and uphill gait after a gastrocnemius or soleus muscle-flap procedure. J Bone Joint Surg Am 2001;83-A:239–46.

[55] Cierny G III, Byrd HS, Jones RE. Primary versus delayed soft tissue coverage for severe open tibial fractures. A comparison of results. Clin Orthop Relat Res 1983;178:54–63.

[56] Godina M. Early microsurgical reconstruction of complex trauma of the extremities. Plast Reconstr Surg 1986;78:285–92.

[57] Worlock P, Slack R, Harvey L, et al. The prevention of infection in open fractures: an experimental study of the effect of fracture stability. Injury 1994;25:31–8.

[58] Henley MB, Chapman JR, Agel J, et al. Treatment of type II, IIIA, and IIIB open fractures of the tibial shaft: a prospective comparison of unreamed interlocking intramedullary nails and half-pin external fixators. J Orthop Trauma 1998;12:1–7.

[59] Tornetta P III, Bergman M, Watnik N, et al. Treatment of grade-IIIb open tibial fractures. A prospective randomised comparison of external fixation and non-reamed locked nailing. J Bone Joint Surg Br 1994;76:13–9.

[60] Brumback RJ, Ellison PS Jr, Poka A, et al. Intramedullary nailing of open fractures of the femoral shaft. J Bone Joint Surg Am 1989;71:1324–31.

[61] Edwards CC, Simmons SC, Browner BD, et al. Severe open tibial fractures. Results treating 202 injuries with external fixation. Clin Orthop Relat Res 1988;230:98–115.

[62] Behrens F, Searls K. External fixation of the tibia. Basic concepts and prospective evaluation. J Bone Joint Surg Br 1986;68:246–54.

[63] Marsh JL, Nepola JV, Wuest TK, et al. Unilateral external fixation until healing with the dynamic axial fixator for severe open tibial fractures. J Orthop Trauma 1991;5:341–8.

[64] Blick SS, Brumback RJ, Lakatos R, et al. Early prophylactic bone grafting of high-energy tibial fractures. Clin Orthop Relat Res 1989;240:21–41.

[65] Malizos KN, Zalavras CG, Soucacos PN, et al. Free vascularized fibular grafts for reconstruction of skeletal defects. J Am Acad Orthop Surg 2004;12:360–9.

[66] Paley D, Maar DC. Ilizarov bone transport treatment for tibial defects. J Orthop Trauma 2000;14:76–85.

INFECTIOUS
DISEASE CLINICS
OF NORTH AMERICA

Infect Dis Clin N Am 19 (2005) 931–946

Antibiotic Prophylaxis in Orthopedic Prosthetic Surgery

Camelia E. Marculescu, MD[a],
Douglas R. Osmon, MD, MPH[b],*

[a]Division of Infectious Disease, Medical University of South Carolina, 100 Doughty Street,
Suite 210, BA/IOP South, PO Box 250752, Charleston, SC 29425, USA
[b]Division of Infectious Disease, Mayo College of Medicine, 200 First Street SW,
Rochester, MN 55905, USA

Prevention of surgical infection encompasses numerous variables, including augmenting the host response, optimizing the wound environment, and decreasing the bacterial load introduced into the surgical wound [1]. Prophylactic measures that achieve these goals can be applied in both the perioperative and postoperative periods. The aim of perioperative prophylaxis is to diminish the quantity and consequences of the bacterial contamination that occurs inevitably during the surgery. Postoperative prophylaxis aims to reduce the risk of joint infection caused by the transient bacteremias associated with infection or instrumentation at remote sites.

Preoperative period

Prophylactic modalities in the preoperative period include antibiotics, surgical site preparation, clean air technology, and optimization of the surgical patient.

Selection of antimicrobial agent

The administration of systemic antibiotics immediately before surgery is the most effective prophylactic measure in the prevention of infection [1]. The optimal antibiotic should have activity against common organisms in prosthetic joint infections (*Staphylococcus* or *Streptococcus* spp); a long half-life; excellent tissue penetration; a lack of toxicity; and be relatively

---

* Corresponding author.
E-mail address: osmon.douglas@mayo.edu (D.R. Osmon).

0891-5520/05/$ - see front matter © 2005 Elsevier Inc. All rights reserved.
doi:10.1016/j.idc.2005.07.002
id.theclinics.com

inexpensive [2]. Cefazolin, a first-generation cephalosporin, meets all the desired criteria [3] and is the most widely used antibiotic at present. Current guidelines for antimicrobial prophylaxis for surgery recommend cefazolin or cefuroxime for patients undergoing total hip arthroplasty [4]. Vancomycin and clindamycin are recommended as alternative agents for patients who have a true type I β-lactam allergy [4], manifested by immediate urticaria, laryngeal edema, or bronchospasm [5]. Penicillin skin testing may be helpful in certain situations to clarify whether the patient has a true penicillin allergy [6].

Current data suggest that the role of vancomycin in orthopedic surgery prophylaxis should be limited. There is ample evidence that vancomycin is an inferior antistaphylococcal agent for methicillin-susceptible strains, compared with cephalosporins and penicillinase-resistant penicillins [7,8]. Routine use of vancomycin for elective orthopedic procedures should be discouraged. There are no prospective comparative data on the clinical efficacy of cephalosporin (cefazolin or cefuroxime) or penicillin (nafcillin or oxacillin) compounds versus vancomycin for prevention of infections associated with surgical implants. Evidence of methicillin-resistant organisms in total joint arthroplasty has already been reported [4,9]. This fact, coupled with the rising prevalence of methicillin-resistant *Staphylococcus aureus* (MRSA), has led surgeons increasingly to use vancomycin prophylaxis [10]. Furthermore, the Hospital Infection Control Practices Advisory Committee guidelines [11] suggest that a high frequency of MRSA infection in an institution should prompt the use of vancomycin for prophylaxis. Wiesel and Esterhai [12] recommend administration of vancomycin in institutions where the prevalence of MRSA is greater than 10% to 20%. There is no consensus about what constitutes a high prevalence of methicillin resistance, however, and no evidence that routine use of vancomycin for prophylaxis in institutions with perceived high risk of MRSA infection results in fewer surgical site infections than the use of cefazolin [4]. Vancomycin is appropriate for surgical prophylaxis for patients with known MRSA colonization [4].

Teicoplanin has proved to be an effective and safe prophylactic agent in prosthetic implant surgery in Europe, but is not available in the United States [13–16]. In a recent review of four comparative trials of the efficacy and safety of teicoplanin for prophylaxis in orthopedic surgery, Periti and coworkers [17] concluded that teicoplanin may be a reasonable choice for orthopedic surgery when there is a high risk of infection with MRSA. Because of the increasing prevalence of vancomycin intermediately resistant *S aureus*, vancomycin-resistant *S aureus*, and vancomycin-resistant enterococci, most authors agree that the use of glycopeptides for prophylaxis should be restricted [1,17,18]. For surgical procedures requiring a tourniquet, such as total knee arthroplasty, regional administration of a single dose of teicoplanin achieved a high concentration in the operative field, and resulted in a rate of postoperative infection similar to those of conventional prophylactic regimens [19]. The use of daptomycin for prophylaxis in orthopedic surgery needs to be investigated. Antimicrobial prophylaxis with third- and fourth-generation cephalosporins is not indicated, because most are less active than cefazolin against staphylococci, their use promotes emergence of resistance, and they are more expensive than more effective alternatives [6].

Timing and dosage of antimicrobial prophylaxis

The goal of antimicrobial prophylaxis is to achieve serum and tissue drug levels that exceed, for the duration of the operation, the minimum inhibitory concentrations for the organisms likely to be encountered. Because peak serum and bone concentration of antibiotics typically occur within 20 minutes of systemic administration [3], it is reasonable to administer a prophylactic antibiotic 30 to 60 minutes before skin incision [4]. Current guidelines recommend that vancomycin infusion should begin within 60 minutes before skin incision, to prevent antibiotic-associated reactions. Arthroplasties that require a tourniquet should have the entire antimicrobial dose before the tourniquet is inflated [4]. For prolonged procedures, or procedures associated with extensive blood loss, an additional intra-operative dose of antibiotic is advised [20,21]. For obese patients, higher doses of cefazolin (2 g) are required [6].

Duration of antimicrobial prophylaxis

The optimal duration has yet to be determined. Several studies have reported no additional benefit when prophylaxis was continued beyond 24 hours [22–26]. The current consensus on the duration of prophylaxis for a routine joint arthroplasty is a single preoperative dose, followed by two to three postoperative doses [27] to minimize toxicity, cost, and antimicrobial resistance. There is no evidence to support prophylactic antibiotics beyond 24 hours after surgery, although some surgeons choose to continue prophylaxis until all indwelling catheters are out [28].

Surgical site preparation

Introduction of a foreign body decreases the number of bacteria required to produce a clinical infection [29]. The risk of infection is also influenced by additional factors, such as patient health, the length of operation, and adequacy of circulation. Strict adherence to aseptic techniques during each case is essential to control the number of infections. Preparation of the patient before operation is important. Several disinfectants can be used to remove bacteria from the patient's skin [28]. Clipping hair immediately before an operation is associated with a lower risk of surgical site infections than shaving or clipping the night before an operation [11]. Appropriate draping of the patient is mandatory, but does not guarantee the prevention of infection.

Clean air technology

Various techniques are used to minimize the number of airborne bacteria in the operating room, such as laminar air flow, ultraviolet light, limitation of traffic, and wearing of surgical facemask under an overlapping hood [27]. Not all of these measures have gained widespread acceptance. Laminar air flow can result in a 90% reduction of bacteria in the wound, and 60% reduction of airborne bacteria in the operating room [30]. Vertical laminar airflow is considered more effective than horizontal airflow in reducing airborne contamination, especially in the absence of body exhaust suits [27,31]. With the use of clean air technology and laminar air flow, various studies have demonstrated a significant reduction in infection rates to 0.5% to 1% [23,32,33]. These studies were not prospective, however, and included confounding factors that were not controlled for, such as concomitant use of prophylactic antibiotics. Other studies did not find a statistically significant difference between the two operating room environments [34]. Currently, the role of laminar airflow in the prophylaxis is controversial if prophylactic antibiotics are used.

Control measures for methicillin-resistant Staphylococcus aureus

MRSA has become an important cause of surgical wound infections, with an increased incidence within both hospitals and the community. Studies on nursing homes in the United States found a monthly bacterial colonization rate between 6.6% and 23%, with an MRSA infection rate of 3% [35,36]. Simple measures, such meticulous hand hygiene, patient screening, careful surveillance of infections, and prompt implementation of isolation policies, are essential components of control [37–39]. Preoperative nasal carriage of *S aureus* represents a risk factor for surgical site infections [11]. Up to 5.3% of orthopedic patients are colonized with methicillin-resistant strains of staphylococci on hospital admission [40]. Current guidelines advocate screening for MRSA carriage in patients at high risk (ie, patients who have spent more than 5 days in acute or long-term care centers) [41].

Intranasal mupirocin has been evaluated in the prevention of surgical site infections. Although intranasal mupirocin reduced nasal carriage of *S aureus,* several studies failed to demonstrate a significant reduction in surgical site infection rates [42–44]. In one study, the rate of endogenous *S aureus* infections was five times lower in the mupirocin group than in placebo group (0.3% and 1.7%, respectively), although this difference was not statistically significant [42]. Other studies have shown a potential benefit in reduction of surgical site infections by using mupirocin. One study that used a historical control group showed a significant reduction in the surgical site infection rate from 2.7% to 1.3%, with a nonsignificant reduction of *S aureus* surgical site infection from 1.1% to 0.7% [45]. Another study that used mupirocin in conjunction with preoperative triclosan shower showed a marked decrease in the incidence of MRSA surgical site infections from

23 per 1000 operations to 3.3 to 4 per 1000 operations, after the introduction of a mupirocin-based protocol [46]. Although a consensus has not been reached regarding the relationship between mupirocin nasal decolonization and the reduction of *S aureus* surgical site infections, identification of patients colonized with MRSA is important, because vancomycin prophylaxis is indicated for these patients [4].

Optimization of the total joint arthroplasty patient

Patients at high risk for infection, such as those with rheumatoid arthritis, the elderly, malnourished, obese, diabetic, or otherwise immunosuppressed, may benefit from the optimization of these risk factors, or may require more intensive prophylaxis to minimize their risk of sepsis [27]. Patients with preoperative lymphocyte counts of less than 1500 cells/mm^3 and an albumin level of less than 3.5 g/dL had five and seven times more frequent major wound complications, respectively [47]. The Rainer-McDonald index may identify nutritionally deficient patients who are at risk for postoperative infections [48]. These patients may benefit from reversal of nutritional deficiencies before elective joint replacement. It is not clear if optimization of obesity is beneficial, because the beneficial effects of its reversal in this setting are unknown, and significant weight loss may result in prolonged immune impairment [49].

The optimal duration of methotrexate in patients with rheumatoid arthritis and the timing of its cessation before surgery are controversial [27]. The most reasonable approach may be to withhold methotrexate for a short time (2 weeks) during the perioperative period [50]. Glycemic control is desirable in diabetic patients undergoing elective implant surgery, although no reports of the effect of normalizing serum glucose levels in the setting of total hip arthroplasty have been published [11,27]. Smoking cessation or abstaining from tobacco for at least 30 days before elective surgery are recommended [11]. Because transfusion of allogeneic blood in the operative period is associated with an increased risk of infection [51], identification of patients who likely require blood after joint arthroplasty is important. Useful transfusion practices include use whenever possible of autologous blood donation, hemodilution, and perioperative blood salvage [27].

Intraoperative period

Surgical technique

Adherence to meticulous surgical technique is essential in reducing the infection rates after joint arthroplasty. There is strong evidence to support the use of impenetrable disposable clothing and drapes, as opposed to using permeable gowns [52]. The operative site should be cleansed with an antiseptic agent, and covered with an antiseptic adhesive tape before incision. A plastic drape impregnated with slow-release iodophor inhibits skin recolonization and lateral migration of bacteria from scrubbed areas not involving the incision [27]. Efforts should be made to minimize the duration of surgery, because prolonged operative time increases the rate of infection [53,54]. Although the method of gloving is controversial, double gloving is still recommended over single gloving [1]. A cloth outer glove significantly reduces the number of punctures to the innermost glove compared with wearing double latex gloves [55]. Surgical staff should wear hoods and masks, although the wearing of masks is controversial [31]. Gore-Tex gowns may prevent dispersion of bacteria up to 1000 times more effectively than cotton gowns [56]. Several operative instruments, such as suction tips and splash basins, are reported as sources of bacterial contamination. Frequent exchanging of the suction tip, and use of a clean suction tip at the time of preparation of the femoral canal, is recommended to minimize bacterial contamination [1]. In addition, delicate tissue handling and prevention of extensive dissection from the underlying fascia help reduce the extent of devitalized tissue [27]. Saline irrigation of the wound contributes to a 12% to 56% reduction of the wound bacterial counts, and prevents tissue desiccation [5,27]. The addition of antibiotics to the irrigation solutions remains controversial [57,58], but may be reasonable during orthopedic procedures [5]. Most commonly used is a triple antibiotic solution of neomycin, polymyxin, and bacitracin, because it provides the most complete coverage against common microorganisms known to cause infection [57]. More studies are needed before routine implementation of this technique. There is insufficient evidence to support or refute the routine use of closed surgical drainage in implant orthopedic surgery [59]. If used, drain removal should be accomplished within 24 to 48 hours to prevent retrograde contamination of the wound [27].

Antibiotic-impregnated bone cement

The use of antibiotic-impregnated cement for primary and revision joint arthroplasty is becoming the standard of practice in Europe and Scandinavia [60]. It has been approved by the Food and Drug Administration in the United States for use only in infected joint arthroplasty. There are no established guidelines for use of these agents for prophylaxis in the United States [4], although the antibiotic-impregnated bone cements have been extensively studied. A large prospective multicenter randomized Swedish study (1688 consecutive total hip arthroplasties) found a statistically significant difference at 5-year follow-up between deep infection rates in patients treated with systemic antibiotics (1.9%) compared with patients who had gentamicin-impregnated cement (0.8%). At 10-year follow-up the difference between the two groups (1.6% versus 1.1%) was not significant [61]. Another small prospective randomized trial comparing the effect of cefuroxime-impregnated cement versus systemic administration of cefuroxime found no statistically significant difference in respect to incidence of superficial or early deep wound infections between the two groups [62]. Two trials (one in patients with diabetes mellitus) in patients undergoing total knee arthroplasty comparing infection rates in patients who received cefuroxime-impregnated bone cement and those who had standard bone cement found a significant reduction in deep infections in the antibiotic cement group [63,64]. A large Norwegian study found that patients who received both systemic prophylaxis and antibiotic-impregnated cement had the lowest risk of revision. Those who received only systemic antimicrobial prophylaxis had a revision rate because of infection that was 1.8 times higher. The authors concluded that systemic antibiotics, combined with antibiotic-impregnated cement, provide the best prophylaxis for total hip arthroplasty [65].

A number of criteria must be met for antibiotics to be effective when mixed with methylmethacrylate: thermal stability, water solubility, bactericidal effect at tissue level, gradual release, minimal or absent development of antimicrobial resistance or allergic reactions, and lack of compromise of mechanical integrity [66]. Concerns about the routine use of antibiotic-impregnated bone cement for prophylaxis of infection include mechanical effects of mixing antibiotics to acrylic bone cement, occurrence of an allergic reaction, emergence of antimicrobial resistance, and cost [5]. Many antibiotics used in bone cement are heat-stable, and demonstrate highly effective bactericidal activity for at least 7 to 10 days, or even up to 10 years [60,67,68]. In addition, low doses of antibiotics may not weaken the bone cement [60]. Allergic reactions are not seen with gentamicin, a commonly used antibiotic in bone cement [60], whereas other antibiotics, such as penicillin or cephalosporins, are best avoided because of their potential allergenicity [66]. In a study of 91 infected total hip arthroplasties caused by coagulase-negative staphylococci, emergence of gentamicin-resistant organisms occurred in 88% of patients who underwent primary hip arthroplasty with gentamicin-impregnated cement, and in only 16% of patients who had not received gentamicin-impregnated cement [69].

In a recent review, Bourne [60] suggested that consideration should be given for use of antibiotic-impregnated bone cements during primary joint arthroplasty. Before the use of antibiotic-impregnated cement can be recommended for routine primary joint arthroplasties, however, randomized trials are needed to study the rate of infection, the risk of antimicrobial resistance, and assessment of cost-benefit [12,60]. Antibiotic-impregnated cement has a more definitive role in high-risk patients, such as the immunocompromised, the elderly, or those requiring revision surgeries [60].

Postoperative prophylaxis

From the moment of implantation, total joint arthroplasty is vulnerable to infection during episodes of transient bacteremia. The risk of hematogenous seeding lasts throughout the lifetime of prosthesis, and may result from infection or manipulation at distant body sites. Some of the more common origins of hematogenous infection are the oral cavity, skin, genitourinary tract, and gastrointestinal tract [27]. The aim of postoperative prophylaxis is to protect the total joint arthroplasty from hematogenous seeding. Currently, there are relatively few generally accepted indications for postoperative prophylaxis.

Antibiotic prophylaxis for dental patients with total joint arthroplasty

In 1997, the American Dental Association and the American Academy of Orthopedic Surgeons have released the first consensus statement on this topic. This advisory statement was revised in 2003 [70]. The advisory statement emphasized that the most critical period for hematogenous seeding is up to 2 years after joint placement [70], occurring at a frequency of 0.14 cases per 1000 joint-years, whereas the annual rate after the first 2 years is only 0.03 cases per 1000 joint-years [71]. The advisory statement does not recommend the routine use of dental prophylaxis for most patients with total joint arthroplasty. Prophylaxis is considered for selected immunocompromised patients (Table 1) undergoing dental procedures with a high bacteremic risk (Box 1). Suggested antibiotic regimens are outlined in Table 2. Any perceived potential benefit of antibiotic prophylaxis must be weighed against the known risk of antibiotic toxicity, allergy and development, selection, and transmission of antimicrobial resistance [70].

Table 1
Dental and urologic patients at increased risk of experiencing hematogenous total joint infection

Patient type	Condition placing patient at risk
All patients during first 2 years following joint replacement	NA[a]
Immunocompromised immunosuppressed patients	Inflammatory arthropathies such as rheumatoid arthritis, systemic lupus erythematosus. Drug or radiation-induced immunosuppression.
Patients with comorbidities[b]	Previous prosthetic joint infections Malnourishment Hemophilia HIV infection Insulin-dependent (type 1) diabetes Malignancy

  [a] Not applicable.
  [b] Conditions shown for patients in this category are examples only; there may be additional conditions that place such patients at risk of experiencing hematogenous total joint infection.
  Adapted from American Dental Association, American Academy of Orthopedic Surgeons. Antibiotic prophylaxis for dental patients with total joint replacements: advisory statement. J Am Dental Assoc 2003;134:895–9; and American Urological Association, American Academy of Orthopaedic Surgeons. Antibiotic prophylaxis for urological patients with total joint replacements. J Urol 2003;169:1796–7; with permission.

Box 1. Incidence stratification of bacteremic dental procedures

Higher incidence[a]
Dental extractions
Periodontal procedure, including surgery, subgingival placement of antibiotic fibers or strips, scaling, root planning, probing, recall maintenance
Dental implant placement and replantation of avulsed teeth
Endodontic (root canal) instrumentation or surgery only beyond the apex
Initial placement of orthodontic bands but not brackets
Intraligamentary and intraosseous local anesthetic injections
Prophylactic cleaning of teeth or implants where bleeding is anticipated

Lower incidence[b,c]
Restorative dentistry[d] (operative or prosthodontic) with or without retraction cord[c]
Local anesthetic injections (nonintraligamentary and nonintraosseous)
Intracanal endodontic treatment: postplacement and buildup
Placement of rubber dam
Postoperative suture removal
Placement of removable prosthodontic and orthodontic appliances
Taking of oral impressions
Fluoride treatments
Taking of oral radiographs
Orthodontic appliance adjustment

---

[a] Prophylaxis should be considered for patients with total joint replacement who meet the criteria in Table 1. No other patients with orthopedic implants should be considered for antibiotic prophylaxis before dental treatment or procedures.
[b] Prophylaxis not indicated.
[c] Clinical judgment may indicate antibiotic use in selected circumstances that may create significant bleeding.
[d] Include restoration of carious (decayed) or missing teeth.
Adapted from Dajani AS, Taubert KA, Wilson WR, et al. Prevention of bacterial endocarditis: recommendations by the American Heart Association. From the Committee on Rheumatic Fever, Endocarditis and Kawasaki Disease, Council on Cardiovascular Disease in the Young. JAMA 1997;277:1794–801; with permission.

Table 2
Suggested antibiotic prophylactic regimens for dental and urologic procedures in patients at risk
with total joint arthroplasty

Procedures	Patient type	Suggested drug	Regimen
Dental	Patients not allergic to penicillin	Cephalexin, cephradine, or amoxicillin	2 g orally 1 h before dental procedure
	Patients not allergic to penicillin and unable to take oral medications	Cefazolin or ampicillin	Cefazolin, 1 g, or ampicillin, 2 g, intramuscularly or intravenously 1 h before the dental procedure
	Patients allergic to penicillin	Clindamycin	600 mg orally 1 h before the dental procedure
	Patients allergic to penicillin and unable to take oral medications	Clindamycin	600 mg intravenously 1 h before the dental procedure[a]
Urologic	Patients allergic to penicillin	Levofloxacin, ciprofloxacin, ofloxacin[a,b] or	Levofloxacin, 500 mg, ciprofloxacin, 500 mg, ofloxacin, 400 mg, orally 1–2 h before procedure.
		Vancomycin plus gentamicin[a,b]	Vancomycin, 1 g intravenously (for 1–2 h) plus gentamicin, 1.5 mg/kg intravenously 30–60 min before procedure
	Patients not allergic to penicillin	Ampicillin plus gentamicin[a,b]	Ampicillin, 2 g intravenously, plus gentamicin, 1.5 mg/kg intravenously, 30–60 min before procedure

[a] No second dosed are recommended for any of these dosing regimens.

[b] For some procedures additional or alternative agents may be considered for prophylaxis against specific organisms. A prophylactic agent is chosen on the basis of its activity against endogenous flora likely to be encountered, its toxicity, and its cost. To prevent bacteriuria, an appropriate dose of a prophylactic agent should be given preoperatively so that effective tissue concentration is present at the time of instrumentation or incision.

Adapted from American Dental Association, American Academy of Orthopedic Surgeons. Antibiotic prophylaxis for dental patients with total joint replacements: advisory statement. J Am Dental Assoc 2003;134:895–9; and American Urological Association, American Academy of Orthopaedic Surgeons. Antibiotic prophylaxis for urological patients with total joint replacements. J Urol 2003;169:1796–7; with permission.

Antibiotic prophylaxis for urologic patients with total joint arthroplasty

In 2003, the American Academy of Orthopedic Surgeons and the American Urological Association released the first consensus statement regarding antibiotic prophylaxis for urologic patients with total joint arthroplasty [72]. The routine use of antibiotic prophylaxis for all urologic patients with total joint arthroplasty is not recommended. Antibiotic prophylaxis is recommended, however, for patients at high risk of hematogenous total joint arthroplasty infections (see Table 1) and for all patients during the first 2 years after prosthetic joint replacement [72]. Prophylaxis for higher-risk patients should be considered for patients with total joint arthroplasty who meet the criteria in Table 1. Risk stratification of bacteremic urologic procedures is listed in Table 3. The recommendations assume the urine is sterile preoperatively. Because the risk of bacteremia is dramatically increased in the presence of bacteriuria, the advisory statement recommends treatment of bacteriuria, if present preoperatively, before the manipulation of the urinary tract [72]. Suggested antibiotic regimens for urologic patients with total joint arthroplasty are outlined in Table 2.

Table 3
Risk stratification of bacteremic urologic procedures

Patients at risk	Procedure
Higher risk[a]	Any stone manipulation (includes shock wave lithotripsy)
	Any procedure with transmural incision into urinary tract (does not include simple ligation with excision or percutaneous drainage procedure)
	Any endoscopic procedures of upper tract (ureter and kidney)
	Any procedure that includes bowel segments
	Transrectal prostate biopsy
	Any procedure with entry into the urinary tract (except for transurethral catheterization) in individuals with higher risk of bacterial colonization
	- Indwelling catheter or intermittent catheterization
	- Indwelling ureteral stent
	- Urinary retention
	- History of recent or recurrent urinary infection or prostatitis
	- Urinary diversion
Lower risk[b]	Endoscopic procedures into urethra and bladder without stone manipulation or incision (includes fulguration and mucosal biopsy, if no incision)
	Open surgical or laparoscopic procedures without stone manipulation or incision into the urinary tract
	Catheterization for drainage or diagnostic instrumentation, including both transurethral and percutaneous access

[a] Prophylaxis for higher-risk patients should be considered for patients with total joint replacement who meet the criteria in Table 1. No other patients should be considered for antibiotic prophylaxis before urologic procedures on the basis of orthopedic implant alone, although antibiotics still may be indicated for prophylaxis against urinary tract or other infections.

[b] Prophylaxis for lower-risk patients not indicated on the basis of the orthopedic implant alone, although antibiotics still may be indicated for prophylaxis against urinary tract or other infections.

Adapted from American Urological Association, American Academy of Orthopedic Surgeons. Antibiotic prophylaxis for urological patients with total joint replacements. J Urol 2003;169:1796–7; with permission.

*Antibiotic prophylaxis for gastrointestinal endoscopy in patients with
total joint arthroplasty*

The frequency and intensity of bacteremia following most gastrointestinal procedures is rather low. The incidence of bacteremia during endoscopy, with or without biopsy, was estimated to be between 0% and 8%, was of short duration, and was not associated with any infectious complications. The incidence of bacteremia associated with flexible sigmoidoscopy varied between 0% and 1%, and the incidence of bacteremia associated with colonoscopy varied between 0% and 25%, with a mean frequency of 4.4% [73]. Because iatrogenic infection of prosthetic joints following endoscopic procedures is extremely rare, there is currently insufficient evidence to recommend antibiotic prophylaxis for patients with total joint arthroplasty undergoing endoscopic procedures [73].

Summary

The problem of prophylaxis in orthopedic implant surgery will become increasingly important and complex as the population ages and requires more arthroplasty procedures, and the prevalence of antimicrobial-resistant bacteria meanwhile also continues to rise. Energy spent preventing prosthetic joint infection is more effective than that expended in treating the infection of a prosthetic joint, once established. Preventive measures encompass a wide array of variables related to host response, wound environment, and microorganisms. Prophylaxis should address these areas in the preoperative, intraoperative, and postoperative periods. Antimicrobial prophylaxis remains the single most effective method of reducing the prevalence of infection after total joint arthroplasty. In the postoperative period, prophylaxis aims to protect the prosthetic joint against hematogenous seeding from oral, urologic, skin, or gastrointestinal sources. Currently, dental and urologic advisory statements provide recommendations for antimicrobial prophylaxis for high-risk patients with total joint arthroplasty undergoing high-risk procedures. Close collaboration between the orthopedic surgeon, urologist, or dentist and the infectious disease specialist is crucial for providing recommendations regarding prophylaxis in special circumstances. In these particular circumstances, individual decisions should be made based on clinical judgment.

References

[1] Hanssen AD, Osmon DR, Nelson CL. Prevention of deep periprosthetic joint infection. J Bone Joint Surg Am 1996;78:458–71.
[2] Fitzgerald JR, Thompson RL. Cephalosporin antibiotics in the prevention and treatment of musculoskeletal sepsis. J Bone Joint Surg Am 1983;65:1201–5.
[3] Wiggins CE, Nelson CL, Clarke R, et al. Concentration of antibiotics in normal bone after intravenous injection. J Bone Joint Surg Am 1978;60:93–6.

[4] Bratzler DW, Houck PM. Antimicrobial prophylaxis for surgery. Clin Infect Dis 2004;38: 1706–15.

[5] Hanssen AD, Osmon DR. The use of prophylactic antimicrobial agents during and after hip arthroplasty. Clin Orthop 1999;369:124–38.

[6] Weed HG. Antimicrobial prophylaxis in the surgical patient. Med Clin North Am 2003;87: 59–75.

[7] Cantoni L, Glauser MP, Bille J. Comparative efficacy of daptomycin, vancomycin and cloxacillin for the treatment of *Staphylococcus aureus* endocarditis in rats and role of test conditions in this determination. Antimicrob Agents Chemother 1990;34:1348–53.

[8] Fishmann NO, Brennan PJ. Optimizing use of antimicrobial agents: pitfalls and consequences of inappropriate therapy. J Clin Outcome Management 1997;4:25–33.

[9] Tanzer M, Miller J, Richards GK. Preoperative assessment of skin colonization and antibiotic effectiveness in total knee arthroplasty. Clin Orthop 1994;299:163–8.

[10] Darouiche RO. Antimicrobial approaches for preventing infections associated with surgical implants. Clin Infect Dis 2003;36:1284–9.

[11] Mangram AJ, Horan TC, Pearson ML. Guideline for prevention of surgical site infections. Hospital Infection Control Practices Advisory Committee. Infect Control Hosp Epidemiol 1999;20:250–78.

[12] Wiesel BB, Esterhai J Jr. Prophylaxis of musculoskeletal infection. In: Calhoun J, Mader JT, editors. Musculoskeletal infections. New York: Marcel Dekker; 2003. p. 115–29.

[13] Mollan RA, Haddock M, Webb CH. Teicoplanin vs cephamandole for antimicrobial prophylaxis in prosthetic joint implant surgery (preliminary results). Eur J Surg 1992;567: 19–21.

[14] Lazzarini L, Pellizzer G, Stecca C, et al. Postoperative infections following total knee replacement: an epidemiological study. J Chemother 2001;13:182–7.

[15] Periti P, Stringa G, Mini E. Comparative multicenter trial of teicoplanin versus cefazolin for antimicrobial prophylaxis in prosthetic joint implant surgery. Italian Study Group for Antimicrobial Prophylaxis in Orthopedic Surgery. Eur J Clin Microbiol Infect Dis 1999;18: 113–9.

[16] Periti P, Stringa G, Donati L, et al. Teicoplanin–its role as systemic therapy of burn infections and as prophylaxis for orthopaedic surgery. Italian Study Groups for Antimicrobial Prophylaxis in Orthopaedic Surgery and Burns. Eur J Surg 1992;567:3–8.

[17] Periti P, Mini E, Mosconi G. Antimicrobial prophylaxis in orthopaedic surgery: the role of teicoplanin. J Antimicrob Chemother 1998;41:329–40.

[18] Garvin KL, Urban JA. Emerging multiresistant strains: recommended precautions in the emergency room and surgical setting. Instr Course Lect 2000;49:605–14.

[19] De Lalla F. Antibiotic prophylaxis in orthopedic prosthetic surgery. J Chemother 2001;13: 48–53.

[20] Dellinger EP, Gross PA, Barrett TL. Quality standard for antimicrobial prophylaxis in surgical procedures. Clin Infect Dis 1994;18:422–7.

[21] Gross PA, Barett TL, Dellinger EP. Purpose of quality standards for infectious diseases. Infectious Disease Society of America. Clin Infect Dis 1994;18:428–30.

[22] Brown WJ. Microbiology of the infected total joint arthroplasty. Semin Arthroplasty 1994;5: 107–13.

[23] Charnley J, Eftekhar N. Postoperative infection in a total prosthetic replacement arthroplasty of the hip joint: with special reference to the bacterial content of the air in the operating room. Br J Surg 1969;56:641–9.

[24] Davies AJ, Lockley RM, Jones A, et al. Comparative pharmacokinetics of cefamandole, cefuroxime, and cephradine during total hip replacement. J Antimicrob Chemother 1986;17: 637–40.

[25] Mauerhan DR, Nelson CL, Smith DL, et al. Prophylaxis against infection in total joint arthroplasty. One day of cefuroxime compared with 3 days of cefazolin. J Bone Joint Surg Am 1994;76:39–95.

[26] Nelson CL, Green RA, Porter RA, et al. One day versus seven days of preventive antibiotic therapy in orthopaedic surgery. Clin Orthop 1983;176:258–63.

[27] Garvin KL, Urban JA. Total hip infections. In: Calhoun JH, Mader JT, editors. Musculoskeletal infections. New York: Marcel Dekker; 2003. p. 241–91.

[28] Stocks G, Janssen HF. Infection in patients after implantation of an orthopedic device. ASAIO J 2000;46:41–6.

[29] Elek SD, Conen PE. The virulence of *Staphylococcus pyogenes* for a man: a study of the problems of wound infection. Br J Exp Pathol 1957;38:573–86.

[30] Ritter MA. Operating room environment. Clin Orthop 1999;369:103–9.

[31] Dharan S, Pittet D. Environmental controls in operating theaters. J Hosp Infect 2002;51: 79–84.

[32] Lidwell OM, Lowburry EJ, Whyte W, et al. Effect of ultraclean air in operating rooms on deep sepsis in the joint after total hip or knee replacement: a randomised study. BMJ 1982; 285:10–4.

[33] Hill C, Flamant R, Mazas F, et al. Prophylactic cefazolin versus placebo in total hip replacement: report of a multicentre double-blind randomized trial. Lancet 1981;1: 795–6.

[34] Fitzgerald JR. Total hip arthroplasty sepsis: prevention and diagnosis. Orthop Clin North Am 1992;23:259–64.

[35] Bradley SF, Terpenning M, Ramsey BS. Methicillin-resistant *Staphylococcus aureus*: colonization and infection in a long term care facility. Ann Intern Med 1991;115:417–22.

[36] Thomas JC, Bridge J, Waterman S. Transmission and control of methicillin-resistant *Staphylococcus aureus* in a skilled nursing facility. Infect Control 1987;8:24–9.

[37] Tai CC, Nirvani AA, Holmes A, et al. Methicillin-resistant *Staphylococcus aureus* in orthopaedic surgery. Int Orthop 2004;28:32–5.

[38] Harvey JR, Benfield EC. Preventing methicillin-resistant *Staphylococcus aureus* infection in joint replacements: a new problem requiring old solutions. Ann R Coll Surg Engl 2004;86: 122–4.

[39] Biant LC, Teare EL, Williams WW, et al. Eradication of methicillin resistant *Staphylococcus aureus* by "ring fencing" of elective orthopaedic beds. BMJ 2004;329:149–51.

[40] Shams WE, Rapp RP. Methicillin-resistant staphylococcal infections: an important consideration for orthopedic surgeons. Orthopedics 2004;27:565–8.

[41] Muto CA, Jernigan JA, Ostrowsky BE, et al. SHEA guideline for preventing nosocomial transmission of multidrug-resistant strains of *Staphylococcus aureus* and enterococcus. Infect Control Hosp Epidemiol 2003;24:362–86.

[42] Kalmeijer MD, Coertjens H, van Nieuwland-Bollen PM, et al. Surgical site infections in orthopedic surgery: the effect of mupirocin nasal ointment in a double-blind, randomized, placebo-controlled study. Clin Infect Dis 2002;35:353–8.

[43] Perl TM, Cullen JJ, Wentzel RP. Intranasal mupirocin to prevent postoperative *Staphylococcus aureus* infections. N Engl J Med 2002;346:1871–7.

[44] Laupland KB, Conly JM. Treatment of *Staphylococcus aureus* colonization and prophylaxis for infection with topical intranasal mupirocin: an evidence-based review. Clin Infect Dis 2003;37:933–8.

[45] Gernaat-van der Sluis AJ, Hoogenboom-Verdegaal A, Edixhoven PJ. Prophylactic mupirocin could reduce orthopedic wound infections. Acta Orthop Scand 1998;69:412–4.

[46] Wilcox MH, Hall JC, Pike H, et al. Use of perioperative mupirocin to prevent methicillin-resistant *Staphylococcus aureus* (MRSA) orthopaedic surgical site infections. J Hosp Infect 2003;54:196–201.

[47] Greene KA, Wilde AH, Stulberg BN. Preoperative nutritional status of total joint patients. J Arthroplasty 1991;6:321–5.

[48] Puskarich CL, Nelson CL, Nusbickel FR, et al. The use of two nutritional indicators in identifying long bone fracture patients who do and do not develop infections. J Orthop Res 1990;8:799–803.

[49] Stallone DD. The influence of obesity and its treatment on the immune system. Nutr Rev 1994;52:37–50.

[50] Bridges SL Jr, Moreland LW. Perioperative use of methotrexate in patients with rheumatoid arthritis undergoing orthopedic surgery. Rheum Dis Clin North Am 1997;23: 981–93.

[51] Biernbaum BE, Callaghan JJ, Galante JO, et al. An analysis of blood management in patients having a total hip or knee arthroplasty. J Bone Joint Surg Am 1999;81:2–10.

[52] Malik MHA, Gambhir AK, Bale L, et al. Primary total hip replacements: a comparison of a nationally agreed guide to best practice and current surgical technique as determined by the North West Regional Arthroplasty Register. Ann R Coll Surg Engl 2004;86:113–8.

[53] Fitzgerald JR. Contamination of the surgical wound in the operating room. Instr Course Lect 1977;27:41–6.

[54] Gherini S, Vaughn BK, Lombardi AVJ, et al. Delayed wound healing and nutritional deficiencies after total hip arthroplasty. Clin Orthop 1993;293:188–95.

[55] Tanner J, Parkinson H. Double gloving to reduce surgical cross-infection. Cochrane Database Syst Rev 2002;3:CD003087.

[56] Wilkins J, Patzakis MJ. Peripheral Teflon catheters: potential source for bacterial contamination of orthopedic implants? Clin Orthop 1990;254:251–4.

[57] Dirschl DR, Wilson FC. Topical antibiotic irrigation in the prophylaxis of the operative wound infections in orthopedic surgery. Orthop Clin North Am 1991;22:419–26.

[58] Bortnem KD, Wetmore RW, Blackburn GW, et al. Analysis of therapeutic efficacy, cost, and safety of gentamicin lavage solution in orthopaedic surgery prophylaxis. Orthop Rev 1990; 19:797–801.

[59] Parker MJ, Roberts C. Closed suction surgical wound drainage after orthopaedic surgery. Cochrane Database Syst Rev 2001;4:CD001825.

[60] Bourne RB. Prophylactic use of antibiotic bone cement. J Arthroplasty 2004;19:69–72.

[61] Josefsson G, Kolmert L. Prophylaxis with systemic antibiotics versus gentamicin bone cement in total hip arthroplasty: a ten-year survey of 1,688 hips. Clin Orthop 1993;292: 210–4.

[62] McQueen MM, Hughes SP, May P, et al. Cefuroxime in total joint arthroplasty: intravenous or in bone cement. J Arthroplasty 1990;5:169–72.

[63] Chiu FY, Lin CF, Lin CF, et al. Cefuroxime-impregnated cement in primary total knee arthroplasty. J Bone Joint Surg Am 2002;84:759–62.

[64] Chiu FY, Lin CF, Chen CM, et al. Cefuroxime-impregnated cement at primary total knee arthroplasty in diabetes mellitus: a prospective, randomized study. J Bone Joint Surg Br 2001;83:691–5.

[65] Engesaeter LB, Espehaug B, Furnes O, et al. Antibiotic prophylaxis in total hip arthroplasty: effects of antibiotic prophylaxis systemically and in bone cement on the revision rate of 22,170 primary hip replacements followed 0 -14 years in the Norwegian Arthroplasty Register. Acta Orthop Scand 2003;74:644–51.

[66] Joseph TN, Chen AL, Di Cesare PE. Use of antibiotic-impregnated cement in total joint arthroplasty. J Am Acad Orthop Surg 2003;11:38–47.

[67] Masari BA, Duncan CP, Beauchamp CP. Long-term elution of antibiotics from bone cement: an in vivo study using the prosthesis of antibiotic-loaded acrylic cement (PROSTALAC) system. J Arthroplasty 1998;13:331–8.

[68] Buchholz HW, Elson RA, Engelbrecht E, et al. Management of deep infection of total hip replacement. J Bone Joint Surg Br 1981;63:342–53.

[69] Hope PG, Kristinsson KG, Norman P, et al. Deep infection of cemented total hip arthroplasties caused by coagulase-negative staphylococci. J Bone Joint Surg Br 1989;71: 851–5.

[70] American Dental Association, American Academy of Orthopedic Surgeons. Antibiotic prophylaxis for dental patients with total joint replacements: advisory statement. J Am Dent Assoc 2003;134:895–9.

[71] Osmon DR, Steckelberg JM, Hanssen AD. Incidence of prosthetic joint infection due to viridans streptococci. Presented at the annual meeting of the Musculoskeletal Infection Society. Snowmass, Colorado, August 20, 1993.

[72] American Urological Association, American Academy of Orthopaedic Surgeons. Antibiotic prophylaxis for urological patients with total joint replacements. J Urol 2003;169:1796–7.

[73] Hirota WK, Petersen K, Baron TH, et al. Standards of Practice Committee of the American Society for Gastrointestinal Endoscopy: guidelines for antibiotic prophylaxis for GI endoscopy. Gastrointest Endosc 2003;58:475–82.

ELSEVIER
SAUNDERS

Infect Dis Clin N Am 19 (2005) 947–961

INFECTIOUS
DISEASE CLINICS
OF NORTH AMERICA

Lyme Arthritis

Linden Hu, MD

Division of Geographic Medicine and Infectious Diseases,
Tufts-New England Medical Center, Tufts University School of Medicine,
750 Washington Street, Boston, MA 02111, USA

Three decades after its first description in the United States, Lyme borreliosis has become the most common vector-borne disease in North America and Europe. The incidence of Lyme borreliosis continues to increase with a near doubling of reported cases in the last decade [1]. In the United States, most Lyme disease is localized to three highly endemic areas: (1) the Northeast (Maine to Maryland); (2) the Midwest (Minnesota and Wisconsin); and (3) the West (Northern California and Oregon). The geographic prevalence of ticks infected with *Borrelia burgdorferi*, the causative agent of Lyme borreliosis, however, has seen steady, contiguous expansion from the epicenters of infection. This article reviews clinical aspects of Lyme borreliosis with a focus on arthritis and current recommendations on the diagnosis, treatment, and prevention of Lyme arthritis.

Borrelia epidemiology and life cycle

Lyme borreliosis is caused by members of the genus *Borrelia*. Three *Borrelia* species are pathogenic for humans: (1) *B burgdorferi* (*sensu stricto*), (2) *B garinii*, and (3) *B afzelii* [2]. *B burgdorferi* is the only definitely pathogenic species found in the United States, although the recently described species, *Borrelia lonestari*, has been implicated in Southern tick-associated rash illness [3,4]. *B afzelii* and *B garinii*, the predominant species infecting humans in Europe and Asia, are less arthritogenic than *B burgdorferi*. As with most vector-borne diseases, there is great specificity of the organisms for a particular tick vector. Pathogenic *Borrelia* are carried and transmitted solely by the *Ixodes ricinus* complex of ticks. These include *Ixodes scapularis* (Northeastern and Midwestern United States); *Ixodes*

E-mail address: lhu@tufts-nemc.org

pacificus (Western United States); *Ixodes ricinus*; and *Ixodes persulcatus* (Europe and Asia).

B burgdorferi may infect many different animals, including small rodents; birds; and larger mammals, such as deer and cows [5–7]. Animals favored as feeding sources by larval and nymphal ticks are the most important for maintaining the cycle of *Borrelia* infection. Animals favored by the adult ticks (which do not transmit infection vertically to their eggs, and do not feed again to pass on the infection) are dead-end hosts for *Borrelia*, but are important in replication and survival of the ticks [8]. In the Northeastern United States, the major reservoir of disease is the white-footed mouse. In Europe and Asia, voles and birds play larger roles as reservoir hosts [9]. Interestingly, the feeding preferences of ticks may also limit the spread of Lyme borreliosis. Lizards, the preferred feeding source of *Ixodes* ticks in the Southeastern United States, are resistant to *B burgdorferi*, and the blood meal from a lizard wipes out the organism in the tick gut by complement-mediated killing [10]. This may explain the lack of penetration of Lyme borreliosis into the Southeastern United States.

Clinical manifestations

The pathognomonic lesion of Lyme disease is the erythema migrans (EM) rash (Fig. 1). The primary EM lesion develops at the site of a tick bite, typically within 5 to 14 days of tick detachment [11]. The rash is erythematous, sometimes with a bull's-eye zone of central clearing, and is usually painless and nonpruritic. Even without therapy, EM lesions spontaneously resolve over days to weeks. Early studies of Lyme disease reported the incidence of EM at approximately 50% to 70% [12]. With better patient education and stricter definitions of Lyme disease, recent studies indicate

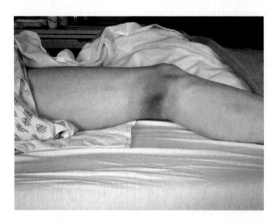

Fig. 1. Erythema migrans rash. (Courtesy of Lucas Wolf, MD.)

a much higher percentage of patients reporting EM lesions (up to 90%) [13,14].

From the original EM lesion, the spirochete disseminates over days to weeks. Common manifestations during this early period after infection include fever; malaise; additional EM lesions at distant sites; facial palsy; aseptic meningitis; radiculoneuropathy (more common in Europe); and carditis with atrioventricular block. Arthralgias and myalgias are common during this period, but true arthritis typically develops only weeks to months after the original infection.

Musculoskeletal manifestations of Lyme disease

Left untreated, approximately 50% to 60% of patients infected with *B burgdorferi* develop true arthritis [15]. The incidence of arthritis in European patients infected with either *B garinii* or *B afzelii* is likely lower. Lyme arthritis is a monoarthritis or oligoarthritis, usually affecting the knee, often with other large joint involvement, and occasionally involving small digital joints. Inflammation may also involve periarticular sites, causing tendonitis, bursitis, and sausage digits. Arthritis is usually intermittent and episodic, with periods of resolution or partial resolution between flares of pain and swelling. Patients have generally resolved their systemic symptoms of fevers, headaches, and malaise, and feel relatively well except for joint pain. Even without antibiotic therapy, flares of arthritis gradually become less severe and more distantly separated until they resolve completely. It is distinctly unusual to have flares of arthritis beyond 5 years.

Effects of therapy on clinical course

Antibiotic therapy early in the course of Lyme disease is very effective in preventing arthritis [16]. Antibiotics hasten recovery from some, but not all of the manifestations of Lyme borreliosis. For example, antibiotics do not affect the course of facial palsy [17]. Antibiotics do shorten the duration of arthritis for most patients, with resolution typically occurring within weeks to months after treatment. A minority of patients continue to have either persistent or intermittent arthritis even after multiple courses of antibiotics. This group of patients is most commonly described as having "antibiotic-resistant chronic Lyme arthritis." Arthritis in patients with antibiotic-resistant Lyme arthritis diminishes over time, and arthritis beyond 5 years is also uncommon in this group of patients. Anecdotally, arthritis in the antibiotic-resistant group of patients tends to be more constant and less intermittent than Lyme arthritis in untreated patients [18].

Mechanisms of disease

Much has been learned about how *B burgdorferi* interacts with its mammalian hosts and how these interactions govern the pathogenesis and manifestations of disease. Studies of disease pathogenesis have been greatly aided by the availability of a murine model, and many of the mechanisms discussed next are extrapolated from data in mice.

Utilization of tick factors by B burgdorferi

As the tick takes its blood meal, spirochetes in the tick midgut undergo changes that enable them to move into a new host. With the influx of nutrients, organisms multiply rapidly. Proteins required for attachment and survival in the tick midgut (eg, outer surface protein A) are down-regulated, and proteins required for colonization of mammalian tissue (eg, outer surface protein C and decorin-binding protein) are up-regulated [19]. The organisms travel from the midgut to the tick salivary glands, and into the vertebrate host. This process typically takes 48 to 72 hours, which explains why ticks attached for less than 24 hours do not transmit *B burgdorferi*.

Invasion by *B burgdorferi* is abetted by tick saliva. Tick saliva impairs inflammatory responses in mammals, including macrophage activation, secretion of the macrophage-associated cytokines interleukin-1 and tumor necrosis factor-α, secretion of the T helper–associated cytokines interleukin-2 and interferon-γ, neutrophil function, and complement activation [20]. These effects last throughout the period of tick attachment, and persist for 3 to 4 days. Administration of tumor necrosis factor-α, interleukin-2, or interferon-γ to mice during the period of tick attachment seems to facilitate early (<21 days) containment of *B burgdorferi* in experimental murine infections, although all mice subsequently did develop chronic infection. The initial response to *B burgdorferi* is mediated by the innate immune system. Toll-like receptors recognize a broad array of bacterial antigens, such as endotoxin, peptidoglycan, CpG nucleic acids, and bacterial lipoproteins. *B burgdorferi* is an unusual organism in that its genome encodes for over 150 known or putative lipoproteins [21]. Bacterial lipoproteins are recognized by toll-like receptor 2 (TLR-2), activating numerous cells, including macrophages, endothelial cells, neutrophils, dendritic cells, B cells, and mast cells. Recognition by TLR-2 causes secretion of cytokines and chemokines that recruit macrophages and neutrophils to areas of spirochete localization [22,23].

Utilization of mammalian factors by B burgdorferi

To disseminate from the original EM lesion, *Borrelia* must traverse extracellular matrix. *B burgdorferi* does not seem to produce its own proteases. Instead, *B burgdorferi* uses host proteases. *B burgdorferi* binds host plasmin and its activator urokinase to its surface, protecting them from inactivation [24–26]. In addition to its fibrinolytic role, plasmin is a broad-spectrum protease, capable of breaking down extracellular matrix. Plasmin also activates matrix metalloproteinase (MMPs), the major proteases involved in extracellular matrix degradation and tissue remodeling.

Infection with *B burgdorferi* induces MMP expression in many different tissues [27–29]. In in vitro and animal models, both MMPs and plasmin facilitate dissemination of the spirochete [25,28]. Plasmin is also important in the movement of spirochetes within the tick, as the tick takes its blood meal [30].

Arthritogenic factors in Borrelia

Different *Borrelia* strains, and even different isolates of the same strain, cause different disease manifestations. *B burgdorferi* is more associated with arthritis, *B garinii* with neurologic disease, and *B afzelii* with the skin lesions of acrodermatitis chronica atrophicans. New York isolates of *B burgdorferi* display significant differences in their ability to cause arthritis in mice [31]. Differences in clinical behavior result from differences in the ability of *Borrelia* strains to localize to specific tissues, and differences in the host response. *B burgdorferi* express surface proteins that attach to integrins, proteoglycans, and glycoproteins on cell surfaces or in extracellular matrix. The best characterized of these proteins include P66, an outer surface membrane protein that mediates binding to two different integrins ($\alpha_{IIb}\beta_3$ and $\alpha_v\beta_3$) found on platelets and other cells [32,33]; *Borrelia* glycosaminoglycan binding protein, which binds to heparin sulfate and dermatan sulfate found commonly on neuronal cells [34,35]; decorin binding proteins A and B, which bind to decorin, a proteoglycan that "decorates" collagen fibers [36]; and a fibronectin binding protein, BBK32, which mediates attachment to fibronectin in the extracellular matrix [37]. In studies with decorin-deficient mice, binding to decorin played an important role in spirochete persistence in the skin and joints, sites with relatively high decorin levels [38].

The host inflammatory response may differ between organs because of differences in the local production of cytokines and chemokines by specific cell populations. For example, inflammatory cardiac infiltrates tend to be monocytic, whereas the synovial inflammatory response is more neutrophilic [39]. These differences are relative, however, and inflammatory cells of all types are present in the different infected organs.

In the joints, recognition by the innate immune system is important in the early host response. Studies of TLR-2–deficient mice, or mice deficient in MyD88, an intermediary signaling protein for most TLRs, however, produced surprising results. Rather than decreased inflammation, TLR-2– and MyD88-deficient mice exhibited equivalent or greatly increased arthritis compared with wild-type mice infected with *B burgdorferi*. This suggests that early recognition of borrelial products also occurs through non–TLR-dependent pathways [40–42]. Despite the increased inflammation, however, these cells fail to control infection in the absence of TLR signaling, because the numbers of spirochetes in TLR-2– and MyD88-deficient mice are much higher than in wild-type. The mechanism by which TLR signaling contributes to the control of the infection is still unknown. At later stages of infection when the adaptive immune response has developed, control of infection is similar in TLR-deficient and wild-type mice, indicating that appropriate antibody responses develop in the absence of TLR signaling.

Factors responsible for progression and persistence of Lyme arthritis

Lyme arthritis progresses in an indolent fashion, compared with other forms of bacterial septic arthritis where joint destruction occurs within days. In Lyme arthritis, irreversible damage occurs only months or years into infection. In this way, Lyme arthritis resembles rheumatoid arthritis. Histologically, the joint damage of Lyme arthritis may be indistinguishable from rheumatoid arthritis. There are several reasons why progression of destructive arthritis is slower in Lyme arthritis. First, *B burgdorferi*, unlike *Staphylococcus aureus* or *Streptococcus pyogenes*, does not produce its own proteases that digest collagen and other extracellular proteins of articular cartilage [24,25]. This suggests that joint damage is caused largely by the host inflammatory response. Joint inflammation is typically moderate, with synovial fluid white blood cells (WBCs) ranging from 1000 to 50,000 cells/ mm^3, also helping to explain the slower progression of disease. In animal and in vitro models of Lyme arthritis, joint destruction is correlated with induction of many of the same MMPs implicated in rheumatoid arthritis, including MMP-1, MMP-3, and MMP-13 [43].

The reasons for the intermittent nature of arthritis in untreated Lyme disease are not fully understood. In murine models, flares in arthritis correlate with increases in spirochete burden, although what triggers these increases is unknown. Borrelial evasion of host immunity has been suggested as one possible mechanism. Several different strategies for immune avoidance have been identified. Although the *B burgdorferi* genome encodes for over 150 putative lipoproteins, only some of these are expressed at any time. On entry into a mammalian host, up to 116 of the lipoprotein genes seem to be transcribed. Under immunologic pressure, however, expression decreases to less than 40 of these lipoproteins by day 30 of infection, giving the host immune response fewer targets [44]. *B burgdorferi* can also change antigenic targets on its outer surface membrane proteins. The *B burgdorferi* VlsE protein undergoes significant antigenic variation, by substituting from 16 different nonexpressed cassettes adjacent to the single expressed locus [45].

In addition to regulation and antigenic variation of outer membrane proteins, *B afzelii* and *B burgdorferi* bind host factors that prevent complement-mediated killing [46–48]. Both organisms can express multiple complement regulator-acquiring surface proteins, which capture host Factor H. Factor H inactivates C3b, protecting the organism from complement-mediated killing in vitro. Binding of factor H may not be essential in survival or dissemination, because borrelial strains that do not express complement regulator-acquiring surface proteins in vitro remain infectious, although it could be possible that they up-regulate these complement regulator-acquiring surface proteins in vivo.

It is unclear why some untreated patients develop arthritis and others do not. Some variability in patient outcome may be accounted for by strain differences. It is also quite likely that host factors may play a role. Different strains of inbred mice exhibit different degrees of arthritis in response to *B burgdorferi* infection [39]. The specific genes involved in the arthritis phenotype have not been identified, but they have been localized to specific chromosomes [49]. The genes governing joint swelling are apparently distinct from the genes controlling the histopathologic development of arthritis in mice. This seems to parallel rheumatoid arthritis, where anti-inflammatory agents that diminish swelling may not affect the progression of synovitis, and conversely, disease-modifying antirheumatic drugs may not decrease swelling, suggesting that there may be pathways common to both Lyme and rheumatoid arthritis.

Causes of chronic Lyme arthritis

In patients not treated with antibiotics, arthritis and other signs of infection resolve spontaneously. It is not known whether the organisms eventually succumb to the host immune system, or whether they persist at low levels without activating inflammatory responses. *Borrelia* have been recovered from skin lesions more than 10 years after the original infection. The mechanism of arthritis in the small group of patients with arthritis after antibiotic therapy remains an area of controversy. The two major hypotheses revolve around the concepts of the continued presence of spirochetes or spirochetal antigens in the joints, or the development of an autoimmune process. There is some evidence to support each of these theories.

In most patients who have antibiotic-resistant chronic Lyme arthritis, live organisms or antigens cannot be detected in synovial fluid more than 3 months after therapy [50]. There have been rare reports from Europe, however, of polymerase chain reaction detection of spirochetal DNA in synovial tissue from patients undergoing synovectomy after long courses of antibiotics [51]. Recovery of spirochetes by xenodiagnosis from *Ixodes* ticks fed on antibiotic-treated mice 3 months after a 1-month course of antibiotics has been documented, but these spirochetes were attenuated and unable to infect new mice [52]. In vitro studies have shown that antibiotic therapy may not completely eradicate organisms cocultured with certain cells, suggesting that bacteria that are sensitive to an antibiotic in vitro may display a resistant phenotype in vivo in the context of host cells [53]. To date, there has been no documented borrelial resistance to commonly used antibiotics.

The hypothesis of autoimmune arthritis in antibiotic-treated patients initially stemmed from the observation that a higher proportion of these patients had antibodies to outer surface protein A [54]. In addition, treatment of patients with antibiotic-resistant chronic Lyme arthritis with immunosuppressive agents does not seem to worsen disease or improve the recovery of organisms. This fact is indirect evidence, however, because patients with Lyme facial palsy who receive corticosteroids, but not antibiotics, also do not worsen their disease. In mouse models, only mice with severe immunodeficiencies (eg, severe combined immunodeficiency or MyD88 knockouts) cannot control borrelial infection. Certain immunodeficiencies (eg, T-cell deficiencies) actually result in decreased inflammation and symptoms.

Patients with antibiotic-resistant Lyme arthritis have an increased incidence of specific HLA haplotypes, including HLA-DRB1*0401, HLA-DRB1*0101, and to a lesser extent HLA-DRB1-0404 [54]. Molecular mimicry of a human antigen, leukocyte adhesion molecule-1 (LFA-1), by borrelial outer surface protein A has been proposed as a potential mechanism for autoimmune arthritis [55]. Although LFA-1 activates T cells directed against amino acids 165-173 of outer surface protein A (which is predicted to be the immunodominant outer surface protein A epitope presented by HLA-DRB1*0401), no definitive evidence that cross-reactions to LFA-1 are involved in arthritis has been found, and the specificity of this response has been called into question [56].

Diagnosis of Lyme arthritis

The tools for the diagnosis of Lyme arthritis are essentially the same as the tools for the diagnosis of early Lyme disease, which have been well described in several reviews [57]. Lyme borreliosis should be considered in patients who present with an acute or subacute oligoarthritis who live in or have traveled to areas endemic for *B burgdorferi*. A history of a rash consistent with EM increases the pretest probability of Lyme borreliosis. Because patients in endemic areas are more aware of Lyme disease and the appearance of EM lesions, however, more patients are being treated early in infection. As a result, the proportion of patients with Lyme arthritis who do not have a history of EM is increasing, and lack of EM should not exclude patients with arthritis in endemic areas from serologic testing for Lyme disease.

Serologic testing remains the mainstay of diagnosis. Most centers use an ELISA for screening, with the Western blot for confirmatory testing. In patients with Lyme arthritis, these tests are expected to be strongly positive. Newer, more specific serologic tests, such as the C6 peptide antibody test, which tests for IgG antibody to a constant region of the VlsE protein, show improved specificity compared with traditional ELISA testing. IgG antibody to the C6 peptide develops as early as IgM antibody in standard ELISA [58]. Whether the sensitivity and specificity of the C6 antibody is sufficient to eliminate the recommendation for two-tiered testing has not been determined. At our institution, we have still been confirming positive C6 antibody tests with Western blot tests interpreted according to Centers for Disease Control and Prevention criteria. Because patients with Lyme arthritis typically present later in the course of Lyme disease, all serologic tests (ELISA, IFA, C6, and Western blots) are generally strongly positive, so the lack of sensitivity and specificity that plague the use of these tests in early Lyme disease are less relevant for Lyme arthritis. Testing in late-stage Lyme disease with either a C6 antibody test or a traditional two-tiered approach results in sensitivity >90% and specificity from 95% to 100%.

Routine blood testing is nonspecific. By the time arthritis develops, peripheral white blood cell counts are typically normal. Erythrocyte sedimentation rates are normal or only slightly increased, which may help distinguish Lyme arthritis from rheumatologic causes of arthritis where erythrocyte sedimentation rates may be high. It is not uncommon to find low titers of nonspecific antinuclear antibodies.

Urine tests for *B burgdorferi* antigens or DNA have been marketed aggressively but are not currently approved by the Food and Drug Administration as tests for Lyme disease. In studies, the Lyme urine antigen test has been shown to provide results that are the equivalent of a random coin toss [59]. Similarly, urine PCRs are neither sensitive nor specific for the diagnosis of Lyme disease [60,61]. Urine tests should not currently be considered part of the diagnostic strategy for Lyme disease.

Synovial fluid should be obtained from all patients with suspected Lyme arthritis. Synovial fluid WBC counts in Lyme arthritis usually range from 1000 to 50,000 cells/mm^3. WBC counts over 100,000 cells/mm^3, however, do not exclude Lyme arthritis. In antibiotic-resistant Lyme arthritis, synovial WBC counts are generally lower, ranging from 500 to 10,000 cells/mm^3. PCR for detecting DNA of *B burgdorferi*, although not yet approved for clinical use, is a useful confirmatory test in active Lyme arthritis, but cannot distinguish live from dead organisms. PCR positivity for *B burgdorferi* DNA most commonly disappears rapidly during the first month of antibiotic therapy, but can persist for a few months after antibiotics. Unfortunately, it has not yet been possible to culture *B burgdorferi* from synovial fluid.

Treatment of Lyme arthritis

Lyme arthritis can be treated successfully with oral or intravenous antibiotic regimens [62]. In patients without evidence of neurologic disease, oral therapy is preferred because of lower cost and complication rates. Doxycycline, 100 mg twice daily, is the agent of choice for its excellent oral absorption, low cost, and anti-inflammatory activity as a matrix metal-loproteinase inhibitor. Doxycycline, unlike many of the other antibiotics used to treat Lyme borreliosis, is also active against *Anaplasma phagocyto-philia*, the cause of human anaplasmosis (formerly known as human granulocytic ehrlichiosis). *A phagocytophilia* is also carried by *Ixodes* ticks, and may be cotransmitted with *B burgdorferi*. Doxycycline is contra-indicated in pregnant or breast-feeding women, and young children, in whom it may cause tooth staining. Alternatives include amoxicillin, cefuroxime axetil, azithromycin, or clarithromycin. When intravenous medication is indicated, ceftriaxone is the drug of choice because of ease of administration. Patients with arthritis are treated initially for 4 weeks.

A small proportion of patients do not respond to the initial course of antibiotics. My approach is to perform repeat arthrocentesis, with synovial fluid PCR testing for *B burgdorferi* DNA. Patients with a positive PCR test should receive continued oral or intravenous antibiotics until symptoms resolve, or PCR testing becomes negative. Patients with a negative PCR test may also receive a single additional 4-week course of antibiotic therapy. If symptoms persist in the face of repeatedly negative PCR tests, however, these patients should be treated for antibiotic-resistant Lyme arthritis. There are no guidelines as to when intravenous antibiotics should be used for Lyme arthritis, and no clear data that intravenous antibiotics are superior to oral antibiotics for Lyme arthritis in the absence of neurologic disease.

If patients do not respond to two courses of antibiotics of 1 month in duration, and their PCR tests on synovial fluid are negative, there is no evidence that continued antibiotic therapy is of benefit. Antibiotic-resistant Lyme arthritis responds well to either steroids or methotrexate. Anticytokine therapy, such as tumor necrosis factor blockers, has been anecdotally reported to be effective, and may become the therapy of choice. Immuno-suppressive medication is continued until patients have had complete suppression of arthritis for 3 months to 1 year, and then gradually tapered off. Synovectomy has a limited role for patients with severe arthritis unresponsive to all other measures. None of these therapies has proved universally to be effective in all patients with antibiotic-resistant arthritis. A summary of my approach to patients with Lyme arthritis is shown in Fig. 2.

Prevention of Lyme disease

Contact avoidance is the primary strategy for prevention. Key measures include the clearing of leaves, tall grass, and brush from contact areas; wearing hats, high boots, and long-sleeved shirts; tucking trouser legs into socks; and wearing light-colored clothing to make ticks more easily visible. Because *Ixodes* ticks cannot transmit Lyme disease before 24 hours of attachment, daily tick checks after exposure are an extremely effective measure for prevention. Ticks should be removed with tweezers by applying gentle, tugging pressure without crushing the tick. After several minutes, the tick's mouth parts fatigue, and the tick releases intact from the skin.

Insecticides containing either DEET or IR3535 are effective tick repellents. Permethrin, a compound toxic to ticks, can be sprayed on clothing but should not be applied directly to skin. Reduction of tick populations has been attempted with some success, with applications of permethrin to mice or deer through the use of special feeding devices. These devices may be used by communities or individual homeowners in endemic areas.

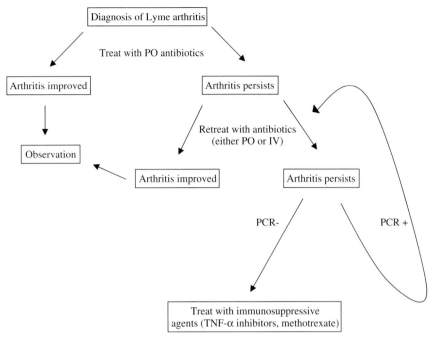

Fig. 2. Flow chart for management of Lyme arthritis. PCR, polymerase chain reaction; TNF-α, tumor necrosis factor-alpha.

A vaccine for Lyme disease, LYMErix, was approved for human use in patients at high risk of exposure to Lyme disease. Vaccine efficacy was approximately 85% [63]. Unfortunately, this vaccine was withdrawn from the market in 2002 because of poor sales. No other vaccine is currently available. Recently, a strategy for vaccinating mice in the wild was shown to reduce carriage of *B burgdorferi* by *Ixodes* ticks, although further development of an appropriate vehicle for vaccine delivery to rodent reservoirs remains necessary [64].

For patients in an endemic area who find an *Ixodes* tick that has been attached for more than 24 hours, antibiotic prophylaxis can be considered. A single dose of doxycycline (200 mg) has been shown to be 87% effective in preventing the development of Lyme disease [65]. Although antibiotic prophylaxis is commonly practiced in many areas endemic for Lyme disease, cost-benefit analyses have not generally supported its use, and careful observation for symptoms after a tick bite is an appropriate alternative [66].

Summary

Lyme borreliosis continues to be a significant public health problem. Because of good public education, the incidence of Lyme arthritis and other late-stage symptoms has not increased in tandem with the increases in early infection. There have been major advances in the understanding of the pathogenesis of Lyme arthritis. The understanding of mechanisms of arthritis in Lyme borreliosis may also shed light on the mechanisms of disease in other infectious and noninfectious arthritides.

Acknowledgments

I appreciate the help of Dr. Jenifer Coburn in review of this manuscript and Dr. Lucas Wolf for donating the picture of erythema migrans.

References

[1] From the Centers for Disease Control and Prevention. Lyme disease—United States, 2000. JAMA 2002;287:1259–60.

[2] Baranton G, Assous M, Postic D. Three bacterial species associated with Lyme borreliosis: clinical and diagnostic implications. Bull Acad Natl Med 1992;176:1075–86.

[3] James AM, Liveris D, Wormser GP, et al. *Borrelia lonestari* infection after a bite by an *Amblyomma americanum* tick. J Infect Dis 2001;183:1810–4.

[4] Masters E, Granter S, Duray P, et al. Physician-diagnosed erythema migrans and erythema migrans-like rashes following Lone Star tick bites. Arch Dermatol 1998;134:955–60.

[5] Telford SR III, Mather TN, Moore SI, et al. Incompetence of deer as reservoirs of the Lyme disease spirochete. Am J Trop Med Hyg 1988;39:105–9.

[6] Burgess EC, Wachal MD, Cleven TC. *Borrelia burgdorferi* infection in dairy cows, rodents, and birds from four Wisconsin dairy farms. Vet Microbiol 1993;35:61–77.

[7] Anderson JF, Magnarelli LA. Avian and mammalian hosts for spirochete-infected ticks and insects in a Lyme disease focus in Connecticut. Yale J Biol Med 1984;57:627–41.

[8] Wilson ML, Levine JF, Spielman A. Effect of deer reduction on abundance of the deer tick (*Ixodes dammini*). Yale J Biol Med 1984;57:697–705.

[9] Gern L, Estrada-Pena A, Frandsen F, et al. European reservoir hosts of *Borrelia burgdorferi sensu lato*. Zentralbl Bakteriol 1998;287:196–204.

[10] Kuo MM, Lane RS, Giclas PC. A comparative study of mammalian and reptilian alternative pathway of complement-mediated killing of the Lyme disease spirochete (*Borrelia burgdorferi*). J Parasitol 2000;86:1223–8.

[11] Nocton JJ, Steere AC. Lyme disease. Adv Intern Med 1995;40:69–117.

[12] Steere AC, Bartenhagen NH, Craft JE, et al. The early clinical manifestations of Lyme disease. Ann Intern Med 1983;99:76–82.

[13] Krause PJ, Telford SR III, Spielman A, et al. Concurrent Lyme disease and babesiosis: evidence for increased severity and duration of illness. JAMA 1996;275:1657–60.

[14] Gerber MA, Shapiro ED, Burke GS, et al. Lyme disease in children in southeastern Connecticut. Pediatric Lyme Disease Study Group. N Engl J Med 1996;335:1270–4.

[15] Steere AC, Schoen RT, Taylor E. The clinical evolution of Lyme arthritis. Ann Intern Med 1987;107:725–31.

[16] Dattwyler RJ, Luft BJ, Kunkel MJ, et al. Ceftriaxone compared with doxycycline for the treatment of acute disseminated Lyme disease. N Engl J Med 1997;337:289–94.

[17] Halperin JJ, Golightly M. Lyme borreliosis in Bell's palsy. Neurology 1992;42:1268–70.

[18] Steere AC. Diagnosis and treatment of Lyme arthritis. Med Clin North Am 1997;81:179–94.

[19] Schwan TG, Piesman J. Temporal changes in outer surface proteins A and C of the Lyme disease-associated spirochete, *Borrelia burgdorferi*, during the chain of infection in ticks and mice. J Clin Microbiol 2000;38:382–8.

[20] Zeidner N, Dreitz M, Belasco D, et al. Suppression of acute Ixodes scapularis-induced *Borrelia burgdorferi* infection using tumor necrosis factor-alpha, interleukin-2, and interferon-gamma. J Infect Dis 1996;173:187–95.

[21] Fraser CM, Casjens S, Huang WM, et al. Genomic sequence of a Lyme disease spirochaete, *Borrelia burgdorferi*. Nature 1997;390:580–6.

[22] Brightbill HD, Libraty DH, Krutzik SR, et al. Host defense mechanisms triggered by microbial lipoproteins through toll-like receptors. Science 1999;285:732–6.

[23] Hirschfeld M, Kirschning CJ, Schwandner R, et al. Cutting edge: inflammatory signaling by *Borrelia burgdorferi* lipoproteins is mediated by toll-like receptor 2. J Immunol 1999;163: 2382–6.

[24] Klempner MS, Noring R, Epstein MP, et al. Binding of human plasminogen and urokinase-type plasminogen activator to the Lyme disease spirochete, *Borrelia burgdorferi*. J Infect Dis 1995;171:1258–65.

[25] Coleman JL, Sellati TJ, Testa JE, et al. *Borrelia burgdorferi* binds plasminogen, resulting in enhanced penetration of endothelial monolayers. Infect Immun 1995;63:2478–84.

[26] Fuchs H, Wallich R, Simon MM, et al. The outer surface protein A of the spirochete *Borrelia burgdorferi* is a plasmin(ogen) receptor. Proc Natl Acad Sci U S A 1994;91:12594–8.

[27] Lin B, Kidder JM, Noring R, et al. Differences in synovial fluid levels of matrix metalloproteinases suggest separate mechanisms of pathogenesis in Lyme arthritis before and after antibiotic treatment. J Infect Dis 2001;184:174–80.

[28] Gebbia JA, Coleman JL, Benach JL. Selective induction of matrix metalloproteinases by *Borrelia burgdorferi* via toll-like receptor 2 in monocytes. J Infect Dis 2004;189: 113–9.

[29] Zhao Z, Chang H, Trevino RP, et al. Selective up-regulation of matrix metalloproteinase-9 expression in human erythema migrans skin lesions of acute Lyme disease. J Infect Dis 2003;188:1098–104.

[30] Coleman JL, Gebbia JA, Peisman J, et al. Plasminogen is required for efficient dissemination of *B. burgdorferi* in ticks and for enhancement of spirochetemia in mice. Cell 1997;89:1111–9.

[31] Wang G, Ojaimi C, Wu H, et al. Disease severity in a murine model of Lyme borreliosis is associated with the genotype of the infecting *Borrelia burgdorferi sensu stricto* strain. J Infect Dis 2002;186:782–91.

[32] Coburn J, Magoun L, Bodary SC, et al. Integrins alpha(v)beta3 and alpha5beta1 mediate attachment of Lyme disease spirochetes to human cells. Infect Immun 1998;66:1946–52.

[33] Coburn J, Leong JM, Erban JK. Integrin alpha IIb beta 3 mediates binding of the Lyme disease agent *Borrelia burgdorferi* to human platelets. Proc Natl Acad Sci U S A 1993;90: 7059–63.

[34] Parveen N, Leong JM. Identification of a candidate glycosaminoglycan-binding adhesin of the Lyme disease spirochete *Borrelia burgdorferi*. Mol Microbiol 2000;35:1220–34.

[35] Leong JM, Wang H, Magoun L, et al. Different classes of proteoglycans contribute to the attachment of *Borrelia burgdorferi* to cultured endothelial and brain cells. Infect Immun 1998;66:994–9.

[36] Guo BP, Brown EL, Dorward DW, et al. Decorin-binding adhesins from *Borrelia burgdorferi*. Mol Microbiol 1998;30:711–23.

[37] Probert WS, Kim JH, Hook M, et al. Mapping the ligand-binding region of *Borrelia burgdorferi* fibronectin-binding protein BBK32. Infect Immun 2001;69:4129–33.

[38] Liang FT, Brown EL, Wang T, et al. Protective niche for *Borrelia burgdorferi* to evade humoral immunity. Am J Pathol 2004;165:977–85.

[39] Barthold SW, Beck DS, Hansen GM, et al. Lyme borreliosis in selected strains and ages of laboratory mice. J Infect Dis 1990;162:133–8.

[40] Bolz DD, Sundsbak RS, Ma Y, et al. MyD88 plays a unique role in host defense but not arthritis development in Lyme disease. J Immunol 2003;173:2003–10.

[41] Wooten RM, Ma Y, Yoder RA, et al. Toll-like receptor 2 is required for innate, but not acquired, host defense to *Borrelia burgdorferi*. J Immunol 2002;168:348–55.

[42] Liu N, Montgomery RR, Barthold SW, et al. Myeloid differentiation antigen 88 deficiency impairs pathogen clearance but does not alter inflammation in *Borrelia burgdorferi*-infected mice. Infect Immun 2004;72:3195–203.

[43] Behera AK, Hildebrand E, Scagliotti J, et al. Induction of host matrix metalloproteinases by *Borrelia burgdorferi* differs in human and murine Lyme arthritis. Infect Immun 2005;73: 126–34.

[44] Liang FT, Yan J, Mbow ML, et al. *Borrelia burgdorferi* changes its surface antigenic expression in response to host immune responses. Infect Immun 2004;72:5759–67.

[45] Zhang JR, Hardham JM, Barbour AG, et al. Antigenic variation in Lyme disease borreliae by promiscuous recombination of VMP-like sequence cassettes. Cell 1997;89:275–85.

[46] Kraiczy P, Skerka C, Kirschfink M, et al. Immune evasion of *Borrelia burgdorferi* by acquisition of human complement regulators FHL-1/reconectin and Factor H. Eur J Immunol 2001;31:1674–84.

[47] Metts MS, McDowell JV, Theisen M, et al. Analysis of the OspE determinants involved in binding of factor H and OspE-targeting antibodies elicited during *Borrelia burgdorferi* infection in mice. Infect Immun 2003;71:3587–96.

[48] Miller JC, Stevenson B. Increased expression of *Borrelia burgdorferi* factor H-binding surface proteins during transmission from ticks to mice. Int J Med Microbiol 2004;293(Suppl 37):120–5.

[49] Weis JJ, McCracken BA, Ma Y, et al. Identification of quantitative trait loci governing arthritis severity and humoral responses in the murine model of Lyme disease. J Immunol 1999;162:948–56.

[50] Carlson D, Hernandez J, Bloom BJ, et al. Lack of *Borrelia burgdorferi* DNA in synovial samples from patients with antibiotic treatment-resistant Lyme arthritis. Arthritis Rheum 1999;42:2705–9.

[51] Priem S, Burmester GR, Kamradt T, et al. Detection of *Borrelia burgdorferi* by polymerase chain reaction in synovial membrane, but not in synovial fluid from patients with persisting Lyme arthritis after antibiotic therapy. Ann Rheum Dis 1998;57:118–21.

[52] Bockenstedt LK, Mao J, Hodzic E, et al. Detection of attenuated, noninfectious spirochetes in *Borrelia burgdorferi*-infected mice after antibiotic treatment. J Infect Dis 2002;186:1430–7.

[53] Girschick HJ, Huppertz HI, Russmann H, et al. Intracellular persistence of *Borrelia burgdorferi* in human synovial cells. Rheumatol Int 1996;16:125–32.

[54] Kalish RA, Leong JM, Steere AC. Association of treatment-resistant chronic Lyme arthritis with HLA-DR4 and antibody reactivity to OspA and OspB of *Borrelia burgdorferi*. Infect Immun 1993;61:2774–9.

[55] Gross DM, Forsthuber T, Tary-Lehmann M, et al. Identification of LFA-1 as a candidate autoantigen in treatment-resistant Lyme arthritis. Science 1998;281:703–6.

[56] Steere AC, Falk B, Drouin EE, et al. Binding of outer surface protein A and human lymphocyte function-associated antigen 1 peptides to HLA-DR molecules associated with antibiotic treatment-resistant Lyme arthritis. Arthritis Rheum 2003;48:534–40.

[57] Steere AC. Lyme disease. N Engl J Med 2001;345:115–25.

[58] Marques AR, Martin DS, Philipp MT. Evaluation of the C6 peptide enzyme-linked immunosorbent assay for individuals vaccinated with the recombinant OspA vaccine. J Clin Microbiol 2002;40:2591–3.

[59] Klempner MS, Schmid CH, Hu L, et al. Intralaboratory reliability of serologic and urine testing for Lyme disease. Am J Med 2001;110:217–9.

[60] Brettschneider S, Bruckbauer H, Klugbauer N, et al. Diagnostic value of PCR for detection of *Borrelia burgdorferi* in skin biopsy and urine samples from patients with skin borreliosis. J Clin Microbiol 1998;36:2658–65.

[61] Lebech AM, Hansen K, Brandrup F, et al. Diagnostic value of PCR for detection of *Borrelia burgdorferi* DNA in clinical specimens from patients with erythema migrans and Lyme neuroborreliosis. Mol Diagn 2000;5:139–50.

[62] Wormser GP, Nadelman RB, Dattwyler RJ, et al. Practice guidelines for the treatment of Lyme disease. The Infectious Diseases Society of America. Clin Infect Dis 2000;31(Suppl 1): 1–14.

[63] Sigal LH, Zahradnik JM, Lavin P, et al. A vaccine consisting of recombinant *Borrelia burgdorferi* outer-surface protein A to prevent Lyme disease. Recombinant Outer-Surface Protein A Lyme Disease Vaccine Study Consortium. N Engl J Med 1998;339:216–22.

[64] Tsao JI, Wootton JT, Bunikis J, et al. An ecological approach to preventing human infection: vaccinating wild mouse reservoirs intervenes in the Lyme disease cycle. Proc Natl Acad Sci U S A 2004;101:18159–64.

[65] Shapiro ED, Gerber MA, Holabird NB, et al. A controlled trial of antimicrobial prophylaxis for Lyme disease after deer-tick bites. N Engl J Med 1992;327:1769–73.

[66] Magid D, Schwartz B, Craft J, et al. Prevention of Lyme disease after tick bites: a cost-effectiveness analysis. N Engl J Med 1992;327:534–41.

ELSEVIER
SAUNDERS

INFECTIOUS
DISEASE CLINICS
OF NORTH AMERICA

Infect Dis Clin N Am 19 (2005) 963–980

Viral Arthritis

Leonard H. Calabrese, DO[a],*, Stanley J. Naides, MD[b]

[a]*Department of Rheumatic and Immunologic Diseases, The Cleveland Clinic,*
9500 Euclid Avenue, Cleveland, OH 44195, USA
[b]*Departments of Medicine, Microbiology, and Immunology, Division of Rheumatology,*
Penn State Milton S. Hershey Medical Center, Arthritis, Bone, & Joint Center,
Suite 400, 500 University Drive, Hershey, PA 17033, USA

The role of viruses in the development of acute and chronic arthritis is complex, because viruses are ubiquitous, and all human beings are occasionally afflicted by viral infections. In general, most viral infections (ie, most respiratory pathogens) are acute and self-limiting and survive by infecting one susceptible host, then moving on to another. Some viruses establish prolonged latency in the host after acute infection, resulting in clinical symptoms after many years of dormancy, such as dermatomal zoster following chicken pox. Still other viral agents produce chronic infections following the primary stage in all (HIV), most (hepatitis C virus), or a minority (hepatitis B virus) of the infected. The mechanisms whereby these infections produce arthritis are diverse and still poorly understood, but are clearly influenced by both host and viral factors. In rubella, viral infection within the joint is probably responsible. For hepatitis B and C, arthritis may result directly from host cellular or humoral immune responses, while other viruses may act indirectly by altering the integrated host defense network, or by inducing frank autoimmunity, as with HIV and HTLV-1. Although viral arthritis is usually self-limited and nondestructive, chronic forms arise in two settings. First, chronic viral arthritis may occur when immunodeficient patients are infected with agents that are short-lived pathogens in normal hosts, leading to chronic or recurrent infection, with arthritis as one sequela. Second, chronic arthritis may also occur with infections that are by their very nature chronic persistent viral illnesses. This review addresses these and other common forms of viral arthritis, such as that caused by parvovirus B19.

* Corresponding author.
E-mail address: calabrl@ccf.org (L.H. Calabrese).

0891-5520/05/$ - see front matter © 2005 Elsevier Inc. All rights reserved.
doi:10.1016/j.idc.2005.09.002
id.theclinics.com

Parvovirus B19

Parovirus B19 causes the common rash illness in children, erythema infectiosum, or fifth disease. It is a member of the family of nonenveloped, single-stranded DNA viruses Parvoviridae. B19 encodes two capsid proteins, VP1 and VP2, and a nonstructural protein, NS1, that plays a pathogenic role in nonerythroid cells not permissive for replication [1]. Although B19 was once thought to be the sole human parvovirus, three human parvovirus genotypes with up to 10% DNA sequence variation have recently been identified [2,3]. The various genotypes have not been associated with variation in clinical presentation [2,3]. B19 remains the prototype human parvovirus. A new human parvovirus has been identified with approximately 80% homology with B19, but its clinical significance, if any, remains unclear [4].

B19 occurs in outbreaks transmitted by respiratory secretions in the late winter and spring, but summer and autumn outbreaks and sporadic cases are also seen. Outbreaks tend to cycle every 3 or 4 years in a community because of the time required for a new cohort of uninfected children to enter school, where the outbreaks are often centered. Up to 50% of all adults are anti-B19 IgG-positive and IgM-negative, indicating past infection [5]. Naive individuals with frequent exposure to school-age children, such as elementary school teachers, pediatric nurses, and daycare workers are at increased risk of B19 infection. During school outbreaks, susceptible teachers may have infection rates as high as 50% [6,7].

The natural history of B19 infection has been elucidated by studying experimental infections and community outbreaks [8]. The incubation period between B19 infection and viremia is 7 to 18 days. Viremia may be intense, with as many as 10^{11} or more viral particles per milliliter of serum. Viremia is associated with a flulike illness and viral shedding by way of nasopharyngeal secretions. After 3 to 4 days of viremia, specific anti-B19 IgM antibodies appear. The appearance of antibodies coincides with the onset of rash and arthralgias or arthritis. Shortly thereafter, acute phase anti-B19 IgG antibodies appear. Both IgM and acute phase IgG antibodies recognize epitopes in the major viral capsid protein, VP2. Within 1 week of antibody response, development of IgG antibodies to epitopes unique to the minor capsid protein, VP1, leads to viral neutralization and clearing of infection. In immunocompromised individuals, such as those with congenital immunodeficiences, prior chemotherapy for lymphoma or leukemia, or AIDS, B19 infection may persist in bone marrow and lead to chronic or recurrent anemia, thrombocytopenia, or leukopenia [9]. Usually, cytopenic episodes are associated with low-level viremia, on the order of 10^4 to 10^6 viral particles per milliliter of serum. B19 is the leading cause of pure red cell aplasia in AIDS patients. Infusion of commercial intravenous immunoglobulin (IVIG) usually clears the viremia and corrects the cytopenia, because IVIG pools contain neutralizing antibodies to B19 [10].

B19 replicates in erythroid precursors. The putative receptor for B19 is the blood group P antigen, or globoside, a neutral glycosphingolipid. Globoside is found on a wide range of cell types in addition to erythrocytes, and B19 may also bind more complex globo-family neutral glycosphingolipids, accounting for the broad clinical presentation of disease [11]. $\alpha5\beta1$ integrins have been reported to be a coreceptor for B19 [12].

B19 was discovered in normal sera in 1975, and was quickly identified as the causative agent of transient aplastic crisis, erythema infectiosum, some cases of hydrops fetalis and spontaneous abortion, a rheumatoid-like arthritis, and chronic or recurrent bone marrow suppression in immunocompromised individuals [13]. Transient aplastic crisis due to B19-induced erythroid maturation arrest may occur in individuals with chronic hemolytic anemias that require constant regeneration of the peripheral erythrocyte pool. Transplacental transmission of B19 can induce a similar anemia in the fetus, sometimes leading to high-output cardiac failure, hydrops fetalis, and spontaneous abortion. B19 also causes the common childhood exanthem, erythema infectiosum, or fifth disease. Classically, children present with bright red, "slapped" cheeks, and a maculopapular or reticular rash. The rash may recur for weeks. Children are usually otherwise well, aside from a flulike illness in some. Ager and colleagues described an outbreak of fifth disease, diagnosed by the typical rash. Arthralgias were present in 5.1% of children under 10 years of age, and 2.8% had joint swelling. Amongst adolescents aged 11 to 19 years, 11.5% had arthralgias, and 5.3% had joint swelling [14].

Less common manifestations of B19 infection include vesiculopustular eruptions, Henoch-Schönlein purpura, and thrombotic thrombocytopenic purpura. An unusual "stocking and glove" acral erythema can occur. Isolated anemia, thrombocytopenia, and leukopenia may occur. A benign acute lymphadenopathy has been reported with B19 infection, as has hemophagocytic syndrome. Paresthesias, sensorineural hearing loss, and aseptic meningitis have been reported [13]. Elevated hepatic enzymes, hepatitis, and acute fulminant liver failure may be encountered. B19 infection in hepatocytes is non-permissive, failing to produce mature capsids. However, the nonstructural protein, NS1, is produced, which may induce hepatocyte apoptosis through intrinsic mitochondrial stress pathways [1].

Parvovirus B19 arthritis

B19 infection in adults is often not associated with rash. If rash is present, it may be subtle. Adults typically present with sudden onset polyarthralgia or polyarthritis. Symptoms may begin in one or a few joints, but involvement is polyarticular within 24 to 48 hours. The pattern of joint involvement mimics that of classic rheumatoid arthritis (RA). Morning stiffness may be severe and prolonged. The key clinical distinction between B19 viral infection and classic RA is the precipitous onset in B19. Joints are tender, often swollen, and occasionally erythematous [15]. Although B19 arthritis may be associated with a low-titer rheumatoid factor, and may mimic RA clinically, there is no definite evidence that B19 plays a role in the pathogenesis of classic RA. Patients may also have positive tests for ANA, anti-DNA antibodies, anti-lymphocyte antibodies, and antiphospholipid antibodies [15]. The association of B19 infection with rash, polyarthritis, cytopenias, and anti-DNA antibodies may also mimic systemic lupus erythematosus.

B19 infection is diagnosed by the finding of anti-B19 IgM antibody or B19 DNA in serum. During the viremic phase, when transient aplastic crisis typically presents, high-titer viremia without anti-B19 IgM antibody may be found. When patients with erythema infectiosum or arthritis typically present, viremia is cleared, and anti-IgM antibody is detected. Anti-B19 IgG becomes positive shortly thereafter. B19 DNA may be assayed by standard DNA hybridization or polymerase chain reaction methods. B19 antibodies have traditionally been detected in radioimmunoassays or enzyme-linked immunoabsorbent assays using virus or recombinant proteins as antigen [15]. A commercial kit test is now available for B19 antibody assay, using recombinant VP2 capsid protein as antigen.

B19 infection is usually treated symptomatically. Patients with transient aplastic crisis may require temporary transfusion support. In immunodeficient patients with B19 persistence and chronic or recurrent bone marrow suppression, intravenous immunoglobulin may be required to clear infection and allow marrow recovery [10]. In most patients with chronic B19 arthritis, viremia is unusual, and IVIG would not be expected to be beneficial. However, B19 may persist in the synovium of normal individuals, and evidence is accumulating that B19 may remain latent in other tissues as well [1,16]. As this form of latent infection is not associated with viremia, IVIG is unlikely to be beneficial. For chronic B19 arthritis, nonsteroidal anti-inflammatory drugs and adjunctive therapy for pain control are appropriate. An experimental vaccine for B19 based on recombinant capsid protein has been developed but is not yet approved for distribution [17].

Rubella

Rubella virus is the sole member of the rubivirus genus of the *Togaviridae* family of enveloped, positive-sense, single-stranded RNA viruses [18]. Spread occurs by way of airborne droplets, with peak incidence in late winter and spring. The success of near universal childhood vaccination has lulled physicians into overlooking rubella in the differential diagnosis of sudden onset arthritis. Before vaccination, rubella occurred in epidemic 6- to 9-year cycles amongst children. Postvaccination, the rate of rubella infection has declined to 10% to 20% of prevaccination rates, with young adults predominating. Outbreaks in college students have prompted many colleges to require revaccination before matriculation.

Viremia appears 7 to 9 days following infection, and is associated with shedding of virus in nasopharyngeal secretions. Posterior cervical and suboccipital lymphadenopathy from local viral replication, often painful in adults, occurs 5 to 10 days before the onset of rash [19]. A maculopapular eruption occurs 14 to 21 days postinfection and is temporally associated with clearing of viremia by antirubella antibody. The rash may last from a few hours or up to 5 days, beginning as a morbilliform facial eruption before appearing on the torso, then the extremities. The rash may be absent or subtle, and be overlooked by the patient [20]. Soft palate petechiae (Forscheimer's spots) may occur, but are not pathognomonic. Constitutional symptoms may precede the rash by 5 days, including fever, rash, coryza, and malaise. Symmetric arthralgias or arthritis are common in adults, especially women, appearing about the onset of rash. Typically, the arthritis has a symmetric RA-like pattern, but it may also be migratory. It usually resolves within 2 weeks, but joint symptoms occasionally persist for months to years, as in B19 infection. Evidence suggests that patients with persistence fail to develop antibodies to select envelope glycoproteins. Virus can be detected in circulating lymphocytes and during flares in synovial fluid [20]. Metacarpophalangeal and proximal interphalangeal joints of the hands, knees, wrists, ankles, and elbows are most frequently affected. Morning stiffness may be prominent. Periarthritis, tenosynovitis, and carpal tunnel syndrome may occur [21,22]. Thrombocytopenia and thrombocytopenic purpura may occur [23]. Encephalitis or encephalomyelitis occurs in approximately 1 of 6000 cases of rubella infection [24].

Rubella may be definitively diagnosed by viral isolation from throat culture. However, because many patients present with rash or arthritis, which often occur after viral clearance, detection of antirubella IgM or anti-IgG seroconversion is the diagnostic test of choice. Antirubella IgM and IgG are usually present at the onset of joint symptoms. IgM antibody levels peak 1 to 2 weeks after infection, then decrease over the next 4 to 6 months to undetectable levels in most patients. Therefore, detection of antirubella IgM indicates recent infection, usually in the last 1 to 2 months. Because antirubella IgG rises rapidly after onset symptoms, a diagnosis of rubella infection based on IgG serology alone can only be made with paired acute and convalescent sera. Antirubella IgG in a single serum sample only documents immunity [25]. Isolated antirubella IgM positivity should be interpreted with caution, because the presence of rheumatoid factor may give a false positive test, but rheumatoid factor may also occur in acute rubella arthritis [26].

Rubella may be prevented by vaccination, but postvaccination complications such as arthralgia, arthritis, myalgia, and paraesthesias have caused some resistance to vaccination. Rubella vaccines are live attenuated rubella strains. The initially used HPV77/DK12 strain was the most arthritogenic of the vaccine strains. Joint involvement in postvaccination arthritis is similar to wild-type infection. Although considered safer than HPV77/DK12 and Cendehill vaccine strains, as many as 15% or more of recipients of the currently used RA27/3 vaccine strain during a rubella outbreak in Canada developed arthropathy [27]. Arthritis usually occurred 2 weeks postinoculation and lasted less than a week. However, in a subset of vaccinees, symptoms persisted for more than a year.

Children may develop two peculiar postvaccination syndromes that underscore potential neurotropism of rubella. A lumbar radiculoneuropathy, dubbed the "catcher's crouch" syndrome, is characterized by popliteal fossa pain on arising in the morning. Knee extension exacerbates the pain, the victim finding relief in the catcher's crouch position. The pain gradually decreases through the day. A brachial radiculoneuropathy known as "arm syndrome" causes arm and hand pain and dysesthesias that are worse at night. Both syndromes occur 1 to 2 months postvaccination. The initial episode may last up to 2 months. Recurrences are usually shorter in duration, occurring for up to 1 year. There are no long-term sequelae [28].

Rubella arthritis is managed conservatively with nonsteroidal anti-inflammatory drugs (NSAIDs). Low to moderate doses of steroids have been used to control symptoms and viremia [29].

Alphaviruses

Chikungunya

Alphaviruses are transmitted to humans by mosquitoes. This genus includes the equine encephalitis viruses, as well as a colorful group of viruses causing dramatic outbreaks of fever, rash, and arthritis in Asia, India, the Pacific, Scandinavia, and South America. Their names often reflect their memorable manifestations [30]. Chikungunya virus was isolated during an epidemic of febrile arthritis in Tanzania in 1952–1953. ("Chikungunya" means "that which twists or bends up" in the local dialect). Epidemics may have occurred in the southern United States from 1779 to 1828 [31,32]. The increasing prevalence of *Aedes* mosquitoes, the major vector of Chikungunya, in the Americas suggests that epidemic reintroduction is possible.

O'nyong-nyong and Igbo Ora viruses

O'nyong-nyong virus, which means "joint breaker" in Acholi, is closely related to Chikungunya virus. It was first described in the Acholi province of northwestern Uganda in February 1959, infecting 2 million people over the next 2 years [33–35]. Following the initial epidemic, there were no reported cases until a 1996 outbreak in south central Uganda [36]. O'nyong-nyong virus vectors are anopheline mosquitoes. Serological surveys show that O'nyong-nyong virus is endemic. Humans are the largest reservoir for Chikungunya and O'nyong-nyong viruses. The nonhuman reservoirs for Chikungunya virus are baboons, monkeys, and bats. The nonhuman vertebrate reservoir for O'nyong-nyong virus is unknown. Another member of the Chikungunya–O'nyong-nyong virus serological group is

Igbo Ora virus. Igbo Ora virus infection, "the disease that breaks your wings," occurred in an Ivory Coast outbreak in 1984, and was isolated from anopheline mosquitoes and patients with febrile arthritis [37].

Ross River and Barmah Forest viruses

An invisible line off the coast of Java and Borneo, defined by the nineteenth-century zoogeographer Alfred Russell Wallace in 1863, separates the Africa-Asia and Pacific biogeographic zones. (Wallace coined the phrase, "survival of the fittest," often erroneously attributed to Charles Darwin) [38]. West of Wallace's line, the Chikungunya–O'nyong-nyong virus serological group is found. East of Wallace's line, Ross River virus is found. Ross River virus causes annual outbreaks and sporadic cases of febrile polyarthritis ("epidemic polyarthritis") [39]. Antibodies to Ross River virus have been found in the sera of endogenous populations in Papua New Guinea, West New Guinea, the Bismarck Archipelago, Rossel Island, and the Solomon Islands [40]. From 1979 to 1980, a major epidemic of febrile polyarthritis occurred in the Fiji Islands, affecting over 40,000 individuals [41]. Australian cases occur in tropical and temperate regions, especially in Queensland and New South Wales. In Queensland, annual disease rates are 31.5 to 288.3 per 100,000 person years [42]. Although infection rates in men and women are similar, women are more likely to develop symptoms. Children are more likely than adults to have asymptomatic infection. Cases occur from the spring through the fall. High rainfall usually precedes epidemics due to increases in mosquito populations [43]. Aedes and culicine mosqitoes are vectors. Domestic animals, rodents, and marsupials may be intermediate hosts. Barmah Forest virus, anther Australian alphavirus, shares epidemiologic and clinical features with Ross River virus [44–46].

Sindbis and Mayaro viruses

Sindbis virus infection is endemic in Sweden, Finland, and Russia's neighboring Karelian isthmus [47]. Aedes, Culex, and Culiseta sp serve as vectors from birds to humans [48]. Outdoor activities and occupations, especially in forested areas, increase infection risk. Sindbis virus infection is less commonly encountered in Africa and Australia [49]. Mayaro virus is endemic in the tropical rainforest shared by Peru, Bolivia, and Brazil. An epidemic in Belterra, Brazil, in 1988 had a clinical attack rate of 80% [50].

Alphavirus pathogensis

Pathogenesis of alphavirus arthritis has not been fully studied. Intense Chikungunya viremia follows the mosquito bite within 48 hours. Chikungunya virus absorbs to and aggregates platelets, and Ross River virus antigens are detected in monocytes and macrophages [51]. During the Chikungunya fever exanthem, erythrocytes extrude from superficial capillaries, and perivascular cuffing occurs. In Ross River virus infections, the perivascular infiltrate predominantly contains T cells. Ross River virus antigen is detected in epithelial cells in skin lesions [51]. Sindbis virus has been detected in skin vesicles that show perivascular edema, lymphocytic infiltrates, hemorrhage, and necrosis [52]. Virus or viral RNA of Chikungunya and Ross River virus have been found in synovium. The persistence of anti-Sindbis IgM over years raises the possibility of long-term viral persistence [48].

After an incubation period of about 1 to 12 days, alphaviruses cause explosive onset of fever up to 40°C with exquisite arthralgias [53,54]. Similarities include constitutional symptoms including pharyngitis, headache, photophobia, retro-orbital pain, anorexia, nausea, vomiting, abdominal pain, and lymphadenopathy [55,56]. Rash appears several days later, often beginning with facial and neck flushing, followed by the appearance of a macular or maculopapular eruption. The eruption may vesiculate before becoming hemorrhagic. Sindbis virus infection is notable for development of large hemorrhagic vesicles on the palms and soles. Fever in Sindbis virus infection may not be as marked, and rash usually begins on the torso, followed by arthralgias and arthritis. In Ross River virus infection, however, joint symptoms may precede rash by 15 days, and fever may not be prominent. Instead, joint symptoms can be incapacitating and are often migratory and asymmetric. Arthralgias can be severe, and are usually more prominent than frank arthritis. In Ross River virus infection, one third of patients have frank synovitis. Joints involved are often the small joints of the hands and feet, wrists, elbows, knees, and ankles. Previously injured joints may be more severely affected. Axial involvement may occur but is not common. Tendonitis of hand extensors and Achilles tendons is common in Sindbis virus infection [30].

Alphavirus arthralgias or arthritis usually resolve in days to weeks, but in severe cases of Chikungunya fever, symptoms may persist for months. Approximately 10% of patients have joint symptoms persisting at least 1 year. Half of Sindbis patients have symptoms $2\frac{1}{2}$ years after onset, and a few are symptomatic for 5 to 6 years [57,58]. Mayaro virus–related joint symptoms may last up to 2 months [50,59,60].

Alphavirus infection should be considered in the differential diagnosis of any febrile polyarthritis, given the appropriate geographic setting. Imported cases of Mayaro virus infection have presented to practitioners in the United States [61]. Travel history should be assessed. Laboratory testing for virus, viral antigen, and specific antibodies should be sought with the aid of national reference laboratories. Reverse transcriptase polymerase chain reaction methods may be used to detect viral genome [62].

Management of alphavirus infection for the most part is supportive. Range of motion exercises may help decrease stiffness. NSAIDs are standard, but aspirin should be avoided given the tendency to develop signs of hemorrhage. Chloroquine phosphate (250 mg/d) has been used in Chunkungunya virus infection when NSAIDs failed [63].

Hepatitis C and rheumatologic disease

Hepatitis C virus (HCV) is an enveloped single-stranded RNA flavivirus. HCV infects an estimated 170 million people worldwide [64]. In the United States alone, it is estimated that 1.8% of the population is chronically infected. HCV is parenterally transmitted, and becomes chronic in about 75% to 80% of patients [65]. Although HCV is a leading cause of end-stage liver disease worldwide, it does not lead directly to death in the majority of infected patients. HCV is also associated with a wide array of extrahepatic manifestations, including rheumatic disorders such as cryoglobulinemic vasculitis and arthritis.

Hepatitis C virus–associated arthritis

Arthritis is common in the setting of HCV infection, but remarkably little is known or agreed upon in terms of precise clinical manifestations, natural history, pathogenesis, or preferred therapy [66]. A small proportion of patients with hepatitis C clearly develop essential cryoglobulinemia, with arthritis, palpable purpura, cryoglobulins, and membranoproliferative glomerulonephritis as possible manifestations. Inflammatory joint disease in HCV-infected patients might also arise through one of three other scenarios. First, HCV and a primary form of inflammatory arthritis, such as rheumatoid disease, may coexist independently given the high prevalence of each disorder in the general population. Even here, however, HCV infection will likely influence treatment selection and potential toxicities of anti-inflammatory and immunosuppressive therapies. In a second scenario, HCV, either directly or indirectly, may initiate or influence the course of an inflammatory arthritis, such as rheumatoid arthritis. Third, HCV infection may be associated with a nosologically distinct form of joint disease.

The prevalence of articular symptoms in HCV infection varies markedly between studies, probably due to major differences in design, with most relying on questionnaires as opposed to detailed physical examinations. French investigators using questionnaires have found that 19% to 29% of infected patients have arthralgias, but only 2% have frank arthritis [67,68]. Buskilla and colleagues [69] using a more rigorous assessment incorporating physical examinations found frank arthritis in only 4%, while 9% had arthralgias.

Whether HCV is associated with a distinct inflammatory arthritis is still unsettled, though a growing number of reports suggest it is. In a recent review by Lovy and Starkebaum, these authors summarize their previous reports of a nonerosive, nonprogressive arthritis associated with tenosynovitis and joint symptoms out of proportion to physical findings [70,71]. Other reports of HCV infection with unusual articular features describe a rheumatoid-like picture, as well as an intermittent mono- and oligoarticular arthritis, all without erosive changes. At present, it is generally agreed that there is a distinct but rare inflammatory arthritis associated with

HCV infection. This disorder is not associated with erosive changes, and the presence of bony destruction should prompt a diagnosis of an inflammatory arthritis unrelated to hepatitis C.

In the HCV-infected population, there is a high prevalence of rheumatoid factor positivity. This has not generally been correlated with articular symptoms, but has led to much confusion in differentiating HCV-infected patients with associated arthralgia and arthritis from those with true rheumatoid arthritis (RA). The presence of characteristic bony erosions is helpful in defining true rheumatoid disease, but these changes are often absent, particularly in early RA. Recently, a novel autoantibody directed at citrullinated proteins (anticyclic citrullinated peptide, or anti-CCP) has been found to have a higher specificity for RA than traditional rheumatoid factor. Recent studies have documented that anti-CCP is absent in HCV-associated articular disease, and thus this test has become a useful tool in diagnosing true RA in the HCV-infected individual [72].

Therapy

The management of rheumatoid arthritis and other forms of primary inflammatory arthritis in the presence of HCV infection, as well as the nonerosive inflammatory HCV-associated arthritis, remain problematic. A recent uncontrolled study and review suggest that HCV-related articular manifestations may indeed respond to aggressive antiviral therapy, but controlled trials and better clinical definitions of disease and response are clearly needed [73].

Hepatitis B virus–associated articular disease

Hepatitis B virus (HBV) is an enveloped, partially double-stranded DNA virus member of the family *Hepadnaviridae*, transmitted by parenteral and sexual routes. An estimated one third of the world's population has been infected with hepatitis B. While infection is self-limited in most, it is chronic in 5% to 10% of those acquiring the infection in adulthood. HBV is a common cause of cirrhosis and hepatocellular carcinoma, as well as being associated with a variety of extrahepatic manifestations [74].

Unlike HCV, HBV is not associated with chronic arthritis unless the patient develops polyarteritis nodosa, a systemic necrotizing vasculitis occasionally complicating chronic HBV infection [75]. Acute HBV is associated with a sudden transient polyarthritis that may mimic the onset of classical RA. The onset is usually during the prodromal phase of viremia, with a symmetric distribution involving the wrists, knees, ankles, and small joints of the hands. It may precede jaundice by days to weeks, and generally subsides at the onset of jaundice or shortly thereafter. No specific therapy is required other than supportive care, since the condition is self-limiting. Recognizing the underlying etiology, however, is of great clinical importance, so as to avoid the use of potentially harmful immunosuppressive drugs that might be used if the arthritis is mistaken for classic RA.

Persistent polyarthritis should raise the suspicion for transformation to a systemic vasculitis, secondary to immune complex formation. Associated urticarial or maculopapular rash may also reflect small vessel immune complex vasculitis.

HIV-related rheumatologic syndromes

Since its original description in 1981, HIV has infected nearly 100 million people worldwide and caused 40 million deaths [76]. The turning point in the HIV epidemic occurred in 1995 with the introduction of highly active anti-retroviral therapy (HAART). With such therapy, there has been a remarkable decline in deaths due to infectious illnesses, and HIV has become a complex but treatable chronic disease in many patients [77]. The complications observed in this population with ever-increasing longevity have also been transformed, including an array of rheumatic, articular, and musculoskeletal syndromes.

HIV and arthritis

Several musculoskeletal syndromes associated with HIV infection have been extensively reviewed [78–82]. The epidemiology of rheumatic disease and HIV infection has been an area of considerable debate. The strength of these associations has varied in clinical reports, and many reports have been anecdotal. Prospective epidemiologic investigations of HIV-related articular disease have reported highly disparate results. From the extremes of these observations, it would appear that HIV might either confer a dramatic risk for the development of certain rheumatic syndromes, or alternatively be protective. The differences between these studies may have several explanations, including radically different types of research design, varying case mix, differing stages of HIV infection among subjects, and possible regional differences in the virus. The frequencies of various rheumatic manifestations in a large number of HIV-positive patients (n = 458) seen in an outpatient rheumatology clinic are shown in Table 1 [83].

Septic arthritis

There are numerous reports of septic arthritis in the setting of HIV disease. However, given the remarkable propensity of HIV-infected patients to infection, the most surprising aspect of this complication is its relative rarity, with most series documenting an incidence of less than 1%. Most cases of septic arthritis reported in the literature were due to *Staphylococcus aureus* [84]. Other frequently encountered agents include *Streptococcus* and *Salmonella* sp, as well as atypical mycobacteria. Opportunistic joint

Table 1
Distribution of diagnoses in HIV-positive patients at an HIV outpatient facility (n = 458)

Diagnosis	No. of patients (%)
Diffuse infiltrative lymphocytosis syndrome	94 (21)
Bursitis/Tenosynovitis	86 (19)
Low back pain	34 (7)
Osteoarthritis	31 (7)
HIV-associated arthralgia	28 (6)
Elevated creatine kinase	26 (6)
Parotid enlargement	21 (6)
Reactive arthritis/psoriatic arthritis	19 (4)
HIV-associated arthritis	17 (4)
Fibromyalgia	17 (4)
Hepatitis B/C syndromes	15 (3)
HIV-associated polymyositis	10 (2)
Gout	8 (2)
Infectious arthritis	6 (1)
Systemic lupus erythematosus	5 (1)
Sicca symptoms	4 (1)
Vasculitis	4 (1)
Ankylosing spondylitis	2 (0.5)

Data from Reveille JD. The changing spectrum of rheumatic disease in human immunodeficiency virus infection. Semin Arthritis Rheum 2000;30:147–66.

infections due to various micro-organisms have sporadically been reported [84]. Despite the rarity of these reports, their presence emphasizes the importance of approaching all new articular disease, especially that which is acute and monoarticular, as potentially infectious with both routine and opportunistic pathogens. In general, the clinical presentation, course, and prognosis of septic arthritis in HIV-positive individuals does not differ from that of septic arthritis in HIV-negative individuals [84].

Nonsuppurative inflammatory arthritis and arthralgia

Nonspecific joint pains are common in the setting of HIV disease, being reported in 12% to 45% of patients [83]. Pain is generally mild, intermittent, and tends to occur later in the course of illness. Increasing arthralgia should always alert to the possibility of other serious underlying problems such as opportunistic infection, drug reactions, and other mimics of articular pain such as peripheral neuropathy and myopathy.

HIV-associated reactive arthritis and psoriatic arthritis

An aseptic peripheral arthritis occurs in HIV-infected individuals and has been reported predominantly among homosexual men. In many of these patients, there are accompanying extra-articular features suggestive of reactive arthritis, including urethritis, ocular inflammation, and skin lesions [83]. The skin disease reported in such individuals ranges from seborrhea to frank keratoderma blennorhagicum. In HIV, there is substantial overlap betweeen reactive and psoriatic arthritis, as shown by the propensity of HIV-infected individuals to have several different skin lesions simultaneously, and for patients with a clinical reactive arthritis syndrome to have fulminant psoriasis.

Many patients with reactive arthritis and undifferentiated spondyloarthropathy develop symptoms after infection with *Shigella flexneri* or *Campylobacter jejuni*, or more rarely *Yersinia* sp. Surprisingly, despite a high frequency of history of urethritis, there are no reported cases of infection with *Chlamydia trachomatis* [85]. Lower extremity involvement of knees, ankles, and feet predominates, though a minority may also have involvement of the hands, wrists, and upper extremities. Axial disease is unusual, and radiographic sacroiliitis is extremely rare. Enthesopathy of the Achilles tendon, plantar fascia, anterior and posterior tibial tendons, and extensor tendons can be seen. The clinical course in such patients is highly variable, and probably reflects underlying clinical heterogeneity. The disease may be relatively mild, unassociated with radiographic changes, and easily controlled by NSAIDs, but at times it may be unusually severe, associated with radiographic periostitis and erosions, and highly refractory to anti-inflammatory medications. A more severe course of reactive arthritis with persistent polyarticular involvement accompanied by erosive changes and progression to joint fusion has been reported recently in African blacks [79].

There is a spectrum of papulosquamous dermopathy associated with HIV infection. These range from seborrheic dermatitis at the mild end through frank psoriasis vulgaris and pustular psoriasis at the severe end. The latter is indistinguishable from keratoderma blennorhagicum. Although its prevalence is apparently not much different than the general population, its severity is increased [84,85]. Regardless of prevalence, the acute onset of papulosquamous dermopathy in an adult with or without arthritis should warrant consideration of possible HIV infection, especially in individuals at high risk.

Arthritis and enthesopathy similar to that of reactive arthritis is also seen with psoriasis. The relative frequency of psoriatic arthritis in HIV patients is a matter of controversy. Although earlier studies did not show a significantly higher prevalence of psoriatic arthritis in Caucasian HIV-infected patients [85], recent studies in black Africans have demonstrated an increased occurrence of psoriatic arthritis [86]. Similar to psoriatic skin disease in the setting of HIV infection, psoriatic arthritis appears to follow a more severe course in these patients. Treatment for both reactive arthritis and psoriatic arthritis is generally symptomatic, and most patients with mild disease can be controlled on NSAIDs. In the pre-HAART era, cases of severe, even fulminant arthritis were commonly seen, and these patients posed complex problems of how to manage aggressive autoimmune or inflammatory disease in a setting of advancing immunodeficiency. As noted below, this scenario has become increasingly uncommon in HIV medicine.

Arthritis and immune reconstitution and the effects of highly active anti-retroviral therapy

Since the introduction of HAART in the mid-1990s, there has been a dramatic change in the patterns of morbidity and mortality in HIV-infected patients with access to such treatment. Attendant to the dramatic fall in death rates due to opportunistic infection has been a rise in other complications, some of which had not previously been recognized. One major effect of HAART has been a dramatic decline in most nonsuppurative rheumatic complications, including reactive arthritis, psoriatic arthritis, and other forms of connective tissue disease [87].

Among new syndromes described in the HAART era is that now commonly referred to as *immune reconstitution syndrome* [88]. In this condition, AIDS patients receiving HAART develop highly inflammatory reactions to occult infections, such as *Mycobacterium avium*, tuberculosis, and cytomegalovirus, as a result of immune resurgence. More recently, immune reconstitution syndrome manifesting as the de novo appearance of a new autoimmune or inflammatory disease, or a flare of a pre-existing similar condition, has been reported. Over 30 such cases have been recently reviewed and include the appearance of disorders such as sarcoidosis, RA-like illnesses, and myositis, among others [87]. Most cases were self-limited, and few required aggressive therapy. Clinicians should become increasingly aware of this complication, and should tend to be conservative in its management.

Finally, among the newly described metabolic complications is the increasing incidence of osteonecrosis of bone, particularly the hip. Risk factors for this complication may include the use of protease inhibitor-based HAART, anabolic or glucocorticoid use, and strength training, among others [89]. Clinicians should be aware that in HIV-infected patients presenting with hip pain, a plain radiograph is inconclusive to rule out this potentially highly morbid complication, and that MRI is the procedure of choice.

HTLV-I

HTLV-I is a human retrovirus endemic to the Caribbean, South America, West Africa, and Japan. It is seen to a far lesser extent in the United States, primarily among intravenous drug users in certain regions. HTLV-I causes T cell leukemia and lymphoma, tropical spastic paraparesis, and an infective dermatitis syndrome. It is also associated with a variety of autoimmune sequelae, including polymyositis, seronegative erosive polyarthritis, and uveitis [90].

References

[1] Poole BD, Karetnyi YV, Naides SJ. Parvovirus B19-induced apoptosis of hepatocytes. J Virol 2004;78:7775–83.

[2] Candotti D, Etiz N, Parsyan A, et al. Identification and characterization of persistent human erythrovirus infection in blood donor samples. J Virol 2004;78:12169–78.

[3] Hokynar K, Norja P, Laitinen H, et al. Detection and differentiation of human parvovirus variants by commercial quantitative real-time PCR tests. J Clin Microbiol 2004;42:2013–9.

[4] Jones MS, Kapoor A, Lukashov VV, et al. New DNA viruses identified in patients with acute viral infection syndrome. J Virol 2005;79:8230–6.

[5] Anderson LJ, Tsou RA, Chorba TL, et al. Detection of antibodies and antigens of human parvovirus B19 by enzyme-linked immunosorbent assay. J Clin Microbiol 1986;24:522–6.

[6] Bell LM, Naides SJ, Stoffman P, et al. Human parvovirus B19 infection among hospital staff members after contact with infected patients. N Engl J Med 1989;321:485–91.

[7] Gillespie SM, Cartter ML, Asch S, et al. Occupational risk of human parvovirus B19 infection for school and day-care personnel during an outbreak of erythema infectiosum. JAMA 1990;263:2061–5.

[8] Anderson MJ, Higgins PG, Davis LR, et al. Experimental parvoviral infection in humans. J Infect Dis 1985;152:257–65.

[9] Kurtzman GJ, Cohen BJ, Field AM, et al. Immune response to B19 parvovirus and an antibody defect in persistent viral infection. J Clin Invest 1989;84:1114–23.

[10] Kurtzman G, Frickhofen N, Kimball J, et al. Pure red-cell aplasia of 10 years' duration due to persistent parvovirus B19 infection and its cure with immunoglobulin therapy. N Engl J Med 1989;321:519–23.

[11] Cooling LLW, Koerner TA, Naides SJ. Multiple glycosphingolipids determine the tissue tropism of parvovirus B19. J Infect Dis 1995;172:1198–205.

[12] Weigel-Kelley KA, Yoder MC, Srivastava A. Alpha5beta1 integrin as a cellular coreceptor for human parvovirus B19: requirement of functional activation of beta1 integrin for viral entry. Blood 2003;102:3927–33.

[13] Naides SJ. Parvoviruses. In: Specter S, Hodinka RL, Young SA, editors. Clinical virology manual. 3rd edition. Washington, DC: ASM Press; 2000. p. 487–500.

[14] Ager EA, Chin TDY, Poland JD. Epidemic erythema infectiosum. N Engl J Med 1966;275: 1326–31.

[15] Naides SJ, Scharosch LL, Foto F, et al. Rheumatologic manifestations of human parvovirus B19 infection in adults. Initial two-year clinical experience. Arthritis Rheum 1990;33: 1297–309.

[16] Söderlund M, von Essen R, Haapasaari J, et al. Persistence of parvoviris B19 DNA in synovial membranes of young patients with and without chronic arthropathy. Lancet 1997;349: 1063–5.

[17] Ballou WR, Reed JL, Noble W, et al. Safety and immunogenicity of a recombinant parvovirus B19 vaccine formulated with MF59C.1. J Infect Dis 2003;187:675–8.

[18] Frey TK. Molecular biology of rubella virus. Adv Virus Res 1994;44:69–160.

[19] Falkensammer B, Walder G, Busch D, et al. Epidemiology of rubella infections in Austria: important lessons to be learned. Eur J Clin Microbiol Infect Dis 2004;23:502–5.

[20] Chantler J, Wolinsky JS, Tingle A. Rubella virus. In: Knipe DM, Howley PM, Griffin DE, et al, editors. Fields virology. 4th edition. Philadelphia: Lippincott Williams & Wilkins; 2001. p. 963–90.

[21] Smith CA, Petty RE, Tingle AJ. Rubella virus and arthritis. Rheum Dis Clin North Am 1987;13:265–74.

[22] Ueno Y. Rubella arthritis. An outbreak in Kyoto. J Rheumatol 1994;21:874–6.

[23] Amitai Y, Granit G. Thrombocytopenic purpura during the incubation period of rubella. Helv Paediatr Acta 1986;41:55–7.

[24] Bechar M, Davidovich S, Goldhammer G, et al. Neurological complications following rubella infection. J Neurol 1982;226:283–7.

[25] Meurman OH. Persistence of immunoglobulin G and immunoglobulin M antibodies after postnatal rubella infection determined by solid-phase radioimmunoassay. J Clin Microbiol 1978;7:34–8.

[26] Thomas HI, Barrett E, Hesketh LM, et al. Simultaneous IgM reactivity by EIA against more than one virus in measles, parvovirus B19 and rubella infection. J Clin Virol 1999; 14:107–18.

[27] Howson CP, Fineberg HV. Adverse events following pertussis and rubella vaccines. Summary of a report to the Institute of Medicine. JAMA 1992;267:392–6.

[28] Schaffner W, Fleet WF, Kilroy AW, et al. Polyneuropathy following rubella immunization: a follow-up study and review of the problem. Am J Dis Child 1974;127:684–8.

[29] Mitchell LA, Tingle AJ, Shukin R, et al. Chronic rubella vaccine-associated arthropathy. Arch Intern Med 1993;153:2268–74.

[30] Laine M, Luukkainen R, Toivanen A. Sindbis viruses and other alphaviruses as cause of human arthritic disease. J Intern Med 2004;256:457–71.

[31] Griffin DE. Alphaviruses. In: Knipe DM, Howley PM, Griffin DE, et al, editors. Fields virology. 4th edition. Philadelphia: Lippincott Williams & Wilkins; 2001. p. 917–62.

[32] Ross RW. The Newala epidemic. III. The virus: isolation, pathogenic properties and relationship to the epidemic. J Hyg (Lond) 1956;54:177–91.

[33] Williams MC, Woodall JP, Corbet PS, et al. O'nyong-nyong fever: an epidemic in east Africa. VIII. Virus isolations from Anopheles mosquitoes. Trans R Soc Trop Med Hyg 1965; 59:300–6.

[34] Williams MC, Woodall JP, Gillett JD. O'nyong-nyong fever: an epidemic in East Africa. VII. Virus isolations from man and serological studies up to July 1961. Trans R Soc Trop Med Hyg 1965;59:186–97.

[35] Williams MC, Woodall JP, Porterfield JS. O'Nyong-nyong fever: an epidemic virus disease in east africa. V. Human antibody studies by plaque inhibition and other serological tests. Trans R Soc Trop Med Hyg 1962;56:166–72.

[36] Lanciotti RS, Ludwig ML, Rwaguma EB, et al. Emergence of epidemic O'nyong-nyong fever in Uganda after a 35-year absence: genetic characterization of the virus. Virology 1998; 252:258–68.

[37] Moore DL, Causey OR, Carey DE, et al. Arthropod-borne viral infections of man in Nigeria, 1964–1970. Ann Trop Med Parasitol 1975;69:49–64.

[38] Winchester S. Kraktoa. The day the world exploded: August 27, 1883. New York: Harper Collins Publishers; 2003.

[39] Mylonas AD, Brown AM, Carthew TL, et al. Natural history of Ross River virus-induced epidemic polyarthritis. Med J Aust 2002;177:356–60.

[40] Scrimgeour EM, Aaskov JG, Matz LR. Ross River virus arthritis in Papua New Guinea. Trans R Soc Trop Med Hyg 1987;81:833–4.

[41] Aaskov JG, Mataika JU, Lawrence GW, et al. An epidemic of Ross River virus infection in Fiji, 1979. Am J Trop Med Hyg 1981;30:1053–9.

[42] Kelly-Hope LA, Purdie DM, Kay BH. Risk of mosquito-borne epidemic polyarthritis disease among international visitors to Queensland, Australia. J Travel Med 2002;9: 211–3.

[43] Woodruff RE, Guest CS, Garner MG, et al. Predicting Ross River virus epidemics from regional weather data. Epidemiology 2002;13:384–93.

[44] Flexman JP, Smith DW, Mackenzie JS, et al. A comparison of the diseases caused by Ross River virus and Barmah Forest virus. Med J Aust 1998;169:159–63.

[45] Kelly-Hope LA, Kay BH, Purdie DM, et al. The risk of Ross River and Barmah Forest virus disease in Queensland: implications for New Zealand. Aust N Z J Public Health 2002;26: 69–77.

[46] Lindsay MDA, Johansen CA, Broom AK, et al. Emergence of Barmah Forest virus in western Australia. Emerging Infect Dis 1995;1:1–6.

[47] Niklasson B, Espmark A, LeDuc JW, et al. Association of a Sindbis-like virus with Ockelbo disease in Sweden. Am J Trop Med Hyg 1984;33:1212–7.

[48] Niklasson B. Sindbis and Sindbis-like viruses. In: Monath TP, editor. The arboviruses: epidemiology and ecology. Boca Raton (FL): CRC Press; 1988. p. 167–76.

[49] Lundstrom JO, Vene S, Saluzzo J-F, et al. Antigenic comparison of Ockelbo virus isolates from Sweden and Russia with Sindbis virus isolates from Europe, Africa, and Australia: further evidence for variation among alphaviruses. Am J Trop Med Hyg 1993;49:531–7.

[50] LeDuc JW, Pinheiro FP, Travassos da Rosa AP. An outbreak of Mayaro virus disease in Belterra, Brazil. II. Epidemiology. Am J Trop Med Hyg 1981;30:682–8.

[51] Fraser JR, Ratnamohan VM, Dowling JP, et al. The exanthem of Ross River virus infection: histology, location of virus antigen and nature of inflammatory infiltrate. J Clin Pathol 1983; 36:1256–63.

[52] Kurkela S, Manni T, Vaheri A, et al. Causative agent of Pogosta disease isolated from blood and skin lesions. Emerg Infect Dis 2004;10:889–94.

[53] Shore H. O'Nyong-nyong fever: an epidemic virus disease in east africa. III. Some clinical and epidemiological observations in the northern province. Trans R Soc Trop Med Hyg 1961;55:361–73.

[54] Tesh RB. Arthritides caused by mosquito-borne viruses. Annu Rev Med 1982;33:31–40.

[55] Halstead SB, Nimmannitya S, Margiotta MR. Dengue and chikungunya virus infection in man in Thailand, 1962–1964. II. Observations on disease in outpatients. Am J Trop Med Hyg 1969;18:972–83.

[56] Nimmannitya S, Halstead SB, Cohen SN, et al. Dengue and chikungunya virus infection in man in Thailand, 1962-1964. I. Observations on hospitalized patients with hemorrhagic fever. Am J Trop Med Hyg 1969;18:954–71.

[57] Laine M, Luukkainen R, Jalava J, et al. Prolonged arthritis associated with sindbis-related (Pogosta) virus infection. Rheumatology (Oxford) 2000;39:1272–4.

[58] Niklasson B, Espmark A. Ockelbo disease: arthralgia 3–4 years after infection with a Sindbis virus related agent. Lancet 1986;1:1039–40.

[59] Hoch AL, Peterson NE, LeDuc JW, et al. An outbreak of Mayaro virus disease in Belterra, Brazil. III. Entomological and ecological studies. Am J Trop Med Hyg 1981;30:689–98.

[60] Pinheiro FP, Freitas RB, Travassos da Rosa JF, et al. An outbreak of Mayaro virus disease in Belterra, Brazil. I. Clinical and virological findings. Am J Trop Med Hyg 1981;30:674–81.

[61] Tesh RB, Watts DM, Russell KL, et al. Mayaro virus disease: an emerging mosquito-borne zoonosis in tropical South America. Clin Infect Dis 1999;28:67–73.

[62] Hasebe F, Parquet MC, Pandey BD, et al. Combined detection and genotyping of Chikungunya virus by a specific reverse transcription-polymerase chain reaction. J Med Virol 2002; 67:370–4.

[63] Brighton SW. Chloroquine phosphate treatment of chronic Chikungunya arthritis. An open pilot study. S Afr Med J 1984;66:217–8.

[64] Alter MJ, Hutin YJ, Armstrong GL. Epidemiology of hepatitis C. In: Liang TJ, Hoofnagle JH, editors. Hepatitis C. San Diego (CA): Academic Press; 2000. p. 169–83.

[65] Hoofnagle JH. Course and outcome of hepatitis C. Hepatology 2002;36:S21–9.

[66] Vassilopoulos D, Calabrese LH. Rheumatic manifestations of hepatitis C infection. Curr Rheumatol Rep 2003;5:200–4.

[67] Cacoub P, Renou C, Rosenthal E, et al. Extrahepatic manifestations associated with hepatitis C virus infection. A prospective multicenter study of 321 patients. The GERMIVIC. Groupe d'Etude et de Recherche en Medecine Interne et Maladies Infectieuses sur le Virus de l'Hepatite C. Medicine (Baltimore) 2000;79:47–56.

[68] Cacoub P, Renou C, Rosenthal E, et al. Extrahepatic manifestations associated with hepatitis C virus infection. The GERMIVIC Groupe d'Etude et de Recherche en Medecine Interne et Maladies Infectieuses sur le Virus de l'Hepatite C. Medicine 2000;79:47–56.

[69] Buskila D. Hepatitis C-associated arthritis. Curr Opin Rheumatol 2000;12:295–9.

[70] Lovy MR, Starkebaum G. Hepatitis C infection presenting with rheumatic manifestations—reply. J Rheumatol 1997;24:1239.

[71] Lovy MR, Starkebaum G, Uberoi S. Hepatitis C infection presenting with rheumatic manifestations: a mimic of rheumatoid arthritis. J Rheumatol 1996;23:979–83.

[72] Wener MH, Hutchinson K, Morishima C, et al. Absence of antibodies to cyclic citrullinated peptide in sera of patients with hepatitis C virus infection and cryoglobulinemia. Arthritis Rheum 2004;50:2305–8.

[73] Zuckerman E, Keren D, Rozenbaum M, et al. Hepatitis C virus-related arthritis: characteristics and response to therapy with interferon alpha. Clin Exp Rheumatol 2000;18:579–84.

[74] Lai CL, Ratziu V, Yuen MF, et al. Viral hepatitis B. Lancet 2003;362:2089–94.

[75] Trepo C, Guillevin L. Polyarteritis nodosa and extrahepatic manifestations of HBV infection: the case against autoimmune intervention in pathogenesis. J Autoimmun 2001;16: 269–74.

[76] UNAIDS/WHO. Report on the global AIDS epidemic 2004. Available at: http://www.unaids.org/bangkok2004/report_pdf.html. Accessed September 1, 2005.

[77] Valdez H, Chowdhry TK, Asaad R, et al. Changing spectrum of mortality due to human immunodeficiency virus: analysis of 260 deaths during 1995–1999. Clin Infect Dis 2001;32: 1487–93.

[78] Calabrese LH. The rheumatic manifestations of infection with the human immunodeficiency virus. Semin Arthritis Rheum 1989;18:225–39.

[79] Cuellar ML, Espinoza LR. Rheumatic manifestations of HIV-AIDS. Baillieres Best Pract Res Clin Rheumatol 2000;14:579–93.

[80] Kaye BR. Rheumatologic manifestations of infection with human immunodeficiency virus (HIV). Ann Intern Med 1989;111:158–67.

[81] Mody GM, Parke FA, Reveille JD. Articular manifestations of human immunodeficiency virus infection. Best Pract Res Clin Rheumatol 2003;17:265–87.

[82] Reveille JD. The changing spectrum of rheumatic disease in human immunodeficiency virus infection. Semin Arthritis Rheum 2000;30:147–66.

[83] Vassilopoulos D, Calabrese LH. Rheumatic aspects of human immunodeficiency virus infection and other immunodeficiency states. In: Hochberg MC, Silman AJ, Smolen JS, et al, editors. Rheumatology. 3rd edition. Edinburgh (UK): Mosby; 2003. p. 1115–29.

[84] Vassilopoulos D, Chalasani P, Jurado RL, et al. Musculoskeletal infections in patients with human immunodeficiency virus infection. Medicine (Baltimore) 1997;76:284–94.

[85] Keat A. HIV and overlap with Reiter's syndrome. Baillieres Clin Rheumatol 1994;8:363–77.

[86] Njobvu P, McGill P. Psoriatic arthritis and human immunodeficiency virus infection in Zambia. J Rheumatol 2000;27:1699–702.

[87] Calabrese L, Kirchner E, Shrestha E. Rheumatic complications of human immunodeficiency virus (HIV) infection in the era of highly active antiretroviral therapy (HAART): emergence of a new syndrome of immune reconstitution and changing patterns of disease. Semin Arthritis Rheum 2005, in press.

[88] DeSimone JA, Pomerantz RJ, Babinchak TJ. Inflammatory reactions in HIV-1-infected persons after initiation of highly active antiretroviral therapy. Ann Intern Med 2000;133: 447–54.

[89] Miller KD, Masur H, Jones EC, et al. High prevalence of osteonecrosis of the femoral head in HIV-infected adults. Ann Intern Med 2002;137:17–25.

[90] Nishioka K, Nakajima T, Hasunuma T, et al. Rheumatic manifestation of human leukemia virus infection. Rheum Dis Clin N Am 1993;19:489–503.

INFECTIOUS
DISEASE CLINICS
OF NORTH AMERICA

Infect Dis Clin N Am 19 (2005) 981–989

Tropical and Temperate Pyomyositis

Lorne N. Small, MD, FRCPC[a],
John J. Ross, MD, CM[b],*

[a]Division of Geographic Medicine and Infectious Diseases, Tufts-New England Medical
Center, 750 Washington Street, Boston, MA 02111, USA
[b]Division of Infectious Diseases, Caritas Saint Elizabeth's Medical Center,
736 Cambridge Street, Boston, MA 02135, USA

Pyomyositis is a primary infection of skeletal muscle not arising from contiguous infection, presumably hematogenous in origin, and often, but not invariably, associated with abscess formation. Classically, pyomyositis is an infection of the tropics, occurring in previously active and healthy young men. Pyomyositis in temperate countries is often regarded as an infection that occurs in hosts who are immunocompromised or otherwise debilitated. However, this distinction may be somewhat artificial, as tropical pyomyositis may be partly related to underlying infection with HIV or parasites, and temperate pyomyositis has been reported in healthy and athletic persons. This article discusses the pathogenesis, clinical presentation, diagnosis, and management of pyomyositis in the tropical and temperate settings.

Pathogenesis and epidemiology

Pyomyositis, as described in 1885 [1,2], is a primary intramuscular infection, usually with abscess formation. This entity is distinct from clostridial myonecrosis and necrotizing fasciitis, which tend to be more acute and lethal processes. By definition, pyomyositis is not secondary to a contiguous infection from another site, probably arising from hematogenous seeding. Multifocal infection affecting more than one muscle group may be present in 10% to 20% of cases [3,4]. Most commonly infection is caused by *Staphylococcus aureus* or group A streptococci [5]. The original descriptions were from tropical areas, and generally referred to the condition as *tropical pyomyositis* or *pyomyositis tropicans* [4,6].

---

* Corresponding author.
E-mail address: jrossmd@cchcs.org (J.J. Ross).

0891-5520/05/$ - see front matter © 2005 Elsevier Inc. All rights reserved.
doi:10.1016/j.idc.2005.08.003
id.theclinics.com

Pyomyositis has been considered common in developing countries and rarer in developed countries [6]. However, in the last 3 decades, similar infections have been reported with increasing frequency in temperate areas, often affecting individuals who are immunocompromised. As the entity is becoming increasingly recognized in nontropical areas and because abscesses are not requisite for diagnosis, alternative terms such as *infectious myositis* and *spontaneous bacterial myositis* have been proposed [7]. There is a trend to consider temperate and tropical pyomyositis as separate entities. However, because pathogenesis is not completely understood, it is difficult to standardize the nomenclature, other than referring to the general geographic location.

In the classic tropical setting, pyomyositis affects all age groups, with a predominance in children [8] and between the ages of 20 and 45 years [1]. In North America, reports of age predominance vary more. The infection appears to be most common in the young adult population, but does occur with some frequency in infants, children, middle-aged adults, and the elderly [8,9]. Reviews and case series generally agree that there is some male predominance [1,8–10]. In temperate areas, up to 75% of cases occur in individuals who have some form of immune compromise [7]. A review of North American cases found that 9% of affected individuals reported recent travel or immigration from tropical areas [8].

The pathogenesis of pyomyositis is not clearly understood. Diminished local resistance in the setting of transient bacteremia is usually invoked. Local predisposition to infection, or "locus minoris resistentiae," may be attributed to antecedent trauma. In a review by Gibson and colleagues [1], predisposing trauma, including strenuous exercise, occurred in 50% of cases in the United States and less than 30% of cases in the tropics. However, in other reviews, very few cases have been associated with trauma [11]. Trauma may facilitate hematogenous access to the muscle and provide a critical bacterial nutritional requirement in the form of iron from myoglobin, which is sequestered under normal circumstances [7]. Formation of a small hematoma may provide a favorable site for the binding of staphylococci and other bacteria, and the surrounding damaged and devitalized tissue might also impede the host immune response. The permissive role of minor muscle damage is suggested by the numerous reports of pyomyositis after vigorous exercise and athletic activity in previously healthy individuals in temperate regions [12–18].

Other possible risk factors for pyomyositis are malnutrition; concurrent viral or parasitic infections; more virulent endemic bacterial strains; or higher local incidences of infection and sepsis. In 1983, Shepherd [10] attempted to characterize epidemiologic factors associated with pyomyositis by visiting endemic tropical sites. His findings were only mildly supportive of these postulated predispositions. Case reports have confirmed bacterial pyomyositis as a complication of parasite infection in some instances [19]. In Brazilian populations and in animal models, toxocariasis is significantly associated with the subsequent development of pyomyositis, perhaps because of predisposing muscle damage and impaired local immunity [20].

More recently, immunodeficiencies, including HIV, have been implicated in the development of pyomyositis in tropical and temperate settings. In a 1996 case-control series performed by Ansaloni and colleagues [21] in Uganda, there was a significant association between pyomyositis and HIV. In North American cases, over half of patients reported an underlying medical condition. In about half of these cases, HIV was the predisposing factor [4,8]. The role of HIV in the development of pyomyositis is unclear, but the compromised immune system may not be the only predisposing factor. Muscle damage from HIV itself; zidovudine treatment; higher incidences of parasite and mycobacterial infections; and increased rates of staphylococcal carriage may also play a role [6].

The most common non-HIV predisposing medical conditions have been diabetes mellitus, malignancies, rheumatologic disease, cirrhosis, renal insufficiency, sickle cell disease, aplastic anemia, and lung disease. Other possible predisposing factors include organ transplantation and iatrogenic immunosuppression by corticosteroids, chemotherapy, or immunomodulating agents [4]. Dysfunction of T cells may also be a significant factor leading to pyomyositis [7].

Intravenous drug use has been implicated in cases of bacterial pyomyositis, perhaps unsurprisingly given the frequency of bacteremia in this condition. Many of these cases may represent local injection site infection and abscess extension into muscle tissue [22,23], and not true primary pyomyositis. However, there are documented cases of pyomyositis occurring in muscle groups distant and unrelated to injection sites [23–25]. Occasionally, such episodes are associated with endocarditis [24].

Risk factors for pyomyositis in children are similar to those in adults. One association reported more commonly in children is an underlying skin condition leading to secondary bacteremia, such as varicella [4,26] or atopic dermatitis [4].

Microscopic analysis of affected muscle tissue reveals edematous separation of muscle fibrils and fibers. No diffuse inflammatory process has been noted in muscles affected by pyomyositis. Rather, patchy myocytolysis ensues and progresses to complete disintegration of muscle fibers [1,7,27]. There is interfiber infiltration by lymphocytes and plasma cells. These muscle fibers may heal or continue to progress to degeneration and suppuration with bacteria and polymorphonuclear infiltration [1,7,27].

Microbiology

Bacteriologic diagnosis of pyomyositis is traditionally made from cultures of surgical specimens, although CT- or ultrasound-guided drainage may be poised to supplant surgery in this regard. Variable rates of bacteremia are reported in pyomyositis. In tropical cases, only 5% to 10% of blood cultures are positive. Temperate cases are associated with bacteremia in approximately 25% to 35% of cases [4,7,10].

The most common causative organisms in hosts who are immunocompetent are staphylococcal and streptococcal species. *S aureus* causes up to 90% of cases in tropical regions, and 75% of those in temperate locales [7]. Recently, virulent strains of community-acquired methicillin-resistant *S aureus* (MRSA) have been reported as causing pyomyositis in the United States [28,29]. Group A streptococci are probably next in frequency. Less common causes include groups B, C, and G streptococci; pneumococci; *Haemophilus influenzae*; *Aeromonas hydrophila*; *Fusobacterium* sp; *Bartonella* sp; gram-negative enteric flora; and anaerobes [9]. Although rare, tuberculous and nontuberculous mycobacterial pyomyositis have been described in individuals who are immunocompromised and immunocompetent [30–35]. There are also occasional reports of *Salmonella* sp [36–38] and gonococci [39] as causative organisms, secondary to disseminated infections with these bacteria.

Patients who have suppressed immune systems or underlying medical conditions, such as diabetes, may be more susceptible to developing infections caused by unusual organisms [4,7]. However, a review of pyomyositis cases in the United States found that the distribution of causative organisms were similar among cohorts that were HIV-positive, HIV-negative with underlying medical conditions, or HIV-negative with no underlying medical conditions [4]. This finding was true of common organisms, such as *S aureus*, and less common organisms, such as mycobacteria.

Clinical manifestations

The most common site of pyomyositis is the thigh, with the calf, buttock, upper extremity, and iliopsoas also commonly involved. The lower extremity is four times more likely than the upper extremity to be involved [4]. The abdominal wall, chest wall, paraspinal muscles, and pelvic muscles are occasionally affected [10]. Distribution of affected muscle groups is similar in children compared with adults, with the possible exception of more frequent involvement of pelvic and psoas muscles in children [26,40,41].

Pyomyositis is heralded by local, crampy muscle pain. These nonspecific symptoms make early diagnosis difficult, and often lead to misdiagnosis until later in the course of infection. Within a few days of onset, the affected area becomes edematous and is often described as having a woody or rubbery quality. At this early point, which some have termed the *invasive stage*, suppuration of the muscle is not yet seen, but mild leukocytosis and low-grade fever may be present [42]. As the infection progresses over 1 to 3 weeks, edema, induration, and tenderness increase. Frequently, significant fever, constitutional symptoms, and leukocytosis will occur. At this point, termed the *suppurative* or *purulent stage*, frank pus is usually present within the muscle on aspiration, but the area is generally not fluctuant [7]. Most patients are diagnosed at this stage [42]. In the late stage, often occurring weeks after initial onset, muscle tissue will contain a large amount of pus, and fluctuation will predominate [6]. Patients may be toxic and have symptoms of sepsis.

Diagnosis

Early diagnosis of pyomyositis is difficult, as the initial symptoms are vague and nonspecific, and a high clinical suspicion is necessary. Initial laboratory data may lack indicators of inflammation or infection. As the infection progresses into the second week, leukocytosis with left shift and elevated erythrocyte sedimentation rate and C-reactive protein are common [11], but nonspecific. Classical descriptions of the infection from tropical regions often report leukocytosis with significant eosinophilia [11], lending credence to parasites as a cofactor. Counterintuitively, creatinine kinase levels are often normal, and frequently remain so throughout the course of infection [9].

Imaging is the most useful method for diagnosing pyomyositis. Plain radiographs are not sensitive, but in a few cases may suggest muscle enlargement, loss of muscle definition, obliteration of deep fat planes, gas in soft tissues, and reactive changes in adjacent bone. Plain radiographs are more useful in excluding other processes, such as osteomyelitis or bone sarcoma [9,11,43]. Ultrasound of the affected area may identify increased muscle volume with associated fluid collections, and hypoechogenicity of fibroadipose septa [43,44].

CT will often detect muscle swelling and well-delineated areas of fluid attenuation (Fig. 1) that display rim enhancement with contrast [43]. However, CT is less sensitive than MRI for evaluating the extent of infection. Typical findings on T1-weighted MRI are higher signal intensity in involved muscles, with a rim of increased intensity at the border of the involved region. On T2-weighted images, this rim is of low intensity with gadolinium enhancement, whereas the affected muscle displays heterogeneous increased intensity. Foci of homogeneous intensity usually correspond to fluid collections. Thickening of fascial planes and reticulation of subcutaneous fat with overlying thickened skin may also be noted [43].

Treatment and outcomes

Appropriate therapy for pyomyositis varies by risk factors, patient demographics, stage of infection, and obviously, microbiologic results, if available.

Although uncommonly diagnosed in the preabscess stage, antibiotics alone are likely effective in this early period. Once an abscess has formed,

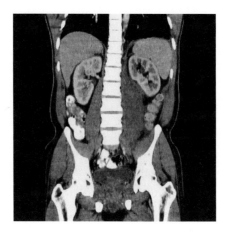

Fig. 1. A 39-year-old man who had HIV, a CD4 count of 278, and poorly controlled insulin-dependent diabetes mellitus presented with several days of high fever and rigors, and left flank pain radiating into the groin. Psoas sign was markedly positive on physical examination. CT images with coronal reconstruction show impressive enlargement of the left psoas, impinging on the left kidney, and causing mild hydronephrosis. Hypodense areas within the psoas likely represent liquefaction and early abscess formation. Blood cultures and cultures of a CT-guided psoas aspiration grew methicillin-sensitive *Staphylococcus aureus*.

drainage is likely required for proper therapy. The extent and method of drainage depends on the size of the affected area and its location. Traditionally, surgical intervention has involved large incisions and wide exposure of affected muscles. Deeper structures, such as the iliopsoas area, require extensive laparotomies. Many of these heavily invasive methods can now be avoided with newer suction methods that allow for primary closure of wounds with continuous suction and drainage [9]. Operative intervention can often be avoided with CT-guided percutaneous drainage. If extensive muscle involvement has occurred and significant necrosis is present, operative intervention is likely still required for recovery. This occurrence is more common when there has been significant delay in diagnosis. Depending on the patient's condition, it may be beneficial to diagnostically drain the abscess before initiating empiric antibiotic therapy so that Gram stain and culture results may direct specific therapy. However, as with most serious infections, initiation of therapy cannot always be delayed, and empiric antimicrobial selection must be guided by clinical judgment.

In uncomplicated cases in patients who are immunocompetent, initial therapy can be directed against staphylococci and streptococci. Oxacillin or nafcillin are appropriate first-line therapies [9], with a first-generation cephalosporin as an alternative [7]. Coverage for MRSA should be considered if the patient is seriously ill or has risk factors for MRSA, such as recent hospitalization, HIV infection, intravenous drug use, or residence in a community with significant MRSA prevalence. In such instances, vancomycin is generally first-line therapy [7].

In individuals who are immunocompromised and HIV-positive, and in severe cases of pyomyositis, broad empiric coverage for resistant gram-positive organisms, gram-negative organisms, and anaerobes should be considered [4,7]. In such instances, vancomycin with antipseudomonal carbapenems or β-lactam/β-lactamase combinations may be appropriate empiric therapies. Other antimicrobials, such as aztreonam, fluoroquinolones, aminoglycosides, or later generation cephalosporins, alone or in combination, have also been used with good results [11].

Intravenous antimicrobial therapy is generally given for at least 7 to 10 days, followed by a variable period of oral antibiotic therapy for a total duration of 4 to 6 weeks, depending on severity and the presence of complications such as osteomyelitis [9]. Patients who have extensive, multifocal, or poorly drained infection may warrant longer courses of therapy. Results of follow-up imaging studies, such as CT scanning, are helpful in assessing response to therapy and delineating length of treatment. Assessment to exclude underlying endocarditis in patients who are bacteremic should be considered, given the obvious impact on duration and route of therapy [7].

In rare cases of infections caused by organisms such as *Bartonella* or mycobacteria, several months of organism-specific antimicrobials are frequently necessary for adequate treatment [4,45].

Unlike the more aggressive necrotizing fasciitis and myonecrosis infections, primary pyomyositis infrequently requires amputation for proper treatment. Surprisingly, even with extensive damage to muscle, there may be little residual deformity and minimal loss of function. Recurrence of the infection can occur in a few cases, especially if the infection is a complication of HIV. Overall mortality rates range from less than 1% to reports of up to 10% [4,7,42].

References

[1] Gibson RK, Rosenthal SJ, Lukert BP. Pyomyositis. Increasing recognition in temperate climates. Am J Med 1984;77(4):768–72.

[2] Patel SR, Olenginski TP, Perruquet JL, et al. Pyomyositis: clinical features and predisposing conditions. J Rheumatol 1997;24(9):1734–8.

[3] Niamane R, Jalal O, El Ghazi M, et al. Multifocal pyomyositis in an immunocompetent patient. Joint Bone Spine 2004;71(6):595–7.

[4] Crum NF. Bacterial pyomyositis in the United States. Am J Med 2004;117(6):420–8.

[5] Heckmann JG, Lang CJ, Haselbeck M, et al. Tropical pyomyositis. Eur J Neurol 2001;8(3): 283–4.

[6] Horn CV, Master S. Pyomyositis tropicans in Uganda. East Afr Med J 1968;45(7):463–71.

[7] Chauhan S, Jain S, Varma S, et al. Tropical pyomyositis (myositis tropicans): current perspective. Postgrad Med J 2004;80(943):267–70.

[8] Christin L, Sarosi GA. Pyomyositis in North America: case reports and review. Clin Infect Dis 1992;15(4):668–77.

[9] Bickels J, Ben-Sira L, Kessler A, et al. Primary pyomyositis. J Bone Joint Surg Am 2002; 84-A(12):2277–86.

[10] Shepherd JJ. Tropical myositis: is it an entity and what is its cause? Lancet 1983;2(8361): 1240–2.
[11] Scharschmidt TJ, Weiner SD, Myers JP. Bacterial Pyomyositis. Curr Infect Dis Rep 2004; 6(5):393–6.
[12] Burkhart BG, Hamson KR. Pyomyositis in a 69-year-old tennis player. Am J Orthop 2003; 32(11):562–3.
[13] Chusid MJ, Hill WC, Bevan JA, et al. Proteus pyomyositis of the piriformis muscle in a swimmer. Clin Infect Dis 1998;26(1):194–5.
[14] Jayoussi R, Bialik V, Eyal A, et al. Pyomyositis caused by vigorous exercise in a boy. Acta Paediatr 1995;84(2):226–7.
[15] King RJ, Laugharne D, Kerslake RW, et al. Primary obturator pyomyositis: a diagnostic challenge. J Bone Joint Surg Br 2003;85(6):895–8.
[16] Koutures CG, Savoia M, Pedowitz RA. Staphylococcus aureus thigh pyomyositis in a collegiate swimmer. Clin J Sport Med 2000;10(4):297–9.
[17] Meehan J, Grose C, Soper RT, et al. Pyomyositis in an adolescent female athlete. J Pediatr Surg 1995;30(1):127–8.
[18] Viani RM, Bromberg K, Bradley JS. Obturator internus muscle abscess in children: report of seven cases and review. Clin Infect Dis 1999;28(1):117–22.
[19] Lambertucci JR, Rayes A, Serufo JC, et al. Visceral larva migrans and tropical pyomyositis: a case report. Rev Inst Med Trop Sao Paulo 1998;40(6):383–5.
[20] Rayes AA, Nobre V, Teixeira DM, et al. Tropical pyomyositis and human toxocariasis: a clinical and experimental study. Am J Med 2000;109(5):422–5.
[21] Ansaloni L, Acaye GL, Re MC. High HIV seroprevalence among patients with pyomyositis in northern Uganda. Trop Med Int Health 1996;1(2):210–2.
[22] Hsueh PR, Hsiue TR, Hsieh WC. Pyomyositis in intravenous drug abusers: report of a unique case and review of the literature. Clin Infect Dis 1996;22(5):858–60.
[23] Ebright JR, Pieper B. Skin and soft tissue infections in injection drug users. Infect Dis Clin North Am 2002;16(3):697–712.
[24] Lo TS, Mooers MG, Wright LJ. Pyomyositis complicating acute bacterial endocarditis in an intravenous drug user. N Engl J Med 2000;342(21):1614–5.
[25] Crossley M. Temperate pyomyositis in an injecting drug misuser. A difficult diagnosis in a difficult patient. Emerg Med J 2003;20(3):299–300.
[26] Gubbay AJ, Isaacs D. Pyomyositis in children. Pediatric Infectious Disease Journal 2000; 19(10):1009–12 [quiz: 1013].
[27] Taylor JF, Templeton AC, Henderson B. Pyomyositis. A clinico-pathological study based on 19 autopsy cases, Mulago Hospital 1964–1968. East Afr Med J 1970;47(10): 493–501.
[28] Martinez-Aguilar G, Avalos-Mishaan A, Hulten K, et al. Community-acquired, methicillin-resistant and methicillin-susceptible Staphylococcus aureus musculoskeletal infections in children. Pediatr Infect Dis J 2004;23(8):701–6.
[29] Ruiz ME, Yohannes S, Wladyka CG. Pyomyositis caused by methicillin-resistant Staphylococcus aureus. N Engl J Med 2005;352(14):1488–9.
[30] Chu CK, Yang TL, Tan CT. Tuberculous pyomyositis of the temporal muscle in a nonimmunocompromised woman: diagnosis by sonography. J Laryngol Otol 2004;118(1):59–61.
[31] Lawn SD, Bicanic TA, Macallan DC. Pyomyositis and cutaneous abscesses due to Mycobacterium avium: an immune reconstitution manifestation in a patient with AIDS. Clin Infect Dis 2004;38(3):461–3.
[32] Wang JY, Lee LN, Hsueh PR, et al. Tuberculous myositis: a rare but existing clinical entity. Rheumatology (Oxford) 2003;42(7):836–40.
[33] Ahmed J, Homans J. Tuberculosis pyomyositis of the soleus muscle in a fifteen-year-old boy. Pediatr Infect Dis J 2002;21(12):1169–71.
[34] Johnson DW, Herzig KA. Isolated tuberculous pyomyositis in a renal transplant patient. Nephrol Dial Transplant 2000;15(5):743.

[35] Shih JY, Hsueh PR, Chang YL, et al. Pyomyositis due to Mycobacterium haemophilum in a patient with polymyositis and long-term steroid use. Clin Infect Dis 1998;26(2):505–7.

[36] Lortholary O, Jarrousse B, Attali P, et al. Psoas pyomyositis as a late complication of typhoid fever. Clin Infect Dis 1995;21(4):1049–50.

[37] Collazos J, Mayo J, Martinez E, et al. Comparison of the clinical and laboratory features of muscle infections caused by Salmonella and those caused by other pathogens. J Infect Chemother 2001;7(3):169–74.

[38] Collazos J, Mayo J, Martinez E, et al. Muscle infections caused by Salmonella species: case report and review. Clin Infect Dis 1999;29(3):673–7.

[39] Haugh PJ, Levy CS, Hoff-Sullivan E, et al. Pyomyositis as the sole manifestation of disseminated gonococcal infection: case report and review. Clin Infect Dis 1996;22(5):861–3.

[40] Romeo S, Sunshine S. Pyomyositis in a 5-year-old child. Arch Fam Med 2000;9(7):653–6.

[41] Peckett WR, Butler-Manuel A, Apthorp LA. Pyomyositis of the iliacus muscle in a child. J Bone Joint Surg Br 2001;83(1):103–5.

[42] Chiedozi LC. Pyomyositis. Review of 205 cases in 112 patients. Am J Surg 1979;137(2):255–9.

[43] Struk DW, Munk PL, Lee MJ, et al. Imaging of soft tissue infections. Radiol Clin North Am 2001;39(2):277–303.

[44] Trusen A, Beissert M, Schultz G, et al. Ultrasound and MRI features of pyomyositis in children. Eur Radiol 2003;13(5):1050–5.

[45] Husain S, Singh N. Pyomyositis associated with bacillary angiomatosis in a patient with HIV infection. Infection 2002;30(1):50–3.

INFECTIOUS
DISEASE CLINICS
OF NORTH AMERICA

Infect Dis Clin N Am 19 (2005) 991–1005

Suppurative Tenosynovitis and Septic Bursitis

Lorne N. Small, MD, FRCPC[a],
John J. Ross, MD, CM[b],*

[a]Division of Geographic Medicine and Infectious Diseases, Tufts-New England
Medical Center, 750 Washington Street, Boston, MA 02111, USA
[b]Division of Infectious Diseases, Caritas Saint Elizabeth's Medical Center,
736 Cambridge Street, Boston, MA 02135, USA

Suppurative tenosynovitis and septic bursitis are closed space infections of the musculoskeletal system. Appropriate antibiotics in combination with incision and drainage are generally recommended. Aggressive surgical management is particularly important in tenosynovitis to prevent tendon necrosis. Empiric antibiotic coverage should be directed toward staphylococci and streptococci. Patient characteristics and epidemiologic exposures may provide clues to unusual causative organisms that are occasionally encountered, such as *Neisseria gonorrhoeae*, *Pasteurella multocida*, atypical mycobacteria, fungi, and protothecosis.

Infectious tenosynovitis

Pathogenesis and epidemiology

Infectious or suppurative tenosynovitis is an infection of the closed synovial sheaths of tendons. These infections occur most frequently in digits of the hand, and most cases involve tendons and tendon sheaths of flexor muscles rather than those of extensors, although there are case reports of the latter [1,2]. The infection is generally associated with trauma and direct inoculation of the affected site. However, tenosynovitis may result from disseminated infection with certain organisms, particularly *N gonorrhoeae* [1].

Knowing the exact nature of antecedent trauma in suppurative tenosynovitis is often helpful in predicting the causative organism. The most

* Corresponding author.
E-mail address: jrossmd@cchcs.org (J.J. Ross).

common causative injuries are likely animal or human bites and scratches [3] because they easily lead to bacterial inoculation. Injuries occurring during fishing or fish handling, thorn injuries, illicit intravenous drug use, and occupational trauma, such as chemical and other injuries, have also been implicated [4,5]. A complete epidemiologic history, including geography, occupation, sexual history, drug use, hobbies, pets, and underlying medical conditions, cannot be overemphasized for the proper diagnosis and treatment of these infections.

The pathogenesis of infectious tenosynovitis depends on the anatomy of the affected site. Most of the reported literature focuses on tenosynovitis of the hand, likely because of its greater frequency and morbidity and the intricacy of surgical intervention. However, tenosynovitis can occur in any extremity, and not only in digits. In the hand, tendons and their synovial sheaths are next to or communicating with structures such as bursae and potential spaces, potentially allowing spread of infection [6], tissue ischemia, and compartment syndrome [7].

The closed nature of the tendon sheaths facilitates infection because the sheaths easily harbor pathogens when contaminated. The sheath consists of an inner visceral layer juxtaposed to the tendon, and an outer parietal layer separating it from other structures [6,8]. The visceral and parietal layers join at their ends to form a closed structure. In the hand, the radial and ulnar bursae are intimately associated with multiple nearby flexor tendons, and up to 80% of individuals have an anatomic communication between these bursae. As such, suppurative tenosynovitis of the thumb or fifth digit may spread to its corresponding bursae, which may then allow the infection access to the opposite side of the hand through the bursal communication [6,8]. This pattern of infection is referred to as a *horseshoe abscess* and must be considered a possibility when evaluating infections that superficially seem well localized. Failure to treat flexor tendon sheath infection promptly may lead to tendon necrosis and proximal spread [6]. Extensor tenosynovitis is much less common, but when extensor structures are involved, there is less propensity for loculated infection and increased tissue pressure, as these tendons lack the retinacular system of the flexors [1].

As with all infections, host immune status is an important factor. Any immunosuppression, whether iatrogenic or secondary to disease state such as HIV, may predispose the individual to these infections and may lead to unusual and severe presentations.

Microbiology

Microbiology of infectious tenosynovitis varies according to exposure. In cases of trauma and punctures caused by clean sources, the offending flora is often that of the skin. In one large recent study, streptococci and *Staphylococcus aureus* were the most common organisms isolated in individuals who were immunocompetent and diabetic, followed by *S epidermidis* and then gram-negative organisms and enterococci. Approximately a quarter of the patients had more than one organism isolated, and there was a significant incidence of methicillin-resistant *S aureus* [9].

Bite wounds vary in their microbiology and are typically polymicrobial. When tissue cultures of human bite infections are collected with good technique and anaerobic cultures, streptococci and staphylococci are common, as are *Eikenella corrodens*, *Haemophilus* sp, *Neisseria* sp, and various anaerobes, including species of *Peptostreptococcus*, *Veillonella*, *Fusobacterium*, and *Bacteroides* [3,10].

Animal bites involve a similar spectra of organisms and high rates of infection with *P multocida* [2,3,10–13]. Other occasionally encountered organisms are *Capnocytophaga* sp, *Bacillus* sp, *Proteus* sp, *Pseudomonas* sp, actinomyces, and *Leptotrichia buccalis*. Although any of these potential bite wound organisms may cause tenosynovitis, most of the more esoteric have been rarely, if ever, reported specifically in tenosynovitis.

Penetrating injuries involving plant thorns may rarely lead to fungal infections, such as sporotrichosis and fusariosis, and sterile inflammatory reactions [14,15].

Infectious tenosynovitis may also occur as secondary hematogenous dissemination, especially *N gonorrhoeae*. It is estimated that disseminated gonococcal infection (DGI) occurs in 1% to 3% of patients who have mucosal gonococcal infections, and of these, up to two thirds have tenosynovitis. Sometimes this may be a reactive process, but there are many documented infectious cases [16–18].

Mycobacterial tenosynovitis is strongly associated with fresh and salt water exposure. However, atypical mycobacterial tenosynovitis has been reported after bites by terrestrial animals, in addition to other environmental exposures [14,19,20]. The prototypical mycobacterium implicated in these cases is *Mycobacterium marinum,* first isolated in 1926 from dead saltwater fish at the Philadelphia Aquarium [21]. Human infections with this organism were documented in 1954 by Linell and Norden and in 1962 by Swift and Cohen, as being associated with swimming pool and tropical aquarium exposure, respectively [21,22]. Less common atypical mycobacteria causing tenosynovitis include *M kansasii*, *M asiaticum*, *M avium*, *M fortuitum*, *M chelonae*, and *M abscessus* [14,19,23–27]. Reports of tuberculous tenosynovitis often, but not always, represent spread from active pulmonary tuberculosis [28–32].

Clinical manifestations

In 1912, Kanavel [6,33] described four classic cardinal signs of flexor tenosynovitis. These signs include tenderness over the course of the flexor sheath, symmetric enlargement of the affected finger (sausage finger), slightly flexed finger at rest, and exquisite pain along the tendon sheath with passive extension of the finger. The less common entity of extensor tenosynovitis has not been characterized as well, and may be more difficult to distinguish from other pathology [1].

Puncture wounds may lead to symptoms and signs of infectious tenosynovitis within hours to days of the initial inoculation [2,11,13]. The time between trauma and the onset of symptoms of infection may vary depending on the type of penetrating injury, depth, overall size, and whether there was direct inoculation into the synovial sheath. After a Siberian tiger bite, one patient presented with classic local symptoms of flexor tenosynovitis and systemic signs within 8 hours of the bite [11]. Along with the classic signs described, there may be other signs and symptoms of local and systemic infection. Localized erythema may occur with lymphangitic streaking. Discharge may occur from the puncture sites [12]. Fever and leukocytosis are also common [11,12].

In tenosynovitis secondary to a disseminated infection such as DGI, systemic and other local signs and symptoms usually precede symptoms of the tenosynovitis [17]. Unlike other causes of bacterial tenosynovitis, gonococcal infection more commonly affects extensor tendons. Skin rash, fever, and arthritis are common manifestations of DGI. Occasionally, tenosynovitis may be the presenting complaint in such infections [18].

Atypical mycobacterial tenosynovitis is a more indolent, chronic process, and its presentation varies depending on the immune status of the patient. In most cases, a history of water exposure coincident with skin breaks can be elicited. However, cases have been reported after bite injury, steroid injection, and soil contamination of wounds [20,34,35]. Some, but not all, affected individuals report an initial nodular cellulitic process which occurs 2 to 4 weeks after initial inoculation [14,21]. This formation represents the classic "fish tank granuloma" or "swimming pool granuloma." The nodules may suppurate or ulcerate [36]. Within weeks to months, there may be new complaints of swelling and pain as the infection involves the synovial sheath. This development is probably most consistent with slow progression of a superficial inoculation to deeper structures, rather than a deep penetrating exposure directly infecting the synovial sheath [14,21,37,38]. Once tenosynovitis develops, often months after initial exposure, the patient presents with local swelling and functional impairment, but pain and tenderness are much less prominent than in tenosynovitis caused by other bacteria [20,21,38]. Untreated, the infection may lead to tendon rupture. Fever is not unusual, and indicators of inflammation such as erythrocyte sedimentation rate and C-reactive protein are often normal [14].

Diagnosis

The diagnosis of bacterial tenosynovitis may be suspected based on clinical history and symptoms at presentation. In extensor involvement, the classic signs of flexor tenosynovitis may be lacking, but the history of a penetrating injury can usually be obtained [2]. Joints should be carefully examined to exclude concomitant septic arthritis. In hematogenous dissemination leading to tenosynovitis, diagnosis may be more difficult given the lack of a history of antecedent local trauma. Fever and mildly elevated leukocyte count with left shift are common, but not invariable [11].

Plain films are of limited use other than to exclude fractures and metallic foreign bodies. Ultrasound evaluation of affected areas may reveal fluid within tendon sheaths, synovial sheath thickening, and sometimes foreign bodies such as thorns, and may guide diagnostic needle aspiration [12]. Effusions caused by infection may be more echogenic than simple effusions. Hypervascularity on Doppler ultrasound may also be a nonspecific indication of local infection. MRI is a useful diagnostic modality for determining extent of infection. CT may be somewhat more limited in evaluation of soft tissues.

Definitive diagnosis is made by Gram stain and culture of synovial sheath fluid, either by needle aspiration or at the time of surgical intervention. Because of the acuity of flexor tenosynovitis and potential morbidity, surgery is often the diagnostic modality, as there is a need for rapid definitive intervention. The presence of clinical findings of DGI, such as hemorrhagic pustules, may aid in the diagnosis of gonococcal tenosynovitis [17,18]. If gonococcal tenosynovitis is suspected, aspirate should be processed appropriately to isolate *N gonorrhea*, such as on Thayer-Martin media.

As opposed to the rapid onset of typical bacterial tenosynovitis, the indolent nature of atypical mycobacterial tenosynovitis may delay accurate diagnosis for several months [14,20,21]. Often the patient will be treated initially for a presumed noninfectious musculoskeletal process or a typical bacterial infection. Imaging, specifically MRI, may be helpful in detecting synovial thickening around tendons. Biopsy of superficial nodules or affected tendon sheaths may be misleading early in the infection, as granulomas, characteristic of mycobacterial infections, may not be present [14,39]. The terms "fish tank granuloma" and "swimming pool granuloma" may be misnomers because these infections may not involve formation of granulomas in the infected tissues until late in the clinical course. Biopsies of affected tissue performed in conjunction with acid-fast staining detect mycobacteria in only 30% of cases [40]. Most frequently, properly performed mycobacterial cultures and a high index of suspicion are required for accurate diagnosis. If *M marinum* is suspected, the microbiology laboratory should be asked to perform mycobacterial cultures at 30°C, as the organism may fail to grow at higher temperatures. Several weeks may elapse before cultures and molecular identification techniques are able to reveal the offending organism [40].

Treatment

The use of prophylactic antibiotics in puncture wounds is fairly common. A meta-analysis of antibiotic prophylaxis in nonbite penetrating injuries revealed no infection prevention benefit [41]. In contrast, it is advised that bite wounds should be treated with antibiotics even in the absence of obvious infection [3]. Because of the high incidence of infection in bites, this is considered active therapy rather than prophylaxis. Objective evidence to support this practice is scanty, but given the high incidence of infection and polymicrobial contamination, it is generally accepted [3]. The exception is those cases presenting 24 hours or more after the bite with no indication of infection. In all cases, local wound care is advisable.

If bacterial tenosynovitis is suspected or objectively diagnosed, empiric antibiotic therapy should be based on the origin of the injury and adjusted according to microbiology results. For simple puncture wounds leading to tenosynovitis, appropriate parenteral staphylococcal and streptococcal therapy may be sufficient [9]. In individuals who have immune compromise or underlying chronic illness, gram-negative coverage may also be advisable. Empiric therapy for methicillin-resistant *S aureus* (MRSA) should also be considered in regions with high community prevalence or in patients who have classic risk factors for MRSA, such as recent hospitalization or intravenous drug use.

In bite wounds with secondary tenosynovitis, broader spectrum antibiotics with additional activity against gram-negative and anaerobic bacteria are indicated [10,41,42]. A β-lactam/β-lactamase inhibitor combination, such as ampicillin/sulbactam, is often first-line therapy. In documented penicillin allergy, alternatives include tetracyclines or trimethoprim/sulfamethoxazole, with additional anaerobic coverage. The newer fluoroquinolones—gatifloxacin and moxifloxacin—may have sufficient inherent anaerobic activity to be adequate as monotherapy. Other alternatives include carbapenems and higher-generation cephalosporins, but these may not be suitable if the patient has documented β-lactam hypersensitivity.

Surgical intervention in acute bacterial flexor tenosynovitis is advocated because of the high risk for morbidity. Severity of these infections may be classified in three stages. Stage one involves serous exudates and congestion of the sheath. Stage two is characterized by murky or cloudy fluid, signs of purulence, and synovial granulation in the sheath. In the third stage, there is overt sheath or tendon necrosis [7,43]. If the infection is in the early stages, antibiotics, elevation, and splinting may be appropriate; however, if no improvement is noted after 24 hours, surgery is advised [6]. Surgery may not be as urgent in cases of extensor synovitis, based on expert clinical assessment [1]. Surgical techniques for treating tenosynovitis include multiple techniques of open drainage or closed-catheter irrigation [6,7,44,45].

Gonococcal tenosynovitis caused by disseminated infection may be successfully treated with intravenous antibiotics and local splinting. Noninvasive therapy is most successful if the patient presents within the first 48 hours of symptoms. Surgical intervention may be necessary if antibiotics alone are not effective after 24 to 48 hours of therapy, or if the patient presents after the first 2 days of symptoms [17,18].

Antimicrobial therapy, surgery, or a combination of the two may be necessary to adequately treat mycobacterial tenosynovitis. *M marinum* and *M kansasii*, the two most common causes of atypical mycobacterial tenosynovitis, have reportedly been successfully treated with antimicrobials or surgery alone [39,40,46,47]. However, evidence suggests that higher cure rates may occur when the two methods are used together, especially in immunocompromised hosts. Extensive tenosynovectomy is recommended, which may be performed at the time of initial biopsy. Repeat debridement may be necessary, depending on the extent of the infection and inflammation. Although amputation is only occasionally indicated in such cases, delay in diagnosis and treatment may increase the risk. Because mycobacterial cultures require weeks for results, clinical suspicion, granulomas on histology, or the presence of acid-fast organisms are indications to begin mycobacterial therapy. Rifampin, isoniazid, and ethambutol are likely to be effective against most slow-growing atypical mycobacteria and are also indicated if a tuberculous process is suspected. If *M marinum* is suspected, clarithromycin is an appropriate addition [14,20,21]. Empiric isoniazid omission may be considered because of toxicity and because some atypical mycobacteria, such as *M marinum*, are inherently resistant. In contrast, rapid-growing atypical mycobacteria, such as *M chelonae*, *M abscessus*, and *M fortuitum*, are not readily susceptible to antituberculous medication, and other antibiotic combinations are usually required, possibly including the carbapenems, aminoglycosides, quinolones, and macrolides [14]. In all cases of mycobacterial infections, monotherapy is inadvisable. Appropriate treatment durations vary, generally ranging from 9 months to 2 years. The duration is determined based on clinical response, host immune status, and organism resistance. A review of such infection recommended at least 9 months of therapy and continuation of treatment until 3 to 4 months after resolution of clinical signs [21,48,49]. In all cases, antimycobacterial agents should be adjusted according to the specific resistance pattern. It is unclear if surgical intervention can decrease the appropriate chemotherapeutic duration.

Septic bursitis

Pathogenesis and epidemiology

More than 150 bursae exist in the human body, some superficial and more vulnerable, whereas others are in deeper, protected locations. The superficial bursae reside in subcutaneous tissues, whereas the deep bursae are found beneath fibrous fascia [50,51]. Bursae are closed sacs with inner synovial linings that produce lubricating fluid, but under normal circumstances very little fluid is present. The bursae act as friction buffers, not unlike ball bearings, to facilitate movement of adjacent connective tissue structures against each other. Bursae may be of the constant type, present at or soon after birth, or the adventitious type, developing in response to recurrent stimuli in one location.

Bursitis, or inflammation of a bursa, may be infectious or a primary inflammatory process. Bursitis of an infectious nature, or septic bursitis, usually involves the superficial bursae because of a predisposition by trauma to these areas [50,51]. In fact, many forms of sterile inflammatory bursitis are popularly named for occupations or activities associated with specific local trauma. These types include housemaid's knee and clergyman's knee, involving the prepatellar bursa and the infrapatellar bursa, respectively. (A clergyman, genuflecting with a more erect upper torso, puts pressure on a different area of the knee, compared with a housemaid scrubbing a floor with the upper torso bent forward.)

The most commonly infected bursae are the olecranon, prepatellar, and superficial infrapatellar bursae because of their subcutaneous locations. The presumed mode of infection is direct percutaneous inoculation of organisms into the bursae caused by trauma, or contiguous spread from cellulitis to a traumatized subcutaneous bursa [51,52]. S aureus and streptococci are by far the most common pathogens associated with septic bursitis. Superficial or deep septic bursitis secondary to hematogenous dissemination of a primary infection is rare. With deep bursae infections, contiguous septic arthritis as the primary site of infection must be excluded [53].

The most important predisposing factor in septic bursitis is trauma. It is estimated that up to 70% of all infectious bursitis is related to preceding trauma [52]. The trauma involved may be chronic, caused by repetitive injury, or acute, and is often occupational or recreational [51,52]. Septic olecranon bursitis has been anecdotally reported in patients who have chronic obstructive pulmonary disease [51,54]. Presumably, the repetitive forward-leaning posture often noted in such patients, along with corticosteroid use, may be a predisposition. A similar postural predisposition may also occur in patients on hemodialysis. Other specific epidemiologic associations include ischial bursitis in individuals who have spinal injuries [55], malleolar bursitis in ice skaters [56], and occasional subacromial or subdeltoid bursitis after local injections [57].

Previous noninfectious inflammation of a bursa, such as in gout, rheumatoid arthritis, or trauma, may also be a risk factor for developing septic bursitis [52,58]. Chronic illnesses such as diabetes mellitus and alcohol abuse may also predispose [59]. Chronic skin conditions, such as atopic dermatitis, may facilitate superficial bursae inoculation and contribute to the incidence of septic bursitis [60]. As for immunocompromised states, such as HIV, some investigators report a higher incidence of septic bursitis, whereas others report no difference compared with individuals who are immunocompetent [51,61]. There does seem to be general agreement that infectious bursitis may be more severe in the individual who is immunocompromised, and often requires lengthier durations of antimicrobial therapy [53,62].

Microbiology

An estimated 80% of cases of septic bursitis are caused by *S aureus* [63]. Most of the remaining cases are caused by streptococci, most commonly the β-hemolytic species [51,52]. Other reported organisms reported are coagulase-negative staphylococci, enterococci, and occasionally gram-negative organisms, including *E coli* and *P aeruginosa* [51,63]. Anaerobes are rarely reported [64].

In chronic or subacute bursitis, various unusual organisms may be considered. In the proper epidemiologic setting, brucellosis may cause recurrent infectious bursitis, especially *Brucella abortus* [65–67]. Tuberculous and atypical mycobacterial bursitis may cause chronic and refractory bursitis [68–72]. There are occasional reports of fungal bursitis caused by *Candida* and molds [51,73,74]. Some of these may represent disseminated infection, rather than localized infection from inoculation.

A more recently recognized, uncommon cause of septic bursitis is *Prototheca wickerhamii* [75,76]. These algae lack chlorophyll, are ubiquitous in nature, and may colonize humans. *Prototheca* may be mistaken for fungi, as they resemble yeasts in tissue biopsy and grow readily on standard mycologic media. Infection mainly occurs in individuals who are immunocompromised and has been best studied in those who have underlying malignancy. The infection ranges from localized skin lesions to disseminated forms, including findings of algae in the blood. Bursal involvement tends to be from direct inoculation, as with most other causes of superficial bursitis. Protothecosis, whether seemingly localized or obviously disseminated, carries a poor prognosis. Treatment is debridement and excision of lesions, where possible, and medication with amphotericin B or azoles.

Clinical manifestations

The most common findings in cases of septic bursitis are erythema and pain over the affected bursa [77]. Patients may recall trauma or there may be abrasions over the affected area. There may be overlying or adjacent cellulitis [78]. Patients may also have a previous history of infectious or noninfectious inflammation of the bursa. The bursa is likely to be locally edematous, and a point of maximal tenderness will be noted at the center of the bursa [52]. Most patients will also have fever. Leukocyte count and sedimentation rate are often mildly to moderately elevated, and neutrophilia with bandemia may be present [53]. Systemic signs of infection and bacteremia occur, but these are more commonly associated with deep bursae infections. Because there is often no direct joint involvement in superficial septic bursitis, some joint mobility may be preserved.

Septic bursitis may also present as a more chronic, indolent process or may recur after treating a presumed acute bacterial or inflammatory bursitis. Frequently, the initial occurrence will be treated with empiric antibiotics or local steroids. In such cases, unusual organisms should be considered. Tuberculous involvement of the trochanteric, subdeltoid, prepatellar, or olecranon bursa has been described [69,70,72,79]. Usually these cases represent systemic infection, and isolated tuberculous bursitis with no evidence of joint or bone involvement is rare [69]. Cases of atypical mycobacterial bursitis occur mostly in individuals who have other underlying chronic illnesses or impaired immunity, and usually represent only local infection [68,71]. Brucella bursitis usually occurs in systemic illness; however, there are case reports of isolated local bursa infection [65–67].

Often the symptoms may subside and recur months to years after the initial complaint. It is not uncommon for these individuals to present with sinus tracts draining cutaneously. Laboratory data may reveal mildly elevated leukocytes and erythrocyte sedimentation rate [67,70]. Vague constitutional symptoms may also be present, especially in cases of brucellar and tuberculous infections.

Diagnosis

A history of recent trauma may be absent in half or more of those who have bursitis, and if present, does not necessarily distinguish primary inflammatory bursitis from septic bursitis [51]. A more intense inflammatory process may be more likely with an infectious cause compared with a purely inflammatory origin. Individuals who have septic bursitis present earlier in the clinical course and have more pain, tenderness, erythema, and warmth compared with those who have an inflammatory process [80].

Diagnosis may be more difficult if there is overlying cellulitis, as it may obscure the bursa. More concerning is that an initial suspicion of bursitis may delay the diagnosis of more serious septic arthritis. Careful evaluation of the nearby joint is therefore prudent. Additionally, an aseptic joint effusion may occur as a consequence of septic bursitis. However, even with a confirmed diagnosis of bursitis, a joint effusion should not be ignored because septic bursitis and arthritis may occur simultaneously [51]. Arthrocentesis should be considered if there is any suspicion of joint involvement. Obviously, inflamed superficial structures should be avoided when performing the arthrocentesis, as iatrogenic bacterial contamination of the joint may occur.

Imaging of suspected septic bursitis may be helpful in identifying bursal or peribursal fluid, a thickened synovium, associated abscesses, or affected adjacent structures [50,57,66–68,70,81]. The most common modalities are MRI and ultrasound. Plain films may be helpful in detecting affected adjacent structures, such as bone [70].

Diagnosis of septic bursitis is made by aspiration of the affected bursa. White blood cell counts from infected bursae are lower than those from infected joints, and counts of less than $20,000/mm^3$ may be consistent with septic bursitis [52]. Grossly purulent fluid is suggestive of infection.

However, other conditions, such as gout and rheumatoid arthritis, may grossly appear purulent but are actually sterile. Conversely, fluid from some infected bursae is only slightly turbid, and may occasionally be hemorrhagic [51]. The sensitivity of detecting organisms by Gram staining the aspirate is highly variable, with reported ranges from 15% to 100% [36,58,59,82]. Aspirates should also be evaluated for crystals when appropriate. If performed with good technique, and providing there has been no partial antibiotic treatment, aspirate cultures are sensitive and specific. There is some evidence that culturing in liquid media can optimize sensitivity [80]. Blood cultures are more likely to be positive when there is infection of deep bursae [51,53].

If a chronic or recurrent infection is suspected, acid-fast staining of bursa aspirates is indicated [68–72,79]. Also, cultures should be specifically incubated for mycobacteria and fastidious organisms, such as *Brucella*. If there is epidemiologic or clinical evidence of brucellosis, serology may be helpful for diagnosis [65–67]. Surgical intervention as a diagnostic procedure may be required for these chronic cases of bursitis. Mycobacterial bursitis, especially tuberculous, may have evidence of granulomas by histology [71]. Systemic infection should be considered in cases of bursitis caused by *Brucella* or *M tuberculosis*.

Treatment

Uncomplicated superficial septic bursitis responds well to appropriate antibiotic therapy. One large review of olecranon septic bursitis found that a short period of intravenous antimicrobials with staphylococcal activity, followed by a variable oral antibiotic course with staphylococcal activity, was sufficient for cure in almost all cases [77]. Total antibiotic duration ranged from approximately 1 to 4 weeks, with no significant difference in outcomes in those who underwent drainage of the bursa compared with those who did not. Only 51% of patients had a drainage procedure, comprised of 43% having incision and drainage and the remaining 8% having only needle aspiration. Only 1 of 118 cases required surgical bursectomy. However, one major methodologic flaw of this study was that the diagnosis of septic bursitis was confirmed by positive culture in only 26% of patients, potentially leading to misdiagnosis of sterile inflammatory bursitis as infection in a large proportion of patients. This study may therefore grossly underestimate the importance of bursal drainage. Fever and leukocytosis were also absent in most patients in the study, again suggesting that many were misdiagnosed with infectious bursitis.

Initial antimicrobial therapy should focus on staphylococci and streptococci. Cefazolin or a penicillinase-resistant penicillin, such as oxacillin, is appropriate initial treatment for most patients. Consideration to empirically cover MRSA or otherwise broaden the microbial spectrum should be given based on host epidemiology and risk factors. Results from bursal fluid

Gram stains and cultures should direct specific therapy. The indications for surgical intervention include failure to adequately drain the bursa through aspiration, bursae inaccessible to aspiration, evidence of foreign body or necrosis, bursectomy for recurrent or refractory bursitis, or the need to evaluate adjacent structures for evidence of infection and possible debridement [51]. Common surgical techniques include incision and drainage with a wick placement or catheter drainage with or without irrigation.

Tuberculous bursitis may be more difficult to treat, and relapse is common with inadequate therapy. Conservative surgical intervention and antituberculous medication have had variable success. Often, full excision of the bursa and surrounding affected tissue is required for complete cure [70]. Antituberculous therapy for 6 to 12 months is generally recommended. Although tuberculous bursitis usually requires aggressive surgery, atypical mycobacterial bursitis tends to respond to appropriate antimicrobial therapy combined with conservative drainage and local debridement procedures [71].

Brucella as the causative organism may be difficult to identify; however, once the cause is determined, there is a good chance of cure with appropriate therapy. Because the organism is difficult to isolate, excision of the bursa may occur as a diagnostic measure or to treat a chronically inflamed bursa. Thus, identification of the organism may only occur after the bursa has already been removed or after debridement of the affected bursa. There have been reports of cure with tetracyclines, with or without rifampin [65–67]. Duration of therapy varies, but generally requires several weeks and may continue for several months until all symptoms are completely resolved.

References

[1] Newman ED, Harrington TM, Torretti D, et al. Suppurative extensor tenosynovitis caused by Staphylococcus aureus. J Hand Surg [Am] 1989;14(5):849–51.
[2] Loncarich D, Shin A. Suppurative extensor tenosynovitis of the extensor carpi ulnalis tendon sheath. Am J Orthop 2002;31:637–9.
[3] Brook I. Human and animal bite infections. J Fam Pract 1989;28(6):713–8.
[4] Dhaliwal AS, Garnes AL. Tenosynovitis in drug addicts. J Hand Surg [Am] 1982;7(6):626–8.
[5] West BC, Vijayan H, Shekar R. Kluyvera cryocrescens finger infection: case report and review of eighteen Kluyvera infections in human beings. Diagn Microbiol Infect Dis 1998; 32(3):237–41.
[6] Hausman MR, Lisser SP. Hand infections. Orthop Clin North Am 1992;23(1):171–85.
[7] Schnall SB, Vu-Rose T, Holtom PD, et al. Tissue pressures in pyogenic flexor tenosynovitis of the finger. Compartment syndrome and its management. J Bone Joint Surg Br 1996;78(5): 793–5.
[8] Tsai E, Failla JM. Hand infections in the trauma patient. Hand Clin 1999;15(2):373–86.
[9] Billings A, Schnall SB, Stine I. Demographics of purulent flexor tenosynovitis: an eleven year review. Presented at the Musculoskeletal Infection Society 14th Annual Open Scientific Meeting. Pittsburgh, PA, August 13–14, 2004.
[10] Brook I. Microbiology and management of human and animal bite wound infections. Prim Care 2003;30(1):25–39.

[11] Isotalo PA, Edgar D, Toye B. Polymicrobial tenosynovitis with Pasteurella multocida and other gram negative bacilli after a Siberian tiger bite. J Clin Pathol 2000;53(11):871–2.

[12] Garcia Triana M, Fernandez Echevarria MA, Alvaro RL, et al. Pasteurella multocida tenosynovitis of the hand: sonographic findings. J Clin Ultrasound 2003;31(3):159–62.

[13] Fahmy FS, Morgan MS, Saxby PJ. Pasteurella tenosynovitis following a dog bite. Injury 1994;25(4):262–3.

[14] Zenone T, Boibieux A, Tigaud S, et al. Non-tuberculous mycobacterial tenosynovitis: a review. Scand J Infect Dis 1999;31(3):221–8.

[15] Flournoy DJ, Mullins JB, McNeal RJ. Isolation of fungi from rose bush thorns. J Okla State Med Assoc 2000;93(7):271–4.

[16] Barr J, Danielsson D. Septic gonococcal dermatitis. BMJ 1971;1(747):482–5.

[17] Craig JG, van Holsbeeck M, Alva M. Gonococcal arthritis of the shoulder and septic extensor tenosynovitis of the wrist: sonographic appearances. J Ultrasound Med 2003;22(2): 221–4.

[18] Schaefer RA, Enzenauer RJ, Pruitt A, et al. Acute gonococcal flexor tenosynovitis in an adolescent male with pharyngitis. A case report and literature review. Clin Orthop Relat Res 1992;(281):212–5.

[19] Southern PM Jr. Tenosynovitis caused by Mycobacterium kansasii associated with a dog bite. Am J Med Sci 2004;327(5):258–61.

[20] Smith DS, Lindholm-Levy P, Huitt GA, et al. Mycobacterium terrae: case reports, literature review, and in vitro antibiotic susceptibility testing. Clin Infect Dis 2000;30(3): 444–53.

[21] Wongworawat MD, Holtom P, Learch TJ, et al. A prolonged case of Mycobacterium marinum flexor tenosynovitis: radiographic and histological correlation, and review of the literature. Skeletal Radiol 2003;32(9):542–5.

[22] Swift S, Cohen H. Granulomas of the skin due to Mycobacterium balnei after abrasions from a fish tank. N Engl J Med 1962;267:1244–6.

[23] Lidar M, Elkayam O, Goodwin D, et al. Protracted Mycobacterium kansasii carpal tunnel syndrome and tenosynovitis. Isr Med Assoc J 2003;5(6):453–4.

[24] Gerster JC, Duvoisin B, Dudler J, et al. Tenosynovitis of the Hands Caused by Mycobacterium kansasii in a patient with scleroderma. J Rheumatol 2004;31(12):2523–5.

[25] Foulkes GD, Floyd JC, Stephens JL. Flexor tenosynovitis due to Mycobacterium asiaticum. J Hand Surg [Am] 1998;23(4):753–6.

[26] Barcat D, Mercie P, Constans J, et al. Disseminated Mycobacterium avium complex infection associated with bifocal synovitis in a patient with dermatomyositis. Clin Infect Dis 1998; 26(4):1004–5.

[27] Anim-Appiah D, Bono B, Fleegler E, et al. Mycobacterium avium complex tenosynovitis of the wrist and hand. Arthritis Rheum 2004;51(1):140–2.

[28] Kriegs-Au G, Ganger R, Petje G. The sequelae of late diagnosis in tuberculous flexor tenosynovitis of the hand–a report of 2 cases. Acta Orthop Scand 2003;74(2):221–4.

[29] Hooker MS, Schaefer RA, Fishbain JT, et al. Tuberculous tenosynovitis of the tibialis anterior tendon: a case report. Foot Ankle Int 2002;23(12):1131–4.

[30] Fukui A, Oshima M, Takakura Y. A case of tuberculous tenosynovitis in a patient with systemic lupus erythematosus. Hand Surg 2004;9(1):109–13.

[31] Aboudola S, Sienko A, Carey RB, et al. Tuberculous tenosynovitis. Hum Pathol 2004;35(8): 1044–6.

[32] Ortiz E, Moro MJ, Diaz-Curiel M. Chronic otitis and tenosynovitis in an elderly diabetic woman. Postgrad Med J 1999;75(880):121–3.

[33] Kanavel AB. Infections of the hand: a guide to the surgical treatment of acute and chronic suppurative processes in the fingers, hand, and forearm. Philadelphia; New York: Lea & Febiger; 1912.

[34] Zenone T, Boibieux A, Tigaud S, et al. Nontuberculous mycobacterial tenosynovitis: report of two cases. Clin Infect Dis 1998;26(6):1467–8.

[35] Lau JH. Hand infection with Mycobacterium chelonei. Br Med J (Clin Res Ed) 1986; 292(6518):444–5.

[36] Smith DL, McAfee JH, Lucas LM, et al. Septic and nonseptic olecranon bursitis. Utility of the surface temperature probe in the early differentiation of septic and nonseptic cases. Arch Intern Med 1989;149(7):1581–5.

[37] Ajmal N, Nanney LB, Wolfort SF. Catfish spine envenomation: a case of delayed presentation. Wilderness Environ Med 2003;14(2):101–5.

[38] Amrami KK, Sundaram M, Shin AY, et al. Mycobacterium marinum infections of the distal upper extremities: clinical course and imaging findings in two cases with delayed diagnosis. Skeletal Radiol 2003;32(9):546–9.

[39] Gunther SF, Levy CS. Mycobacterial infections. Hand Clin 1989;5(4):591–8.

[40] Kozin SH, Bishop AT. Atypical Mycobacterium infections of the upper extremity. J Hand Surg [Am] 1994;19(3):480–7.

[41] Cummings P, Del Beccaro MA. Antibiotics to prevent infection of simple wounds: a meta-analysis of randomized studies. Am J Emerg Med 1995;13(4):396–400.

[42] Taplitz RA. Managing bite wounds. Currently recommended antibiotics for treatment and prophylaxis. Postgrad Med 2004;116(2):49–52, 55–46, 59.

[43] Juliano PJ, Eglseder WA. Limited open-tendon-sheath irrigation in the treatment of pyogenic flexor tenosynovitis. Orthop Rev 1991;20(12):1065–9.

[44] Gutowski KA, Ochoa O, Adams WP Jr. Closed-catheter irrigation is as effective as open drainage for treatment of pyogenic flexor tenosynovitis. Ann Plast Surg 2002; 49(4):350–4.

[45] Lille S, Hayakawa T, Neumeister MW, et al. Continuous postoperative catheter irrigation is not necessary for the treatment of suppurative flexor tenosynovitis. J Hand Surg [Br] 2000; 25(3):304–7.

[46] Neviaser RJ. Tenosynovitis. Hand Clin 1989;5(4):525–31.

[47] Hellinger WC, Smilack JD, Greider JL Jr, et al. Localized soft-tissue infections with Mycobacterium avium/Mycobacterium intracellulare complex in immunocompetent patients: granulomatous tenosynovitis of the hand or wrist. Clin Infect Dis 1995;21(1):65–9.

[48] Lacy JN, Viegas SF, Calhoun J, et al. Mycobacterium marinum flexor tenosynovitis. Clin Orthop Relat Res 1989;(238):288–93.

[49] Kiely JL, O'Riordan DM, Sheehan S, et al. Tenosynovitis due to mycobacteria other than tuberculosis: a hazard of water sports and hobbies. Respir Med 1995;89(1):69–71.

[50] Chartash EK, Good PK, Gould ES, et al. Septic subdeltoid bursitis. Semin Arthritis Rheum 1992;22(1):25–9.

[51] Zimmermann B III, Mikolich DJ, Ho G Jr. Septic bursitis. Semin Arthritis Rheum 1995; 24(6):391–410.

[52] Valeriano-Marcet J, Carter JD, Vasey FB. Soft tissue disease. Rheum Dis Clin North Am 2003;29(1):77–88.

[53] Garcia-Porrua C, Gonzalez-Gay MA, Ibanez D, et al. The clinical spectrum of severe septic bursitis in northwestern Spain: a 10 year study. J Rheumatol 1999;26(3):663–7.

[54] Enzenauer RJ, Pluss JL. Septic olecranon bursitis in patients with chronic obstructive pulmonary disease. Am J Med 1996;100(4):479–80.

[55] Rubayi S, Montgomerie JZ. Septic ischial bursitis in patients with spinal cord injury. Paraplegia 1992;30(3):200–3.

[56] Brown TD, Varney TE, Micheli LJ. Malleolar bursitis in figure skaters. Indications for operative and nonoperative treatment. Am J Sports Med 2000;28(1):109–11.

[57] Drezner JA, Sennett BJ. Subacromial/subdeltoid septic bursitis associated with isotretinoin therapy and corticosteroid injection. J Am Board Fam Pract 2004;17(4):299–302.

[58] Ho G Jr, Tice AD, Kaplan SR. Septic bursitis in the prepatellar and olecranon bursae: an analysis of 25 cases. Ann Intern Med 1978;89(1):21–7.

[59] Canoso JJ, Yood RA. Reaction of superficial bursae in response to specific disease stimuli. Arthritis Rheum 1979;22(12):1361–4.

[60] Narula A, Khatib R. Characteristic manifestations of clostridium induced spontaneous gangrenous myositis. Scand J Infect Dis 1985;17(3):291–4.

[61] Soderquist B, Hedstrom SA. Predisposing factors, bacteriology and antibiotic therapy in 35 cases of septic bursitis. Scand J Infect Dis 1986;18(4):305–11.

[62] Roschmann RA, Bell CL. Septic bursitis in immunocompromised patients. Am J Med 1987; 83(4):661–5.

[63] Cea-Pereiro JC, Garcia-Meijide J, Mera-Varela A, et al. A comparison between septic bursitis caused by Staphylococcus aureus and those caused by other organisms. Clin Rheumatol 2001;20(1):10–4.

[64] Fischer PA, Kopp A, Massarotti EM. Anaerobic septic bursitis: case report and review. Clin Infect Dis 1996;22(5):879.

[65] Davis JM, Broughton SJ. Prepatellar bursitis caused by Brucella abortus. Med J Aust 1996; 165(8):460.

[66] Guiral J, Reverte D, Carrero P. Iliopsoas bursitis due to Brucella melitensis infection–a case report. Acta Orthop Scand 1999;70(5):523–4.

[67] McDermott M, O'Connell B, Mulvihill TE, et al. Chronic Brucella infection of the suprapatellar bursa with sinus formation. J Clin Pathol 1994;47(8):764–6.

[68] Rutten MJ, van den Berg JC, van den Hoogen FH, et al. Nontuberculous mycobacterial bursitis and arthritis of the shoulder. Skeletal Radiol 1998;27(1):33–5.

[69] Kim RS, Lee JY, Jung SR, et al. Tuberculous subdeltoid bursitis with rice bodies. Yonsei Med J 2002;43(4):539–42.

[70] Ihara K, Toyoda K, Ofuji A, et al. Tuberculous bursitis of the greater trochanter. J Orthop Sci 1998;3(2):120–4.

[71] Friedman ND, Sexton DJ. Bursitis due to Mycobacterium goodii, a recently described, rapidly growing mycobacterium. J Clin Microbiol 2001;39(1):404–5.

[72] Crespo M, Pigrau C, Flores X, et al. Tuberculous trochanteric bursitis: report of 5 cases and literature review. Scand J Infect Dis 2004;36(8):552–8.

[73] Ornvold K, Paepke J. Aspergillus terreus as a cause of septic olecranon bursitis. Am J Clin Pathol 1992;97(1):114–6.

[74] Wall BA, Weinblatt ME, Darnall JT, et al. Candida tropicalis arthritis and bursitis. JAMA 1982;248(9):1098–9.

[75] Ahbel DE, Alexander AH, Kleine ML, et al. Protothecal olecranon bursitis. A case report and review of the literature. J Bone Joint Surg Am 1980;62(5):835–6.

[76] Torres HA, Bodey GP, Tarrand JJ, et al. Prototothecosis in patients with cancer: case series and literature review. Clin Microbiol Infect 2003;9(8):786–92.

[77] Laupland KB, Davies HD. Calgary Home Parenteral Therapy Program Study Group. Olecranon septic bursitis managed in an ambulatory setting. Clin Invest Med 2001;24(4):171–8.

[78] Coste N, Perceau G, Leone J, et al. Osteoarticular complications of erysipelas. J Am Acad Dermatol 2004;50(2):203–9.

[79] King AD, Griffith J, Rushton A, et al. Tuberculosis of the greater trochanter and the trochanteric bursa. J Rheumatol 1998;25(2):391–3.

[80] Stell IM, Gransden WR. Simple tests for septic bursitis: comparative study. BMJ 1998; 316(7148):1877.

[81] Brocq O, Euller-Ziegler L, Petit E, et al. First reported case of infection of the suprapatellar bursa of the knee due to Streptococcus pneumoniae. Arthritis Rheum 1990;33(7):1063–4.

[82] Ho G Jr, Tice AD. Comparison of nonseptic and septic bursitis. Further observations on the treatment of septic bursitis. Arch Intern Med 1979;139(11):1269–73.

**INFECTIOUS
DISEASE CLINICS**
OF NORTH AMERICA

ELSEVIER
SAUNDERS

Infect Dis Clin N Am 19 (2005) 1007–1022

Musculoskeletal Gene Therapy and its Potential Use in the Treatment of Complicated Musculoskeletal Infection

Wei Shen, MD, MS[a,b], Yong Li, MD, PhD[a,c],
Johnny Huard, PhD[a,b,c,d],*

[a]*Growth and Development Laboratory of Children's Hospital of Pittsburgh,
4100 Rangos Research Center, 3460 Fifth Avenue, Pittsburgh, PA 15213–2583, USA*
[b]*Department of Bioengineering, University of Pittsburgh, 4100 Rangos Research Center,
3460 Fifth Avenue, Pittsburgh, PA 15213–2583, USA*
[c]*Department of Orthopaedics, University of Pittsburgh, 4100 Rangos Research Center,
3460 Fifth Avenue, Pittsburgh, PA 15213–2583, USA*
[d]*Department of Molecular Genetics and Biochemistry, University of Pittsburgh,
4100 Rangos Research Center, 3460 Fifth Avenue, Pittsburgh, PA 15213–2583, USA*

Gene therapy is used to introduce exogenous genes into cells. Transferred DNA material enters the nucleus, where it either integrates into host chromosomes or remains separate in the form of an episome. Consequently, the modified cell serves as a reservoir of the desired protein product. The delivery of genes into target tissues allows the persistent local expression of therapeutic products.

Virus-mediated and non–virus-mediated delivery methods can be used to deliver genetic material into cells [1–3]. The non–virus-mediated delivery methods are usually easier to manipulate and result in lower toxicity and immunogenicity, but a low transfection rate hinders the efficiency of gene delivery. The use of viral vectors enables much more efficient gene delivery because, over time, viruses have naturally evolved the most efficient mechanism of entering a cell, and integrating their own genetic material into the DNA of the infected cell. Researchers genetically modify viral vectors to remove the genes that code for pathogenic protein products, and insert the gene of interest. The most commonly used viruses are adenovirus, retrovirus, adeno-associated virus, and herpes simplex virus; the different

* Corresponding author. Growth and Development Laboratory of Children's Hospital of Pittsburgh, 4100 Rangos Research Center, 3460 Fifth Avenue, Pittsburgh, PA 15213–2583.
E-mail address: jhuard@pitt.edu (J. Huard).

0891-5520/05/$ - see front matter © 2005 Elsevier Inc. All rights reserved.
doi:10.1016/j.idc.2005.07.005   *id.theclinics.com*

properties of these viruses dictate their use in certain conditions [1]. Scientists are working to develop new generations of viral vectors, characterized by reduced cytotoxicity and immunogenicity.

Various gene transfer strategies have been used to treat musculoskeletal diseases [1–3]. Systemic delivery involves injecting the vector into the bloodstream and allowing it to disseminate throughout the body. This strategy is used when the target tissue cannot be reached directly or when broad dissemination is desired. There are drawbacks, however, to systemic delivery. Systemic delivery usually requires a high vector concentration, and the lack of blood supply in some tissues, especially tissues of the musculoskeletal system (eg, cartilage and meniscus), makes this strategy inappropriate. Furthermore, the nonspecific dissemination of the vectors to all areas of the body raises safety concerns. In most orthopedic applications, tissue-specific local delivery is more desirable.

Direct and indirect gene delivery

Researchers have investigated two basic strategies for local gene delivery in the musculoskeletal system: in vivo and ex vivo [1–3]. The in vivo approach involves direct injection of the vectors containing DNA into the targeted host tissue. In the ex vivo strategy, cells are removed from the injured tissue, genetically modified, and injected back into the target site. Although the direct (in vivo) method is technically simpler, the indirect (ex vivo) gene delivery technique is safer and easier to control. The ex vivo strategy also enables the delivery of growth factors by endogenous cells that can also participate in the healing process in injured tissue. Specific cell types can be used for specific clinical problems. Stem cells of different origins are now receiving the most attention, because of their differentiation potential. Under proper growth factor induction, such stem cells can differentiate into desired cell types and form musculoskeletal tissues (Fig. 1). Selection of the appropriate strategy is influenced by various factors, however, including the cell source, the size of the gene of interest, and the pathophysiology of certain diseases.

Two major potential strategies for gene therapy in musculoskeletal infection are control of infection by bacterial inhibition or immune augmentation, or repair of tissue damage arising from infection.

Gene therapy for infectious diseases

Gene therapy for infection could involve the introduction of genes to block gene expression or the function of gene products by pathogens. Alternatively, gene therapy could inhibit an infectious agent at the extracellular level by the sustained expression of a secreted inhibitory protein, or elicit a specific immune response in vivo. Antisense DNA or RNA [4,5] can block gene expression by pathogens in a sequence-specific fashion based

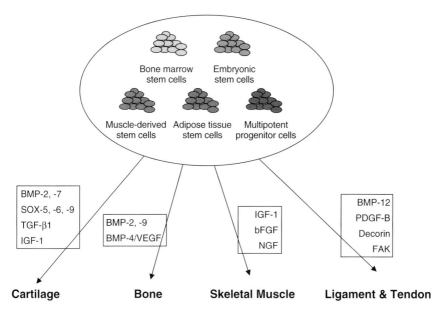

Fig. 1. Potential use of stem cells of different origins in orthopedic gene therapy. Stem cells from different origins can be used for ex vivo gene therapy to regenerate musculoskeletal tissues. Different molecules promote different differentiation pathways of stem cells.

on the concept of base-pairing. RNA decoys [6,7] can prevent the binding of *trans* activators to their corresponding *cis*-acting elements in the viral genome. Protein product-based strategies, such as transdominant negative proteins [8] and single-chain antibodies [9], also can inhibit the replication of infectious agents. Another strategy involves the use of genetic vaccines [10,11] that elicit an immune response to native proteins of the infectious agent by transferring plasmid DNA into cells. Gene therapy has received attention as a possible alternative treatment for a wide range of infectious diseases that do not respond to standard clinical management, particularly HIV, hepatitis viruses, herpes simplex virus, and tuberculosis [12–18]. So far, the use of gene therapy to treat complicated musculoskeletal infections has been very limited. Most of the gene therapy studies have been focused on the repair of damaged musculoskeletal tissues rather than on the alleviation of the infectious disease itself. Because the final outcome of complicated musculoskeletal infections is tissue damage, the development and use of gene therapies to repair damaged tissue is appropriate. Direct interference with the infectious pathogen and the infectious process may be another approach, however, by which to treat complicated musculoskeletal infections effectively in the future.

Gene therapy poses special safety and efficacy issues, especially when used to treat infection. The viral vectors used in gene therapy often elicit a host immune response that may hinder their effectiveness. Researchers have used transient immunosuppression to promote bone repair when using adenoviral gene transfer strategies, because the first-generation adenoviral vectors induce an immune response that decreases gene expression over time and limits the effectiveness of repeat dosing [19,20]. Okubo and coworkers [21,22] evaluated osteoinduction in the calf muscles of rats treated with cyclophosphamide (125 mg/kg) and found that the injection of an adenovirus vector encoding for bone morphogenetic protein (BMP)-2 (Ad.BMP-2) led to ectopic bone formation. Systemic administration of an immunosuppressive agent may not be an acceptable option for the treatment of otherwise healthy patients, however, and could have deleterious effects on the target tissue itself, especially if infection is present. For these reasons, gene therapy targeted directly at bacterial pathogens or infectious conditions warrants extra caution.

Gene therapy for bone repair

Studies have examined different gene therapy strategies designed to repair bone defects. Using plasmids as a nonviral delivery method, Bonadio and coworkers [23] implanted a collagen sponge containing parathyroid hormone cDNA in a critical-sized canine tibial bone defect model. Although the researchers observed protein production 6 weeks after implantation, bone production was insufficient. The results suggest that either the local transfection efficiency was low, or parathyroid hormone has limited osteoinductive potential under such conditions. This study did demonstrate, however, the importance of identifying the optimal combination of matrix material and osteoinductive agent when trying to induce bone formation.

Using an in vivo technique, Baltzer and coworkers [24,25] injected Ad.BMP-2 into a femoral bone defect created in a rabbit model. They reported that osseous tissue filled the critical-sized defects treated with the adenovirus, whereas fibrotic tissue filled most of each control defect. Musgrave and coworkers [26] also used Ad.BMP-2 to induce bone formation. They observed ectopic bone formation in the thigh muscles of mice after injection. Significantly less bone formed in immunocompetent animals, however, than in immunocompromised animals. This finding likely reflected decreased gene expression over time, and the limited effectiveness of repeat dosing because of the immune response elicited by the first-generation adenovirus [19,20].

The cells that have received the most interest as ex vivo delivery vehicles are mesenchymal stem cells (MSCs) and muscle-derived stem cells. These cells not only secrete an osteoinductive protein, but also respond to it. The genetic manipulation of stem cells to overexpress an osteoinductive protein could further enhance the bone repair response. Lieberman and coworkers [27] transduced bone marrow cells with an Ad.BMP-2 vector, injected them into a critical-sized femoral bone defect, and observed a robust pattern of bone formation. Engineered muscle-derived stem cells also have osteogenic potential. Peng and coworkers [28] demonstrated that muscle-derived stem cells genetically engineered to express human BMP-4, and muscle-derived stem cells genetically engineered to express vascular endothelial growth factor acted synergistically to enhance bone formation significantly and accelerate cartilage resorption. In addition to MSCs and muscle-derived stem cells, adipose-derived stem cells [29,30] and skin fibroblasts also have been used as cell gene delivery vehicles to heal bone defects [31].

Gene therapy for osteomyelitis

Osteomyelitis is an acute or chronic inflammatory disease of the bone and its structures, caused by pyogenic organisms. It may be localized or may spread through the periosteum, cortex, marrow, and cancellous tissue. With appropriate antibiotic treatment, the outcome of acute osteomyelitis is usually good. Chronic cases of the infection usually require surgical removal of dead bone tissue, however, resulting in large bone defects. Although physicians view conventional bone grafting as the method of choice for the treatment of segmental fractures, the need for a bone source and other complications limit the usefulness of the procedure [32–34].

Researchers have investigated the use of gene therapy to treat osteomyelitis. Using Ad.BMP-2, Southwood and coworkers [35] tried to improve fracture healing in rabbits modeling infected femur fractures. Forty-eight hours after surgically creating a 10-mm femoral defect, the investigators percutaneously injected 0.5×10^7 colony-forming units/0.5 mL *Staphylococcus aureus* into the defect. They also applied a sclerosing agent to the defect to facilitate the development and persistence of osteomyelitis. The results suggest that Ad.BMP-2 can accelerate the early stages of fracture healing in this model. The results were not as favorable, however, as those obtained through the use of noninfection models [25]. The lack of ossification could be attributed to the infection or the use of the sclerosing agent, which could cause cell death and damage the adenoviral vector.

Gene therapy for cartilage

Damaged or diseased cartilage lacks a natural repair mechanism. Compared with other methods, gene therapy provides the advantage of continuous localized presentation of gene products within cartilage defects. Among the list of cDNAs that may be useful for cartilage repair, transforming growth factor-β superfamily [36,37], BMPs [38,39], insulin-like growth factor (IGF)-1 [40,41], fibroblast growth factors [42], and epidermal growth factor [43] are the most important. The transcription factors Sox-9 [44,45], L-Sox 5, and Sox-6 [45] can promote chondrogenesis or maintenance of the chondrocytic phenotype. Signal transduction molecules, such as SMADs [46,47], also play important roles in chondrocyte differentiation. Proteins, such as interleukin-1 (IL-1) and tumor necrosis factor-α, are elevated within arthritic joints, and are important mediators of cartilage degradation. Administration of proteins, such as IL-1 receptor antagonist (IL-1Ra) [48], soluble tumor necrosis factor receptors, or inhibitors of matrix metalloproteinase, may effectively reduce cartilage loss.

Direct intra-articular injection of a vector or genetically modified cells into the joint space is the simplest method of gene transfer to joint tissues. Researchers have intensively evaluated the ability of different vectors to deliver genes to the synovial lining cells. Of the viral vectors, adenovirus [49,50] and lentivirus [51,52] seem to be highly effective for in vivo gene delivery. The injection of adenovirus containing IGF-1 cDNA increases matrix synthesis in both rabbit and horses models [53,54]. This strategy does not seem to work, however, for the delivery of transforming growth factor (TGF)-β1 [55]. Some researchers have turned their attention to localizing the transgene to the site of cartilage damage.

Some success has been reported using ex vivo delivery of genetically modified chondrocytes to cartilage defects to maintain the expression of transgene products at biologically relevant levels. Kang and coworkers [56] have confirmed that this strategy leads to transgene expression in full-thickness cartilage defects. Moreover, the transduction of chondrocytes with adenovirus carrying transforming growth factor-β1 cDNA [57,58], IGF-1 cDNA [58,59], BMP-2 cDNA [58], or BMP-7 cDNA [60] dramatically enhanced matrix synthesis, even in the presence of IL-1, a strong inhibitor of matrix synthesis [57,58]. Clinical ex vivo repair based on this strategy, however, is tedious and expensive. Alternatively, genetically modified MSCs and other marrow cells could be implanted into the repair site in one surgical procedure, avoiding the need for long-term cell culture. This approach supplies chondroprogenitor cells and genes to the targeted site. After transfecting plasmid DNA encoding either BMP-2 or BMP-4 into the mesenchymal progenitor cell line C3H10T1/2 and growing the cells in monolayer, Ahrens and coworkers [61] reported that most of the cells underwent osteogenic differentiation, whereas some cells developed into adipocytes or chondrocytes. Human MSCs transduced to express human BMP-2 and injected into mice have formed ectopic bone and cartilage [62]. These reports support the concept that the delivery and expression of cDNAs encoding chondroinductive proteins can influence the differentiation of MSCs.

Gene therapy of inflammatory arthritis

Septic (infective) arthritis can result from the direct invasion of joint space by a variety of microorganisms. Reactive arthritis, a sterile inflammatory process, results from an infectious process elsewhere in the body.

Although any infectious agent may cause arthritis, bacterial pathogens are the most rapidly destructive. The major consequence of bacterial invasion is damage to joint cartilage. Infiltrating immune cells induce the synthesis of cytokines and other inflammatory products, resulting in the hydrolysis of essential collagen and proteoglycans. As the destructive process continues, pannus formation and cartilage erosion occur.

Gene therapy for inflammatory arthritis has been studied in animal models. Van de Loo and coworkers [63] designed an inflammation-inducible adenoviral expression system for the local treatment of arthritis. Because IL-1 and IL-6 are early inflammatory responsive genes, the researchers designed a replication-deficient adenovirus with luciferase controlled by IL-1–IL-6 promoter (Ad5.IL-1–IL-6_luc) [64,65]. Three days and 21 days after the intrajoint injection of Ad5.IL-1–IL-6_luc, the investigators injected zymosan (from *Saccharomyces cerevisiae*) and streptococcal cell walls (from *Streptococcus pyogenes*) directly into the joint cavity of mice. Both injections increased Luc activity significantly in treated animals, compared with the control group injected with constitutive cytomegalovirus promoter, or the control group of IL-6$^{-/-}$ and IL-1$^{-/-}$ gene knockout mice. By injecting streptococcal cell wall peptidoglycan-polysaccharide complexes intraperitoneally, Song and coworkers [66] created a rat arthritis model. Plasmid DNA containing transforming growth factor-β1, administered intramuscularly at the peak of the acute inflammatory phase, suppressed the development of chronic erosive disease. When delivered during the late inflammatory phase, this treatment essentially eliminated the signs and symptoms of chronic disease.

To create an arthritis animal model for the study of gene therapy, most researchers have used pathogenic compartments isolated from bacteria [63,66] or type II collagen [67–69], which are injected into joints, the abdomen, or the circulatory system to induce an inflammatory response of articular cartilage. These systems generally provide good models of rheumatoid arthritis or other types of aseptic arthritis, because they induce an immune response rather than a direct invasion of live organisms. The future study of gene therapy for septic arthritis requires models based on the injection of live organisms.

Gene therapy for tendon and ligament

Several investigators have studied gene transfer to tendon and ligament tissues. To study tendon gene transfer, researchers have used three model systems: (1) the patellar tendon [70,71], (2) the digital flexor tendon [72,73], and (3) the Achilles tendon [74]. Most studies focusing on ligament gene transfer used the medial collateral ligament [75,76] and the anterior cruciate ligament [75–77] as models. Before attempting to manipulate the tendon [70–72,74,78] and ligament [75,77] healing environments, researchers successfully transferred β-galactosidase by different techniques in various animal models, and demonstrated the feasibility of gene transfer to tendon and ligament tissue.

Studies of tendon repair

Very few studies have focused on promoting the healing of tendon tissue. In addition to the common problems of gene therapy discussed previously, the formation of scar tissue and adhesions poses particularly challenging problems that are specific for tendon and ligament healing. Lou and coworkers [79] constructed an adenovirus containing the focal adhesion kinase gene, an intracellular kinase involved with cell dissemination and mobility. They injected these adenoviral constructs into the flexor profundus tendon of the long toe of chickens. Four weeks later, immunostaining showed overexpression of focal adhesion kinase in treated chickens compared with controls. Biomechanical testing revealed a significantly greater work-of-flexion value in the adenovirus containing the focal adhesion kinase gene group than in the control groups. Lou's research group [73] also studied the effect of BMP-12 on tendon healing. Using an adenoviral construct of BMP-12 (Ad.BMP-12), they transduced tendon cells in vitro and tendons in vivo to investigate its effect on tendon composition. The in vitro results revealed a 30% increase in collagen type I synthesis by cells transduced with the Ad.BMP-12 construct, compared with control cells or cells transduced with an adenovirus-β-galactosidase construct. The in vivo model used by these researchers involved complete bilateral laceration of the middle toe flexor digitorum profundus, followed by surgical repair of the tendon. Immediately after wound closure, one toe received Ad.BMP-12 injections, whereas the contralateral toe received adenovirus-β-galactosidase injections. Comparisons of treated animals with controls revealed no significant differences 2 weeks after surgery, but significantly higher ultimate failure force, and significantly lower stiffness in the treated animals 4 weeks after surgery.

Researchers have used rat patellar tendons to investigate the implantation of platelet-derived growth factor-B cDNA [80]. They transected the mid-portion of the medial half of the patellar tendon, and injected hemagglutinating virus of Japan-conjugated liposomes suspension, containing platelet-derived growth factor-B cDNA, into the wound site and the fascial pocket over the patellar tendon at the injury site. Platelet-derived growth factor-B gene transfer caused increased expression of platelet-derived growth factor-B for up to 4 weeks after transfection. There was also a significant increase in the vascularity of platelet-derived growth factor-B–treated patellar tendon wounds compared with control tissues 1 week after surgery, but the researchers observed no significant differences between the two groups 4 and 8 weeks after surgery. Collagen deposition increased with time in both groups. Tendons from the platelet-derived growth factor-B group contained significantly more collagen than controls at the 4-week time point, but there was no significant difference between the groups 1 and 8 weeks after surgery. The enhanced angiogenesis and extracellular matrix deposition observed in the platelet-derived growth factor-B–treated animals indicate that this technique could be used to improve tendon repair, at least during the early phase.

Studies of ligament repair

Using a well-established model of medial collateral ligament healing in an adult female rabbit knee, researchers created and marked a 4-mm gap in the ligament. Two weeks after surgery, they injected the scar that filled the gap with hemagglutinating virus of Japan-conjugated liposomes containing antisense oligodeoxynucleotides to decorin [76,81,82]. Decorin is a small leucine-rich proteoglycan that plays a role in collagen fibrillogenesis; specifically, there is an association between increased levels of decorin and decreased diameters of collagen fibrils. Reverse transcription–polymerase chain reaction revealed a significant decrease in decorin mRNA levels in the antisense group, compared with the sense group. Evaluation of the scars in both groups by electron microscopy showed both small- and large-diameter fibrils in the antisense group that were similar to normal medial collateral ligaments, but only small-diameter fibrils in the sense group. Using hematoxylin and eosin staining, Nakamura and coworkers [81] observed scars with a more normal appearance in the antisense group, and polarized light microscopy revealed some return of the normal crimp pattern. The failure stresses in the antisense group 4 weeks after injection (6 weeks after original injury), however, were still only approximately 20% of failure stresses in the normal medial collateral ligament group. The distribution of large-diameter fibrils in the antisense scars was patchy, likely caused by the difficulty associated with delivering the vector through the ligament tissue.

Several studies have demonstrated gene intervention in tendon and ligament tissue. No such study has been performed, however, in an infectious disease model. Acute tenosynovitis is an orthopedic emergency that is caused predominantly by *S aureus* or *S pyogenes*, and most frequently involves the tendon sheaths of the digital flexor muscles [83]. This condition, which usually results from a penetrating injury, can be complicated by the presence of foreign bodies. Devastating complications, such as tendon necrosis and contamination of other palmar spaces or adjacent joints, can arise without proper early diagnosis and treatment [84]. Because the transfer of genes to tendons seems feasible, this method could provide a new option for the treatment of complications caused by acute tenosynovitis.

Gene therapy for skeletal muscle

Sports-related muscle injuries may be direct (ie, attributed to laceration, contusion, or strain) or indirect (ie, related to ischemia or neurologic dysfunction). Severe injuries typically culminate in the formation of scar tissue and functional impairment. Because IGF-1 can promote muscle regeneration [85,86], researchers have evaluated the ability of an adenovirus carrying the IGF-1 gene (Ad.IGF-1) to improve muscle healing after injury. Myoblast-mediated ex vivo gene transfer of Ad.IGF-1 into lacerated muscle improved muscle healing more effectively than direct injection of Ad.IGF-1. The functional recovery remained incomplete, however, and scar tissue still developed in the injured area [87]. Barton-Davis and coworkers [88] showed that direct injection of adeno-associated virus containing IGF-1 into skeletal muscle stimulated muscle regeneration. Research has shown that the basal lamina surrounding mature myofibers contains pores that are approximately 40 nm in diameter [89], and acts as a barrier to direct gene transfer [90]. The smaller size of the adeno-associated virus particle should give it an advantage over adenovirus and herpes simplex virus in penetrating the basal lamina [91,92].

Duchenne muscle dystrophy is the most frequent lethal inheritable childhood disease: approximately 1 in every 3500 boys are born with Duchenne muscle dystrophy [93–95]. The X-linked dystrophin gene is one of the largest of the 30,000 genes that encode proteins in the human genome. The size of the dystrophin gene has presented a challenge to gene therapy for Duchenne muscle dystrophy. Delivery of the 14-kb dystrophin cDNA requires the use of vectors with high capacities. The generation and use of the high-capacity adenovirus, an adenovirus devoid of all adenoviral genes, improved the persistence of transgene expression in skeletal muscle [96,97]. Adenoviral vectors generally are too large to penetrate the basal lamina, and this fact has hampered their therapeutic applicability in muscle. Although researchers have investigated the use of the herpes simplex virus to carry the dystrophin gene [98,99], immunogenicity and cytotoxicity have restricted its effectiveness. More recently, researchers have developed a minidystrophin and microdystrophin strategy to ameliorate the dystrophic histopathology and increase muscle force and resistance to mechanical stress [100,101]. This approach is based on the fact that large parts of the dystrophin gene are not vital to its function [102–104]. The smallest microconstruct was only 3.6 kb in size, and was highly effective in restoring nearly normal skeletal muscle structure and function [100]. Utrophin is a homolog of dystrophin; although utrophin is approximately one third the size of the dystrophin gene, its transcript is almost as large as dystrophin [105]. Researchers have evaluated gene transfer of utrophin as an alternative strategy by which to treat DMD [106,107] because the structure and function of these two proteins are similar [108].

The inflammatory myopathies are characterized by immune-mediated chronic inflammation of the skeletal muscle tissue, resulting in progressive weakness. Pyomyositis is a pyogenic muscle infection occurring in tropical countries, immunocompromised patients, and drug abusers. Myopathy also results from drugs and viral infection. Although no gene therapy studies have been focused on these infectious and inflammatory diseases, possible target gene products have been identified, including IL-1α and -β and transforming growth factor-β1–3 [109,110]. In an in vitro study evaluating the transfer of HLA-G, a nonclassical MHC class I molecule, to myoblasts, Wiendl and coworkers [111] showed that ectopic expression of HLA-G could help prevent inflammation progression.

Summary

Tissue repair is a major issue in orthopedics. Many musculoskeletal tissues, including cartilage, meniscus, and the anterior cruciate ligament, heal poorly after injury. Recent studies have led to the identification of numerous growth factors and other gene products that can promote the regeneration of damaged musculoskeletal tissues. In the last century, the discovery and evolving use of antibiotics has significantly decreased the prevalence and severity of infectious diseases. In many orthopedic scenarios, however, treatment of infections can be difficult, and often involves a prolonged course of antibiotics with concomitant surgical interventions and loss of tissue. Although studies have demonstrated the successful transfer of target genes and the associated manipulation of the musculo-skeletal tissue environment, researchers have made few attempts designed to use gene therapy to treat infectious musculoskeletal diseases in animal models. Before it is possible to use gene-based approaches to treat such diseases effectively, researchers must perform more studies to investigate the potential problems that may arise when using gene therapy in an infectious environment.

Acknowledgments

The authors thank Ryan Sauder, University of Pittsburgh, for his excellent editorial assistance with the manuscript.

References

[1] Hannallah D, Peterson B, Lieberman JR, et al. Gene therapy in orthopaedic surgery. Instr Course Lect 2003;52:753–68.
[2] Robbins PD, Ghivizani SC. Viral vectors for gene therapy. Pharmacol Ther 1998;80:35–47.
[3] Evans CH, Robbins PD. Possible orthopaedic applications of gene therapy. J Bone Joint Surg Am 1995;77:1103–14.
[4] Lisziewicz J, Sun D, Klotman M, et al. Specific inhibition of human immunodeficiency virus type 1 replication by antisense oligonucleotides: an in vitro model for treatment. Proc Natl Acad Sci U S A 1992;89:11209–13.
[5] Gervaix A, Li X, Kraus G, et al. Multigene antiviral vectors inhibit diverse human immunodeficiency virus type 1 clades. J Virol 1997;71:3048–53.
[6] Sullenger BA, Gallardo HF, Ungers GE, et al. Overexpression of TAR sequences renders cells resistant to human immunodeficiency virus replication. Cell 1990;63:601–8.

[7] Sullenger BA, Gallardo HF, Ungers GE, et al. Analysis of trans-acting response decoy RNA-mediated inhibition of human immunodeficiency virus type 1 transactivation. J Virol 1991;65:6811–6.

[8] Herskowitz I. Functional inactivation of genes by dominant negative mutations. Nature 1987;329:219–22.

[9] Duan L, Bagasra O, Laughlin MA, et al. Potent inhibition of human immunodeficiency virus type 1 replication by an intracellular anti-Rev single-chain antibody. Proc Natl Acad Sci U S A 1994;91:5075–9.

[10] Tang DC, DeVit M, Johnston SA. Genetic immunization is a simple method for eliciting an immune response. Nature 1992;356:152–4.

[11] Ulmer JB, Donnelly JJ, Parker SE, et al. Heterologous protection against influenza by injection of DNA encoding a viral protein. Science 1993;259:1745–9.

[12] Davis HL, McCluskie MJ, Gerin JL, et al. DNA vaccine for hepatitis B: evidence for immunogenicity in chimpanzees and comparison with other vaccines. Proc Natl Acad Sci U S A 1996;93:7213–8.

[13] Heslop HE, Brenner MK, Rooney C, et al. Administration of neomycin-resistance-gene-marked EBV-specific cytotoxic T lymphocytes to recipients of mismatched-related or phenotypically similar unrelated donor marrow grafts. Hum Gene Ther 1994;5:381–97.

[14] Morgan RA, Walker R. Gene therapy for AIDS using retroviral mediated gene transfer to deliver HIV-1 antisense TAR and transdominant Rev protein genes to syngeneic lymphocytes in HIV-1 infected identical twins. Hum Gene Ther 1996;7:1281–306.

[15] Tascon RE, Colston MJ, Ragno S, et al. Vaccination against tuberculosis by DNA injection. Nat Med 1996;2:888–92.

[16] Tokushige K, Wakita T, Pachuk C, et al. Expression and immune response to hepatitis C virus core DNA-based vaccine constructs. Hepatology 1996;24:14–20.

[17] Walter EA, Greenberg PD, Gilbert MJ, et al. Reconstitution of cellular immunity against cytomegalovirus in recipients of allogeneic bone marrow by transfer of T-cell clones from the donor. N Engl J Med 1995;333:1038–44.

[18] Manickan E, Yu Z, Rouse RJ, et al. Induction of protective immunity against herpes simplex virus with DNA encoding the immediate early protein ICP 27. Viral Immunol 1995; 8:53–61.

[19] Christ M, Lusky M, Stoeckel F, et al. Gene therapy with recombinant adenovirus vectors: evaluation of the host immune response. Immunol Lett 1997;57:19–25.

[20] Yang Y, Nunes FA, Berencsi K, et al. Cellular immunity to viral antigens limits E1-deleted adenoviruses for gene therapy. Proc Natl Acad Sci U S A 1994;91:4407–11.

[21] Okubo Y, Bessho K, Fujimura K, et al. In vitro and in vivo studies of a bone morphogenetic protein-2 expressing adenoviral vector. J Bone Joint Surg Am 2001;83(Suppl 1, Pt 2): S99–104.

[22] Okubo Y, Bessho K, Fujimura K, et al. Osteoinduction by bone morphogenetic protein-2 via adenoviral vector under transient immunosuppression. Biochem Biophys Res Commun 2000;267:382–7.

[23] Bonadio J, Smiley E, Patil P, et al. Localized, direct plasmid gene delivery in vivo: prolonged therapy results in reproducible tissue regeneration. Nat Med 1999;5:753–9.

[24] Baltzer AW, Lattermann C, Whalen JD, et al. Potential role of direct adenoviral gene transfer in enhancing fracture repair. Clin Orthop 2000;379:S120–5.

[25] Baltzer AW, Lattermann C, Whalen JD, et al. Genetic enhancement of fracture repair: healing of an experimental segmental defect by adenoviral transfer of the BMP-2 gene. Gene Ther 2000;7:734–9.

[26] Musgrave DS, Bosch P, Ghivizzani S, et al. Adenovirus-mediated direct gene therapy with bone morphogenetic protein-2 produces bone. Bone 1999;24:541–7.

[27] Lieberman JR, Daluiski A, Stevenson S, et al. The effect of regional gene therapy with bone morphogenetic protein-2-producing bone-marrow cells on the repair of segmental femoral defects in rats. J Bone Joint Surg Am 1999;81:905–17.

[28] Peng H, Wright V, Usas A, et al. Synergistic enhancement of bone formation and healing by stem cell-expressed VEGF and bone morphogenetic protein-4. J Clin Invest 2002;110: 751–9.

[29] Dragoo JL, Choi JY, Lieberman JR, et al. Bone induction by BMP-2 transduced stem cells derived from human fat. J Orthop Res 2003;21:622–9.

[30] Peterson B, Zhang J, Iglesias R, et al. Healing of critically sized femoral defects, using genetically modified mesenchymal stem cells from human adipose tissue. Tissue Eng 2005; 11:120–9.

[31] Rutherford RB, Moalli M, Franceschi RT, et al. Bone morphogenetic protein-transduced human fibroblasts convert to osteoblasts and form bone in vivo. Tissue Eng 2002;8:441–52.

[32] Zaslav KR, Meinhard BP. Management of resistant pseudarthrosis of long bones. Clin Orthop 1988;233:234–42.

[33] Albertson KS, Medoff RJ, Mitsunaga MM. The use of periosteally vascularized autografts to augment the fixation of large segmental allografts. Clin Orthop 1991;269:113–9.

[34] Bostrom M, Lane JM, Tomin E, et al. Use of bone morphogenetic protein-2 in the rabbit ulnar nonunion model. Clin Orthop 1996;327:272–82.

[35] Southwood LL, Frisbie DD, Kawcak CE, et al. Evaluation of Ad-BMP-2 for enhancing fracture healing in an infected defect fracture rabbit model. J Orthop Res 2004;22:66–72.

[36] Moses HL, Serra R. Regulation of differentiation by TGF-beta. Curr Opin Genet Dev 1996;6:581–6.

[37] Izumi T, Scully SP, Heydemann A, et al. Transforming growth factor beta 1 stimulates type II collagen expression in cultured periosteum-derived cells. J Bone Miner Res 1992;7: 115–21.

[38] Sellers RS, Peluso D, Morris EA. The effect of recombinant human bone morphogenetic protein-2 (rhBMP-2) on the healing of full-thickness defects of articular cartilage. J Bone Joint Surg Am 1997;79:1452–63.

[39] Sato K, Urist MR. Bone morphogenetic protein-induced cartilage development in tissue culture. Clin Orthop 1984;183:180–7.

[40] Nixon AJ, Saxer RA, Brower-Toland BD. Exogenous insulin-like growth factor-I stimulates an autoinductive IGF-I autocrine/paracrine response in chondrocytes. J Orthop Res 2001;19:26–32.

[41] Fortier LA, Mohammed HO, Lust G, et al. Insulin-like growth factor-I enhances cell-based repair of articular cartilage. J Bone Joint Surg Br 2002;84:276–88.

[42] Ellsworth JL, Berry J, Bukowski T, et al. Fibroblast growth factor-18 is a trophic factor for mature chondrocytes and their progenitors. Osteoarthritis Cartilage 2002;10:308–20.

[43] Osborn KD, Trippel SB, Mankin HJ. Growth factor stimulation of adult articular cartilage. J Orthop Res 1989;7:35–42.

[44] Majumdar MK, Wang E, Morris EA. BMP-2 and BMP-9 promotes chondrogenic differentiation of human multipotential mesenchymal cells and overcomes the inhibitory effect of IL-1. J Cell Physiol 2001;189:275–84.

[45] de Crombrugghe B, Lefebvre V, Behringer RR, et al. Transcriptional mechanisms of chondrocyte differentiation. Matrix Biol 2000;19:389–94.

[46] Watanabe H, de Caestecker MP, Yamada Y. Transcriptional cross-talk between Smad, ERK1/2, and p38 mitogen-activated protein kinase pathways regulates transforming growth factor-beta-induced aggrecan gene expression in chondrogenic ATDC5 cells. J Biol Chem 2001;276:14466–73.

[47] Osaki M, Tsukazaki T, Ono N, et al. cDNA cloning and chromosomal mapping of rat Smad2 and Smad4 and their expression in cultured rat articular chondrocytes. Endocr J 1999;46:695–701.

[48] Arend WP. Physiology of cytokine pathways in rheumatoid arthritis. Arthritis Rheum 2001;45:101–6.

[49] Ghivizzani SC, Lechman ER, Kang R, et al. Direct adenovirus-mediated gene transfer of interleukin 1 and tumor necrosis factor alpha soluble receptors to rabbit knees with

experimental arthritis has local and distal anti-arthritic effects. Proc Natl Acad Sci U S A 1998;95:4613–8.

[50] Roessler BJ, Allen ED, Wilson JM, et al. Adenoviral-mediated gene transfer to rabbit synovium in vivo. J Clin Invest 1993;92(2):1085–92.

[51] Gouze E, Pawliuk R, Gouze JN, et al. Lentiviral-mediated gene delivery to synovium: potent intra-articular expression with amplification by inflammation. Mol Ther 2003;7: 460–6.

[52] Gouze E, Pawliuk R, Pilapil C, et al. In vivo gene delivery to synovium by lentiviral vectors. Mol Ther 2002;5:397–404.

[53] Mi Z, Ghivizzani SC, Lechman ER, et al. Adenovirus-mediated gene transfer of insulin-like growth factor 1 stimulates proteoglycan synthesis in rabbit joints. Arthritis Rheum 2000;43: 2563–70.

[54] Saxer RA, Bent SJ, Brower-Toland BD, et al. Gene mediated insulin-like growth factor-I delivery to the synovium. J Orthop Res 2001;19:759–67.

[55] Mi Z, Ghivizzani SC, Lechman E, et al. Adverse effects of adenovirus-mediated gene transfer of human transforming growth factor beta 1 into rabbit knees. Arthritis Res Ther 2003;5:R132–9.

[56] Kang R, Marui T, Ghivizzani SC, et al. Ex vivo gene transfer to chondrocytes in full-thickness articular cartilage defects: a feasibility study. Osteoarthritis Cartilage 1997;5: 139–43.

[57] Shuler FD, Georgescu HI, Niyibizi C, et al. Increased matrix synthesis following adenoviral transfer of a transforming growth factor beta1 gene into articular chondrocytes. J Orthop Res 2000;18:585–92.

[58] Smith P, Shuler FD, Georgescu HI, et al. Genetic enhancement of matrix synthesis by articular chondrocytes: comparison of different growth factor genes in the presence and absence of interleukin-1. Arthritis Rheum 2000;43:1156–64.

[59] Nixon AJ, Brower-Toland BD, Bent SJ, et al. Insulinlike growth factor-I gene therapy applications for cartilage repair. Clin Orthop 2000;379:S201–13.

[60] Hidaka C, Quitoriano M, Warren RF, et al. Enhanced matrix synthesis and in vitro formation of cartilage-like tissue by genetically modified chondrocytes expressing BMP-7. J Orthop Res 2001;19:751–8.

[61] Ahrens M, Ankenbauer T, Schroder D, et al. Expression of human bone morphogenetic proteins-2 or -4 in murine mesenchymal progenitor C3H10T1/2 cells induces differentiation into distinct mesenchymal cell lineages. DNA Cell Biol 1993;12:871–80.

[62] Turgeman G, Pittman DD, Muller R, et al. Engineered human mesenchymal stem cells: a novel platform for skeletal cell mediated gene therapy. J Gene Med 2001;3:240–51.

[63] van de Loo FA, de Hooge AS, Smeets RL, et al. An inflammation-inducible adenoviral expression system for local treatment of the arthritic joint. Gene Ther 2004;11:581–90.

[64] van de Loo AA, Arntz OJ, Bakker AC, et al. Role of interleukin 1 in antigen-induced exacerbations of murine arthritis. Am J Pathol 1995;146:239–49.

[65] van de Loo FA, Joosten LA, van Lent PL, et al. Role of interleukin-1, tumor necrosis factor alpha, and interleukin-6 in cartilage proteoglycan metabolism and destruction: effect of in situ blocking in murine antigen- and zymosan-induced arthritis. Arthritis Rheum 1995;38: 164–72.

[66] Song XY, Gu M, Jin WW, et al. Plasmid DNA encoding transforming growth factor-beta1 suppresses chronic disease in a streptococcal cell wall-induced arthritis model. J Clin Invest 1998;101:2615–21.

[67] Bloquel C, Bessis N, Boissier MC, et al. Gene therapy of collagen-induced arthritis by electrotransfer of human tumor necrosis factor-alpha soluble receptor I variants. Hum Gene Ther 2004;15:189–201.

[68] Parks E, Strieter RM, Lukacs NW, et al. Transient gene transfer of IL-12 regulates chemokine expression and disease severity in experimental arthritis. J Immunol 1998;160: 4615–9.

[69] Kageyama Y, Koide Y, Uchijima M, et al. Plasmid encoding interleukin-4 in the amelioration of murine collagen-induced arthritis. Arthritis Rheum 2004;50:968–75.

[70] Nakamura N, Horibe S, Matsumoto N, et al. Transient introduction of a foreign gene into healing rat patellar ligament. J Clin Invest 1996;97:226–31.

[71] Ozkan I, Shino K, Nakamura N, et al. Direct in vivo gene transfer to healing rat patellar ligament by intra-arterial delivery of haemagglutinating virus of Japan liposomes. Eur J Clin Invest 1999;29:63–7.

[72] Goomer RS, Maris TM, Gelberman R, et al. Nonviral in vivo gene therapy for tissue engineering of articular cartilage and tendon repair. Clin Orthop 2000;379:S189–200.

[73] Lou J, Tu Y, Burns M, et al. BMP-12 gene transfer augmentation of lacerated tendon repair. J Orthop Res 2001;19:1199–202.

[74] Dai Q, Manfield L, Wang Y, et al. Adenovirus-mediated gene transfer to healing tendon–enhanced efficiency using a gelatin sponge. J Orthop Res 2003;21:604–9.

[75] Hildebrand KA, Deie M, Allen CR, et al. Early expression of marker genes in the rabbit medial collateral and anterior cruciate ligaments: the use of different viral vectors and the effects of injury. J Orthop Res 1999;17:37–42.

[76] Nakamura N, Timmermann SA, Hart DA, et al. A comparison of in vivo gene delivery methods for antisense therapy in ligament healing. Gene Ther 1998;5:1455–61.

[77] Menetrey J, Kasemkijwattana C, Day CS, et al. Direct-, fibroblast- and myoblast-mediated gene transfer to the anterior cruciate ligament. Tissue Eng 1999;5:435–42.

[78] Lou J, Manske PR, Aoki M, et al. Adenovirus-mediated gene transfer into tendon and tendon sheath. J Orthop Res 1996;14:513–7.

[79] Lou J, Kubota H, Hotokezaka S, et al. In vivo gene transfer and overexpression of focal adhesion kinase (pp125 FAK) mediated by recombinant adenovirus-induced tendon adhesion formation and epitenon cell change. J Orthop Res 1997;15:911–8.

[80] Nakamura N, Shino K, Natsuume T, et al. Early biological effect of in vivo gene transfer of platelet-derived growth factor (PDGF)-B into healing patellar ligament. Gene Ther 1998;5:1165–70.

[81] Nakamura N, Hart DA, Boorman RS, et al. Decorin antisense gene therapy improves functional healing of early rabbit ligament scar with enhanced collagen fibrillogenesis in vivo. J Orthop Res 2000;18:517–23.

[82] Hart DA, Nakamura N, Marchuk L, et al. Complexity of determining cause and effect in vivo after antisense gene therapy. Clin Orthop 2000;379:S242–51.

[83] Canoso JJ, Barza M. Soft tissue infections. Rheum Dis Clin North Am 1993;19:293–309.

[84] Jeffrey RB Jr, Laing FC, Schechter WP, et al. Acute suppurative tenosynovitis of the hand: diagnosis with US. Radiology 1987;162:741–2.

[85] Kasemkijwattana C, Menetrey J, Bosch P, et al. Use of growth factors to improve muscle healing after strain injury. Clin Orthop 2000;370:272–85.

[86] Menetrey J, Kasemkijwattana C, Day CS, et al. Growth factors improve muscle healing in vivo. J Bone Joint Surg Br 2000;82:131–7.

[87] Lee CW, Fukushima K, Usas A, et al. Biological intervention based on cell and gene therapy to improve muscle healing after laceration. J Musculoskel Res 2000;4:265–77.

[88] Barton-Davis ER, Shoturma DI, Musaro A, et al. Viral mediated expression of insulin-like growth factor I blocks the aging-related loss of skeletal muscle function. Proc Natl Acad Sci U S A 1998;95:15603–7.

[89] Yurchenco PD. Assembly of basement membranes. Ann N Y Acad Sci 1990;580:195–213.

[90] Huard J, Feero WG, Watkins SC, et al. The basal lamina is a physical barrier to herpes simplex virus-mediated gene delivery to mature muscle fibers. J Virol 1996;70:8117–23.

[91] Pruchnic R, Cao B, Peterson ZQ, et al. The use of adeno-associated virus to circumvent the maturation-dependent viral transduction of muscle fibers. Hum Gene Ther 2000;11:521–36.

[92] Wang Z, Zhu T, Qiao C, et al. Adeno-associated virus serotype 8 efficiently delivers genes to muscle and heart. Nat Biotechnol 2005;23:321–8.

[93] Brooks AP, Emery AE. The incidence of Duchenne muscular dystrophy in the South East of Scotland. Clin Genet 1977;11:290–4.

[94] van Essen AJ, Busch HF, te Meerman GJ, et al. Birth and population prevalence of Duchenne muscular dystrophy in The Netherlands. Hum Genet 1992;88:258–66.

[95] Tangsrud SE, Halvorsen S. Child neuromuscular disease in southern Norway: the prevalence and incidence of Duchenne muscular dystrophy. Acta Paediatr Scand 1989;78: 100–3.

[96] Kochanek S, Clemens PR, Mitani K, et al. A new adenoviral vector: replacement of all viral coding sequences with 28 kb of DNA independently expressing both full-length dystrophin and beta-galactosidase. Proc Natl Acad Sci U S A 1996;93:5731–6.

[97] Chen HH, Mack LM, Kelly R, et al. Persistence in muscle of an adenoviral vector that lacks all viral genes. Proc Natl Acad Sci U S A 1997;94:1645–50.

[98] Akkaraju GR, Huard J, Hoffman EP, et al. Herpes simplex virus vector-mediated dystrophin gene transfer and expression in MDX mouse skeletal muscle. J Gene Med 1999; 1:280–9.

[99] Huard J, Krisky D, Oligino T, et al. Gene transfer to muscle using herpes simplex virus-based vectors. Neuromuscul Disord 1997;7:299–313.

[100] Harper SQ, Hauser MA, DelloRusso C, et al. Modular flexibility of dystrophin: implications for gene therapy of Duchenne muscular dystrophy. Nat Med 2002;8:253–61.

[101] Watchko J, O'Day T, Wang B, et al. Adeno-associated virus vector-mediated minidystrophin gene therapy improves dystrophic muscle contractile function in mdx mice. Hum Gene Ther 2002;13:1451–60.

[102] Warner LE, DelloRusso C, Crawford RW, et al. Expression of Dp260 in muscle tethers the actin cytoskeleton to the dystrophin-glycoprotein complex and partially prevents dystrophy. Hum Mol Genet 2002;11:1095–105.

[103] Crawford GE, Faulkner JA, Crosbie RH, et al. Assembly of the dystrophin-associated protein complex does not require the dystrophin COOH-terminal domain. J Cell Biol 2000; 150:1399–410.

[104] Yuasa K, Miyagoe Y, Yamamoto K, et al. Effective restoration of dystrophin-associated proteins in vivo by adenovirus-mediated transfer of truncated dystrophin cDNAs. FEBS Lett 1998;425:329–36.

[105] Tinsley JM, Blake DJ, Roche A, et al. Primary structure of dystrophin-related protein. Nature 1992;360:591–3.

[106] Tinsley J, Deconinck N, Fisher R, et al. Expression of full-length utrophin prevents muscular dystrophy in mdx mice. Nat Med 1998;4:1441–4.

[107] Perkins KJ, Burton EA, Davies KE. The role of basal and myogenic factors in the transcriptional activation of utrophin promoter A: implications for therapeutic up-regulation in Duchenne muscular dystrophy. Nucleic Acids Res 2001;29:4843–50.

[108] Mizuno Y, Nonaka I, Hirai S, et al. Reciprocal expression of dystrophin and utrophin in muscles of Duchenne muscular dystrophy patients, female DMD-carriers and control subjects. J Neurol Sci 1993;119:43–52.

[109] Lundberg I, Ulfgren AK, Nyberg P, et al. Cytokine production in muscle tissue of patients with idiopathic inflammatory myopathies. Arthritis Rheum 1997;40:865–74.

[110] Lundberg IE. The role of cytokines, chemokines, and adhesion molecules in the pathogenesis of idiopathic inflammatory myopathies. Curr Rheumatol Rep 2000;2:216–24.

[111] Wiendl H, Mitsdoerffer M, Hofmeister V, et al. The non-classical MHC molecule HLA-G protects human muscle cells from immune-mediated lysis: implications for myoblast transplantation and gene therapy. Brain 2003;126(pt 1):176–85.

ELSEVIER
SAUNDERS

INFECTIOUS
DISEASE CLINICS
OF NORTH AMERICA

Infect Dis Clin N Am 19 (2005) 1023–1043

Cumulative Index 2005

Note: Page numbers of article titles are in **boldface** type.

A

Abscess(es), Brodie's, osteomyelitis with, 781

Abstinence, in genital herpes management, 436

Abuse, sexual, childhood, sexual behavior effects of, 306–307

N-Acetylcysteine, for malaria, 234

Acidosis, in malaria, management of, 227–228

Acquired immunodeficiency syndrome (AIDS), travelers with, 36–39

Acute lung injury, in malaria, management of, 228–229

Acute myocardial infarction, in expatriates in Ghana, 86–89

Acute otitis media, in children, pneumococcus and, 633–634

Acute renal failure, in malaria, management of, 230–231

Acute respiratory distress syndrome (ARDS), in malaria, management of, 228–229

Adult osteomyelitis, **765–786.** See also *Osteomyelitis, adult.*

African trypanosomiasis
  from Tanzania, detection of, 10–11
  HIV infection and, 126–128

Age
  as factor in adverse effects of yellow fever vaccine, 156
  as factor in malaria in travelers, 213

AIDS. See *Acquired immunodeficiency syndrome (AIDS).*

Air travel. See also *Air travelers.*
  crib death due to, 78
  during pregnancy, 79–80
  sickness due to, 79

Air travelers. See also *Air travel.*
  aspirin use by, 74–75
  cardiovascular problems in, automated external defibrillators for, 73–75
  child safety seats for, 77
  face masks for, 67–69
  health risks to, **67–84**
    peanuts, 75–77
    travel delay recommended for, 72–73
  in-flight oxygen for, 69–72
  SARS in, 68
  tuberculosis in, 69

Airway hyperreactivity, genetics of, 673–674

Alphavirus(es)
  pathogenesis of, 969–970
  viral arthritis due to, 968–970

Amphotericin B
  for cutaneous leishmaniasis in returning travelers, 257
  lipid preparations of, for neonatal candidiasis, 607–608

Amphotericin B deoxycholate, for neonatal candidiasis, 606–607

Amputation
  for open fractures, 917–918
  for prosthetic joint infections, 900

Anemia, in malaria, management of, 231–232

Anidulafungin, for neonatal candidiasis, 610–611

Animal bites, septic arthritis due to, 807

Anthrax, children exposed to, treatment of, 733–736

Antibiotic(s)
  for orthopedic prosthetic surgery, **931–946.** See also *Orthopedic prosthetic surgery, antibiotic prophylaxis in.*
  for prosthetic joint infections, 901–905
  in open fracture management, 920–922

Changing Your Address?

Make sure your subscription changes too! When you notify us of your new address, you can help make our job easier by including an exact copy of your Clinics label number with your old address (see illustration below.) This number identifies you to our computer system and will speed the processing of your address change. Please be sure this label number accompanies your old address and your corrected address—you can send an old Clinics label with your number on it or just copy it exactly and send it to the address listed below.

We appreciate your help in our attempt to give you continuous coverage. Thank you.

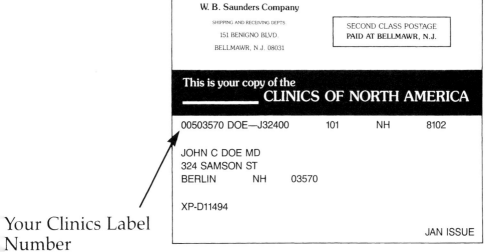

Your Clinics Label Number

Copy it exactly or send your label along with your address to:
W.B. Saunders Company, Customer Service
Orlando, FL 32887-4800
Call Toll Free 1-800-654-2452

Please allow four to six weeks for delivery of new subscriptions and for processing address changes.

United States Postal Service
Statement of Ownership, Management, and Circulation

1. Publication Title	2. Publication Number	3. Filing Date
Infectious Disease Clinics of North America	0 8 9 1 - 5 5 2 0	9/15/05

4. Issue Frequency	5. Number of Issues Published Annually	6. Annual Subscription Price
Mar, Jun, Sep, Dec	4	$165.00

7. Complete Mailing Address of Known Office of Publication (Not printer) (Street, city, county, state, and ZIP+4)

Elsevier Inc.
6277 Sea Harbor Drive
Orlando, FL 32887-4800

Contact Person: Gwen C. Campbell
Telephone: 215-239-3685

8. Complete Mailing Address of Headquarters or General Business Office of Publisher (Not printer)

Elsevier Inc., 360 Park Avenue South, New York, NY 10010-1710

9. Full Names and Complete Mailing Addresses of Publisher, Editor, and Managing Editor (Do not leave blank)

Publisher (Name and complete mailing address)
Tim Griswold, Elsevier Inc., 1600 John F. Kennedy Blvd., Suite 1800, Philadelphia, PA 19103-2899

Editor (Name and complete mailing address)
Carin Davis, Elsevier Inc., 1600 John F. Kennedy Blvd., Suite 1800, Philadelphia, PA 19103-2899

Managing Editor (Name and complete mailing address)
Heather Cullen, Elsevier Inc., 1600 John F. Kennedy Blvd., Suite 1800, Philadelphia, PA 19103-2899

10. Owner (Do not leave blank. If the publication is owned by a corporation, give the name and address of the corporation immediately followed by the names and addresses of all stockholders owning or holding 1 percent or more of the total amount of stock. If not owned by a corporation, give the names and addresses of the individual owners. If owned by a partnership or other unincorporated firm, give its name and address as well as those of each individual owner. If the publication is published by a nonprofit organization, give its name and address.)

Full Name	Complete Mailing Address
Wholly owned subsidiary of	4520 East-West Highway
Reed/Elsevier Inc., US holdings	Bethesda, MD 20814

11. Known Bondholders, Mortgagees, and Other Security Holders Owning or Holding 1 Percent or More of Total Amount of Bonds, Mortgages, or Other Securities. If none, check box ▶ ☐ None

Full Name	Complete Mailing Address
N/A	

12. Tax Status (For completion by nonprofit organizations authorized to mail at nonprofit rates) (Check one)
The purpose, function, and nonprofit status of this organization and the exempt status for federal income tax purposes:
☐ Has Not Changed During Preceding 12 Months
☐ Has Changed During Preceding 12 Months (Publisher must submit explanation of change with this statement)

(See Instructions on Reverse)

PS Form 3526, October 1999

---

13. Publication Title	14. Issue Date for Circulation Data Below
Infectious Disease Clinics of North America	June 2005

15. Extent and Nature of Circulation		Average No. Copies Each Issue During Preceding 12 Months	No. Copies of Single Issue Published Nearest to Filing Date
a. Total Number of Copies (Net press run)		3050	2900
b. Paid and/or Requested Circulation	(1) Paid/Requested Outside-County Mail Subscriptions Stated on Form 3541. (Include advertiser's proof and exchange copies)	1831	1744
	(2) Paid In-County Subscriptions Stated on Form 3541 (Include advertiser's proof and exchange copies)		
	(3) Sales Through Dealers and Carriers, Street Vendors, Counter Sales, and Other Non-USPS Paid Distribution	392	430
	(4) Other Classes Mailed Through the USPS		
c. Total Paid and/or Requested Circulation [Sum of 15b. (1), (2), (3), and (4)]	▶	2223	2174
d. Free Distribution by Mail (Samples, complimentary, and other free)	(1) Outside-County as Stated on Form 3541	55	62
	(2) In-County as Stated on Form 3541		
	(3) Other Classes Mailed Through the USPS		
e. Free Distribution Outside the Mail (Carriers or other means)			
f. Total Free Distribution (Sum of 15d. and 15e.)	▶	55	62
g. Total Distribution (Sum of 15c. and 15f)	▶	2278	2236
h. Copies not Distributed		772	664
i. Total (Sum of 15g. and h.)	▶	3050	2900
j. Percent Paid and/or Requested Circulation (15c. divided by 15g. times 100)		98%	97%

16. Publication of Statement of Ownership
☐ Publication required. Will be printed in the **December 2005** issue of this publication.   ☐ Publication not required

17. Signature and Title of Editor, Publisher, Business Manager, or Owner	Date
[signature] Paul Fanucci – Executive Director of Subscription Services	9/15/05

I certify that all information furnished on this form is true and complete. I understand that anyone who furnishes false or misleading information on this form or who omits material or information requested on the form may be subject to criminal sanctions (including fines and imprisonment) and/or civil sanctions (including civil penalties).

Instructions to Publishers

1. Complete and file one copy of this form with your postmaster annually on or before October 1. Keep a copy of the completed form for your records.
2. In cases where the stockholder or security holder is a trustee, include in items 10 and 11 the name of the person or corporation for whom the trustee is acting. Also include the names and addresses of individuals who are stockholders who own or hold 1 percent or more of the total amount of bonds, mortgages, or other securities of the publishing corporation. In item 11, if none, check the box. Use blank sheets if more space is required.
3. Be sure to furnish all circulation information called for in item 15. Free circulation must be shown in items 15d, e, and f.
4. Item 15h., Copies not Distributed, must include (1) newsstand copies originally stated on Form 3541, and returned to the publisher, (2) estimated returns from news agents, and (3), copies for office use, leftovers, spoiled, and all other copies not distributed.
5. If the publication had Periodicals authorization as a general or requester publication, this Statement of Ownership, Management, and Circulation must be published; it must be printed in any issue in October or, if the publication is not published during October, the first issue printed after October.
6. In item 16, indicate the date of the issue in which this Statement of Ownership will be published.
7. Item 17 must be signed.

Failure to file or publish a statement of ownership may lead to suspension of Periodicals authorization.

PS Form 3526, October 1999 (Reverse)